Workbook for

Merrill's Atlas of Radiographic Positioning & Procedures

14th edition

Bruce W. Long, MS, RT(R)(CV), FASRT, FAEIRS
Jeannean Hall Rollins, MRC, BSRT(R)(CV)
Barbara J. Smith, MS, RT(R)(QM), FASRT, FAEIRS
Tammy Curtis, PhD, RT(R)(CT)(CHES)

ELSEVIER

ELSEVIER

3251 Riverport Lane
St. Louis, Missouri 63043

WORKBOOK FOR MERRILL'S ATLAS OF RADIOGRAPHIC
POSITIONING & PROCEDURES, FOURTEENTH EDITION

ISBN: 978-0-323-59704-3

Notices

Practitioners and researchers must always rely on their own experience and knowledge in evaluating and using any information, methods, compounds or experiments described herein. Because of rapid advances in the medical sciences, in particular, independent verification of diagnoses and drug dosages should be made. To the fullest extent of the law, no responsibility is assumed by Elsevier, authors, editors or contributors for any injury and/or damage to persons or property as a matter of products liability, negligence or otherwise, or from any use or operation of any methods, products, instructions, or ideas contained in the material herein.

Content Strategist: Sonya Seigafuse
Content Development Manager: Lisa Newton
Content Development Specialist: Betsy McCormac
Publishing Services Manager: Shereen Jameel
Project Manager: Nadhiya Sekar
Designer: Gopalakrishnan Venkatraman

Printed in United States of America

Last digit is the print number: 9 8 7 6 5 4 3 2 1

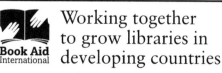

Working together
to grow libraries in
developing countries

www.elsevier.com • www.bookaid.org

Preface

This workbook has been developed to accompany *Merrill's Atlas of Radiographic Positioning and Procedures* (commonly referred to as *Merrill's Atlas* or just *Merrill's*). The chapters in this workbook supplement the 25 chapters of *Merrill's Atlas of Radiographic Positioning and Procedures* and provide a thorough review for students, helping them to learn and retain the content presented in the atlas. The workbook is also a useful companion to *Mosby's Radiography Online: Anatomy and Positioning for Merrill's Atlas of Radiographic Positioning & Procedures*. In addition, the material presented in this workbook can function as a useful review for any anatomy and positioning course or as a review for the American Registry of Radiologic Technologists (ARRT) certification examination. The exercises found in this workbook are designed to test the student's knowledge and understanding of osteology, anatomy, physiology, arthrology, pathology, radiographic examinations, and image evaluation.

FEATURES

The chapters containing essential projections are divided into two sections: an anatomy section and a positioning section.

- The anatomy sections consist of various exercises such as labeling and identification diagrams, short-answer and multiple-choice questions, matching exercises, and crossword puzzles.
- The positioning sections include short-answer and multiple-choice questions, true-false statements, fill-in-the-blank statements, matching exercises, identification exercises, and comparisons of standard radiographic projections.
- At the end of each chapter are self-assessments in the format of multiple-choice questions that review the entire chapter.
- Answers are provided in the instructor's resources, giving the instructors the flexibility to share the answers with their students.

NEW TO THIS EDITION

- New questions were added to 16 chapters.
- Several questions were revised to reflect the content presented in the textbook.

- Terminology for imaging has been updated to match Content Specifications for the ARRT Radiography Examination and the American Society of Radiologic Technologists (ASRT) Radiography Curriculum.
- Selected images were replaced to match new images in the textbook.
- Similar content was merged and rearranged to better reflect the order in which the majority of students learn radiographic positioning and procedures.
- Chapters were removed to coincide with those removed from the atlas.
- Relevant material was updated to current practice and integrated into appropriate chapters.

Some of the radiographic projections included and described in *Merrill's Atlas* are for reference purposes only and are no longer routinely performed in radiologic imaging facilities. Therefore we have chosen to focus on essential terminology, anatomy, and positioning information for the projections identified as necessary by the ARRT competencies, the Merrill's Advisory Board, and the authors' research.

Some chapters of *Merrill's Atlas* have limited radiographic applications or consist of radiographic procedures rarely performed today because of technologic advances in adjunct medical imagery modalities (e.g., computed tomography, magnetic resonance imaging, and sonography). Because those chapters do not include radiographic examinations deemed essential for entry-level competency, this workbook provides only cursory coverage for those chapters.

This workbook is one of three learning aids for students. The review exercises and assessments in this workbook along with related exercises in *Merrill's Atlas* and *Mosby's Radiography Online* and review of procedures in *Merrill's Pocket Guide to Radiography* will help students to master the theory and concepts presented in *Merrill's Atlas*.

Tammy Curtis

Acknowledgments

Special recognition to Steven G. Hayes, Sr., M.Ed., BSRT, (R), who was the original author of this workbook. Steven was also responsible for revising the second and third editions. I recently met Steven at a national conference and caught him browsing through the workbook only to discover his original puzzles and other material still printed as he designed. Steven's vision for creating a study tool that supports the content in the *Merrill's Atlas* continues to help radiography students today. Reflecting back as a radiography student, the workbook was a vital tool that reinforced my learning. I completed every exercise and then completed the end of the chapter self-tests. I knew that if I passed the self-tests without cheating, I could most likely pass my course examinations. Since the last edition, I have surveyed my students each year concerning how helpful they perceived the workbook to be for studying for their tests. Unanimously, the students responded that the workbook is their top study tool.

Special appreciation to Eugene Frank MA, RT(R), FASRT, FAEIRS, who took a chance and invited me to contribute to the textbook which later led to this once-in-a-life time opportunity to join the Merrill's team as a coauthor. I am honored to have worked with Gene, and I am forever grateful. Thank you Gene.

Special thanks to the current authors of the Merrill's team, Bruce Long, Barb Smith, and Jeannean Rollins who made me feel that I had a special place on the team during the revision of this edition. I continue to learn from their expertise. Thanks to each of you.

Special thanks to previous author Philip W. Ballinger, PhD, RT(R), FASRT, FAEIRS, who continues to be inspirational and share his experiences over the years at professional conferences.

Special appreciation to my friend Jon T. Williams, who is Miss Vinita Merrill's great nephew. He has inspired me to continue in his aunt's footsteps and contribute to the profession.

I would also like to thank my radiography students who pointed out areas of improvement in the workbook even though they were encouraged to do so by awarding them bonus points.

Special thanks to my husband who never complained as I spent hours working on this project, even though I spoiled him with a new truck and big boy toys along the way.

Most importantly, I would like to thank my Lord and Savior Jesus Christ who gave me favor, imparted wisdom, and opened doors that led me to this project.

Tammy Curtis

Contents

1 Preliminary Steps in Radiography

REVIEW

New and different important factors must be considered every time a radiograph is obtained. This exercise provides a comprehensive review of those important areas. Items require you to fill in missing words, select answers from a list, provide a short answer, or choose true or false (provide an explanation for any statement you believe to be false).

1. Define *image receptor* (IR).

2. List the four types of IRs used in diagnostic radiology.

3. Define the following radiographic terms:

   a. Positive beam limitation: _____

   _____

   b. Brightness: _____

   _____

   c. Spatial resolution: _____

   _____

   d. Distortion: _____

   _____

   e. Magnification: _____

   _____

   f. Contrast resolution: _____

   _____

4. What should the radiographer do if he or she notices a potentially serious or life-threatening condition of the patient when reviewing an image that was just performed?
   a. Tell the patient about the suspected condition
   b. Do nothing
   c. Instruct the patient to go to the emergency department
   d. Notify the radiologist before the patient is released

5. Fig. 1.1 shows two images demonstrating differences in the range of brightness between anatomic structures of varying tissue densities. Compare these images and identify which image was exposed using a compensating filter and which image was exposed without a compensating filter. (The choices are "with filter" and "without filter.")

   a. Image A: _____

   b. Image B: _____

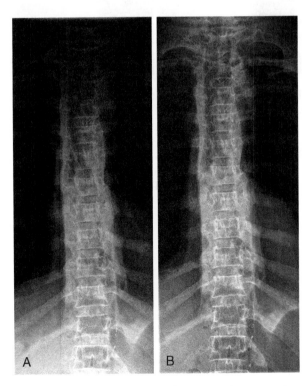

Fig. 1.1 Two images showing differences in range of brightness.

6. What exposure factor controls radiographic contrast?

7. Fig. 1.2 shows two images with different radiographic contrast. Compare the images, and identify each according to its contrast (short scale [high contrast] or long scale [low contrast]).

   a. Image A: _____

   b. Image B: _____

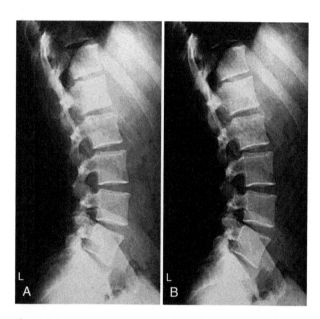

Fig. 1.2 Two images showing different scales of radiographic contrast.

8. From the following list, circle the six factors that control spatial resolution.
   a. Image Plate (IP) phosphor (digital)
   b. Flat panel detector
   c. Motion
   d. Distance
   e. Exposure
   f. Geometry
   g. Focal spot size
   h. mA
   i. kVp

9. Fig. 1.3 shows two images with different levels of spatial resolution. Compare the images, and identify each according to its spatial resolution (sharp image or unsharp image).

   a. Image A: _____

   b. Image B: _____

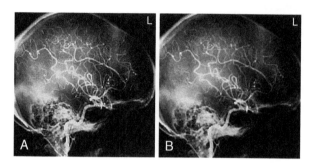

Fig. 1.3 Two images showing different levels of spatial resolution.

10. From the following list, circle the two factors that control radiographic magnification.
    a. Time, in second(s)
    b. mA
    c. kVp
    d. Object-to-image receptor distance (OID)
    e. Source-to-image receptor distance (SID)

11. True or false. All radiographs yield some degree of magnification.

12. Fig. 1.4 shows two images with different degrees of magnification. Assuming that both patients are average-size adults, which image (A or B) shows the most magnification?

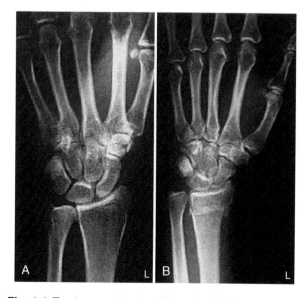

Fig. 1.4 Two images showing different levels of magnification.

13. True or false. If washable gowns are used, they should be starched; starch is radiolucent, which means it can be penetrated easily by x-rays.

14. Define and describe the anatomic position.

15. Describe how a posteroanterior (PA) projection radiograph of the chest should be oriented on the display monitor.

16. Fig. 1.5 shows two images of a PA projection of a chest. Which image (A or B) is correctly displayed?

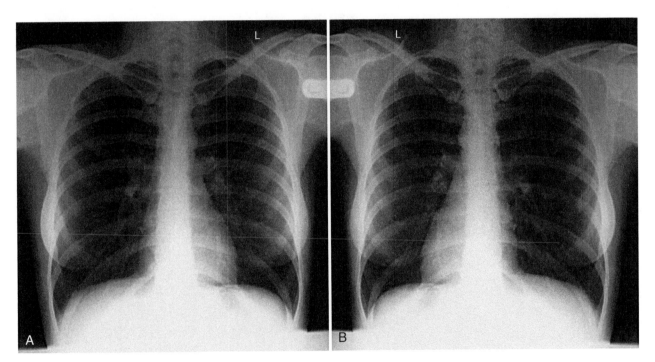

Fig. 1.5 Two images of a PA chest.

17. Describe how lateral projection radiographs should be displayed.

18. Fig. 1.6 shows two lateral projection chest radiographs. Which image (A or B) is correctly displayed as a left lateral chest radiograph?

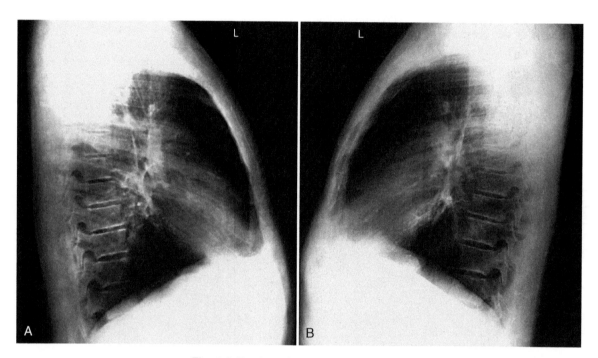

Fig. 1.6 Two lateral projections of a chest.

19. Describe how hand and foot radiographs should be displayed.

20. Fig. 1.7 shows two images of a PA left hand radiograph. Which image (A or B) is correctly displayed?

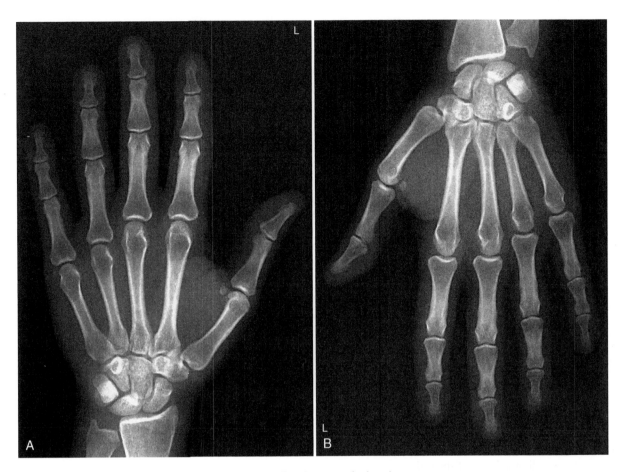

Fig. 1.7 Two images of a hand.

21. Fig. 1.8 shows two images of an anteroposterior (AP) right knee radiograph. Which image (A or B) is correctly displayed?

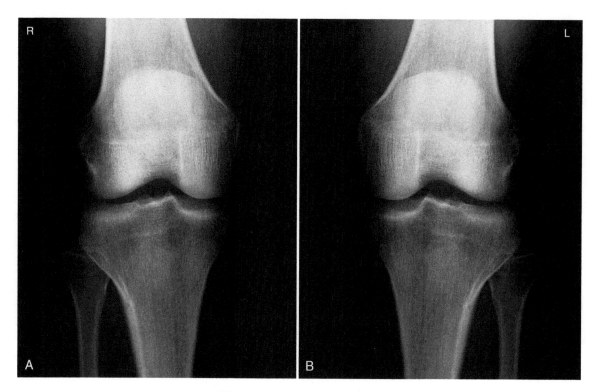

Fig. 1.8 Two images of a knee.

22. Describe the two most common ways that lateral decubitus radiographs are displayed.

23. Fig. 1.9 shows two AP chest radiographs with the patient in a lateral decubitus position. The patient has fluid present in the right lung. Correctly identify each image as either left lateral decubitus or right lateral decubitus.

a. Image A: _____

b. Image B: _____

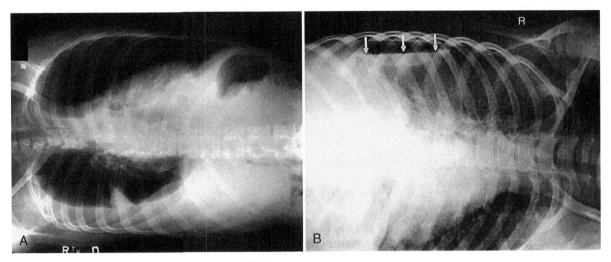

Fig. 1.9 Two anteroposterior chest radiographs, lateral decubitus position.

24. When the radiologist is unable to see the patient, who is responsible for ensuring that an adequate clinical history accompanies the radiographs?

25. What is the easiest and most convenient method to prevent the spread of microorganisms?

26. When using a free IR to perform an examination on an isolation patient, the IR should be placed _____ the sheet (on top of or under).

27. What protective apparel should radiographers wear if the possibility of touching blood exists?

28. What procedure should be followed to dispose of used hypodermic needles properly?

29. List procedures that require aseptic technique when performed in the radiology department.

30. True or false. When performing an examination in the operating room (OR), position the C-arm next to the operating table on the same side as the surgeon.

31. What information should be included in a procedure (or protocol) book that identifies each examination performed in the radiography department?

32. List the three ways a patient's colon may be cleansed for an abdominal examination.

33. Identify the three types of muscular tissue, and state the type of motion (voluntary or involuntary) associated with each.

34. The rhythmic motion of smooth muscle structures is

    called _____.

35. What exposure factor is used to control involuntary motion?

36. What body system controls the movement of voluntary muscles?

37. From the following list, circle the four ways voluntary motion can be controlled by a radiographer.
    a. Increase mAs
    b. Decrease mAs
    c. Apply immobilization
    d. Give clear instructions
    e. Adjust support devices
    f. Increase exposure time
    g. Decrease exposure time
    h. Provide patient comfort

38. Why is it necessary to ensure that any folds in cloth gowns are straightened out before making the radiographic exposure?

39. What devices must be removed from the patient within the area of interest when the skull is examined?

40. Before beginning a radiographic examination, what should the radiographer do to gain the cooperation of a coherent patient?

41. What is the minimum number of personnel that should be used to transfer a helpless patient from a gurney to the radiographic table?

42. From the following list, circle the four items of identification information that should be on every radiograph.
    a. Patient's name
    b. Patient's diagnosis
    c. Date of examination
    d. Institutional identity
    e. Patient's marital status
    f. Side marker (right or left)
    g. Requesting physician's name

43. Some examinations require an additional marker to

    indicate the _____ after the introduction of a contrast medium.

44. From the following list, indicate which of the following *is **not recommended*** or ***unacceptable*** for right and left side marker placement.
    a. Use of electronic insertion of the side marker in digital imaging
    b. Placement of the marker in the anatomy of interest
    c. Placement of the marker on the border of the collimated field
    d. Placing the marker directly on the body part

For Questions 45 to 54, for each projection in Column A, select from Column B the best choice for how side markers should be used for that particular projection (R = right side; L = left side).

Column A

_____ 45. PA hand

_____ 46. PA chest

_____ 47. AP forearm

_____ 48. Lateral skull

_____ 49. PA skull

_____ 50. AP cervical spine

_____ 51. Lateral lumbar spine

_____ 52. Lateral decubitus chest

_____ 53. AP oblique lumbar spine

_____ 54. Bilateral AP knees (side-by-side on one IR)

Column B

a. R marker typically used

b. L marker typically used

c. Appropriate R or L marker used

d. Mark side closer to the IR

e. Mark side farther from the IR

f. Mark the side up (opposite of side laid on)

g. Use both R and L marker to identify both sides

AP, Anteroposterior; *IR,* image receptor; *PA,* posteroanterior.

55. What adjustment can be made by the radiographer to compensate for an increase in OID?

56. List four reasons why it would become necessary to angle the central ray.

57. List two purposes of collimation when restricted to irradiate only the anatomy of interest.

58. When using computed radiography imaging plates, how is the field size limited to prevent overexposing the patient?

59. True or false. In a direct digital image, the field size or collimation must be manually adjusted.

60. True or false. Creating an image using a larger than required (necessary) field size is a violation of the American Society of Radiologic Technologists (ASRT) Code of Ethics.

61. True or false. Shuttering of direct digital images is an acceptable substitution for proper collimation.

62. List the three guidelines for determining when gonadal shielding should be used.

For Questions 63 to 74, match the patient conditions in Column A with the appropriate radiation exposure compensation necessary to provide a diagnostic image listed in Column B.

Column A

_____ 63. Ascites

_____ 64. Edema

_____ 65. Old age

_____ 66. Atrophy

_____ 67. Emaciation

_____ 68. Pneumonia

_____ 69. Emphysema

_____ 70. Enlarged heart

_____ 71. Pneumothorax

_____ 72. Hydrocephalus

_____ 73. Pleural effusion

_____ 74. Degenerative arthritis

Column B

a. Requires a decrease in radiation exposure

b. Requires an increase in radiation exposure

9

75. What are the two phases of respiration?

76. What respiration phase is requested when the goal is to expand lung fields to the maximum extent possible?

77. What respiration procedure provides for lung motion but not rib motion?

For Questions 78 to 89, define the following abbreviations:

78. AP: _____

79. AEC: _____

80. ASRT: _____

81. IR: _____

82. CR: _____
    (imaging method)

83. CR: _____
    (x-ray field reference)

84. mAs: _____

85. DR: _____

86. APR: _____

87. ARRT: _____

88. ASIS: _____

89. BMI: _____

Questions 90 to 94 pertain to "Working Effectively with Obese Patients."

90. How have equipment manufacturers responded to the growing obesity problem in the United States?

91. What is the major risk factor in transportation and transfer of obese patients?

92. Which body parts are most affected, in terms of increased size, by morbid obesity?

93. What bony landmark(s) are usually palpable on obese patients?
    a. Jugular notch
    b. Xiphoid process
    c. ASIS
    d. Iliac crest

94. What is the approximate distance of the pubic symphysis from the jugular notch on a patient who measures 5 feet, 3 inches (160 cm) tall?

CHAPTER 1: SELF-TEST: PRELIMINARY STEPS IN RADIOGRAPHY

Answer the following questions by selecting the best choice.

1. _____ elevates the diaphragm and abdominal viscera, shortens the lung fields, depresses the sternum, and lowers the ribs and increases their angle near the spine.
   a. Inspiration
   b. Expiration

2. _____ depresses the diaphragm and abdominal viscera, lengthens and expands the lung fields, elevates the sternum and pushes it anteriorly, and elevates the ribs.
   a. Inspiration
   b. Expiration

3. Which of the following factors controls shape distortion?
   a. Alignment
   b. mA
   c. Milliampere-time (mAs)
   d. SID

4. When imaging an obese patient, which landmarks are difficult to palpate? (Select all that apply)
   a. Jugular notch
   b. Anterior-superior iliac spine (ASIS)
   c. Iliac crest
   d. Greater trochanter

5. Based on the exterior dimensions of obese patients, larger IRs are needed to image these patients.
   a. True
   b. False

6. A PA projection radiograph of the hand should be displayed:
   a. from the perspective of the x-ray tube and with the fingers pointing upward.
   b. from the perspective of the x-ray tube and with the fingers pointing downward.
   c. with the patient in the anatomic position and with the fingers pointing upward.
   d. with the patient in the anatomic position and with the fingers pointing downward.

7. Who is responsible for obtaining a necessary clinical history when the radiologist is unable to see the patient?
   a. Radiographer
   b. Radiology nurse
   c. Chief technologist
   d. Department receptionist

8. To dispose of a hypodermic needle properly, it should be:
   a. bent.
   b. recapped.
   c. broken to prevent its reuse.
   d. placed in a puncture-proof container.

9. Which of the following technical factors is most important to adjust and increase when imaging an obese patient?
   a. mAs
   b. kVp
   c. Focal spot
   d. Automatic exposure control (AEC)

10. Within the OR, who should remove sterile items that are in the way of the radiographer?
   a. Surgeon
   b. Radiographer
   c. Anesthesiologist
   d. Circulating nurse

11. To prepare the patient for a radiographic examination of the abdomen, what are the three methods used for cleansing the patient's bowel?
   a. Laxatives, enemas, and exercise
   b. Limited diet, enemas, and exercise
   c. Limited diet, laxatives, and enemas
   d. Limited diet, laxatives, and exercise

12. Which type of muscle tissue produces peristalsis?
   a. Cardiac
   b. Striated
   c. Smooth

13. Which type of muscle tissue comprises skeletal muscle?
   a. Cardiac
   b. Striated
   c. Smooth

14. Which pathologic condition requires a decrease in exposure factors from the routine procedure?
   a. Edema
   b. Pneumonia
   c. Emphysema
   d. Pleural effusion

15. Which change in exposure factors should be used to control voluntary motion that is a result of the patient's age or mental illness?
   a. Increase the mA
   b. Decrease the mA
   c. Increase the exposure time
   d. Decrease the exposure time

16. Which procedure best reduces the possibility of patient-controlled motion?
    a. Increase the mA.
    b. Increase the exposure time.
    c. Give understandable instructions to the patient.
    d. Use shorter SID.

17. Which side marker placement rule applies when performing an AP oblique radiograph of the cervical spine?
    a. The R marker is typically used.
    b. The L marker is typically used.
    c. Always mark the side closest to the IR.
    d. Always mark the side farthest from the IR.

18. Which piece of information is *not* required as part of the identification of radiographs?
    a. Name of the patient
    b. Date of the examination
    c. Name of the radiographer
    d. Name of the medical facility

19. What is the primary purpose of collimating to the area of interest?
    a. Lengthens the scale of contrast
    b. Reduces the required mA
    c. Reduces patient exposure
    d. Compensates for an increase in OID

20. How is radiographic image quality affected when the radiation field is restricted to the area under examination only?
    a. Increased image brightness
    b. Increased radiographic contrast resolution
    c. Reduced magnification
    d. Decreased radiographic contrast resolution

21. Which of the following is a consideration for determining when to use gonadal shielding?
    1. The patient has a reasonable reproductive potential.
    2. The gonads lie within or close (approximately 2 inches [5 cm]) to the primary x-ray field.
    3. The patient is aware of the application of the gonadal shield.

    a. 1 and 2 only
    b. 1 and 3 only
    c. 2 and 3 only
    d. 1, 2, and 3

22. Which change most improves spatial resolution when the sternum is imaged?
    a. Increasing the OID
    b. Decreasing the SID
    c. Decreasing the source-to-object distance
    d. Increasing the SID

23. For which examination is the use of gonadal shielding most important for a patient of childbearing age?
    a. Wrist
    b. Skull
    c. Chest
    d. Lumbosacral region

24. Which computed radiography accessory houses the image storage phosphors that acquire the latent image?
    a. Image reader
    b. Control panel
    c. Imaging plate
    d. Video monitor

25. What is the IR in direct digital radiography?
    a. Phosphor imaging plate
    b. Intensifying screen
    c. Solid-state detector
    d. Computer monitor

26. In direct digital imaging, how is collimation (field size) controlled?
    a. Manually by the radiographer
    b. Automatically by an automatic collimator
    c. Electronically by shuttering
    d. All of these control field size in direct digital imaging

27. Reasons to avoid using electronic side marker placement (annotation) in digital imaging include:
    1. increased potential for errors in marking the correct side.
    2. increased legal implications.
    3. eliminating anatomy being obscured by the marker.

    a. 1 and 2 only
    b. 1 and 3 only
    c. 2 and 3 only
    d. 1, 2, and 3

28. The knowledge, skills, ability, and behaviors that are essential for providing optimal care to *defined groups* of patients is termed:
    a. functional competence.
    b. age-specific competence.
    c. patient care competence.
    d. chronologic competence.

29. When imaging obese patients, all of the following should be taken into consideration *except for*:
    a. locating landmarks such as the jugular notch and pubic symphysis.
    b. setting the collimator to the smallest dimensions.
    c. selecting standard IR sizes and standard collimation settings for DR.
    d. selecting larger IR sizes and larger collimation settings for DR.

30. The approximate distance from the jugular notch to the pubic symphysis on a patient who is more than 6 feet (183 cm) tall is:
    a. 15 inches (38 cm).
    b. 21 inches (53 cm).
    c. 22 inches (56 cm).
    d. 24 inches (61 cm).

For Questions 31 to 35, match the functions in Column A with the appropriate organization in Column B.

Column A

_____ 31. Maintain Radiography Practice Standards

_____ 32. Maintain the Standard of Ethics

_____ 33. Describe necessary education and certification

_____ 34. Radiographer Scope of Practice can be found on their website

_____ 35. Provides directives for infection control

Column B

a. ASRT

b. ARRT

c. Centers for Disease Control and Prevention (CDC)

2 General Anatomy and Radiographic Positioning Terminology

Exercise 1: General Anatomy

No one can succeed in a profession without first mastering its terminology. This exercise reviews the terminology unique to radiography. Items require you to identify illustrations, fill in missing words, provide a short answer, match columns, or select answers from a list.

1. Define the following terms:

   a. Anatomy: _____

   _____

   b. Physiology:_____

   _____

   c. Osteology: _____

   _____

2. Describe the anatomic position.

3. List the four fundamental planes of the body.

4. Any plane passing vertically through the body from front to back and dividing the body into right and left segments is called a(n) _____ plane.

5. Any plane passing vertically through the body from side to side and dividing the body into anterior and posterior segments is called a(n) _____ plane.

6. The plane that passes vertically through the midline of the body from side to side and divides the body into equal anterior and posterior segments is called the

   _____ plane.

7. The plane passing through the midline of the body and dividing it into equal right and left halves is known as the _____ plane.

8. A plane that passes crosswise through the body and divides the body into superior and inferior segments is a(n) _____ plane or

   _____ plane.

9. Identify the four body planes shown in Fig. 2.1.

   A. _____

   B. _____

   C. _____

   D. _____

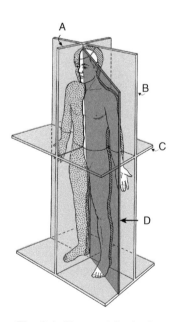

Fig. 2.1 Planes of the body.

10. List the two major cavities of the torso.

For questions 11 to 20, match the structures (Column A) with the body cavities in which they are found (Column B).

Column A

_____ 11. Liver

_____ 12. Lungs

_____ 13. Heart

_____ 14. Uterus

_____ 15. Spleen

_____ 16. Rectum

_____ 17. Ureters

_____ 18. Trachea

_____ 19. Ovaries

_____ 20. Esophagus

Column B

a. Thoracic

b. Abdominal

c. Pelvic

21. Identify each body cavity shown in Fig. 2.2.

A. _____

B. _____

C. _____

D. _____

E. _____

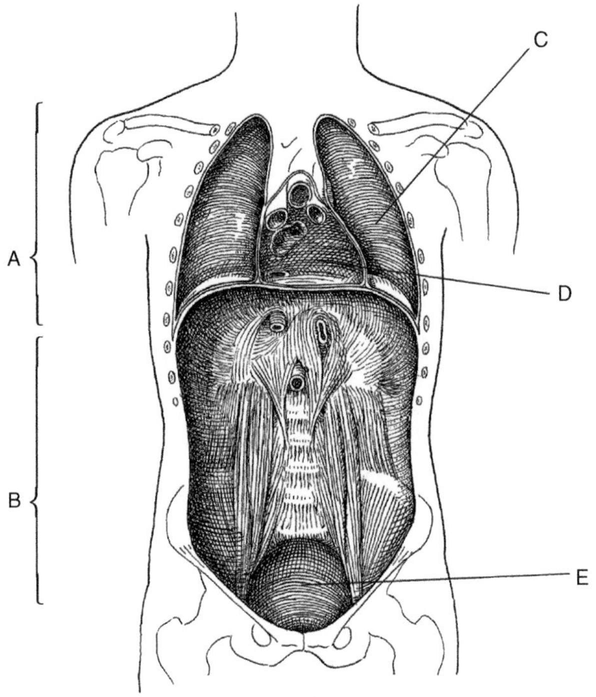

Fig. 2.2 Anterior view of the torso.

22. Identify the four quadrants of the body shown in Fig. 2.3.

A. _____

B. _____

C. _____

D. _____

23. Identify the nine regions of the abdomen shown in Fig. 2.4.

A. _____

B. _____

C. _____

D. _____

E. _____

F. _____

G. _____

H. _____

I. _____

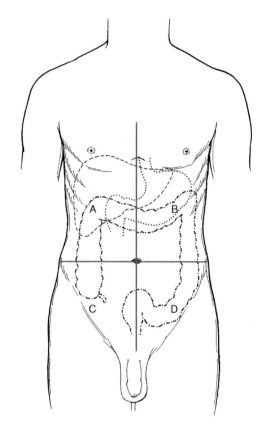

Fig. 2.3 Clinical divisions of the four quadrants of the abdomen.

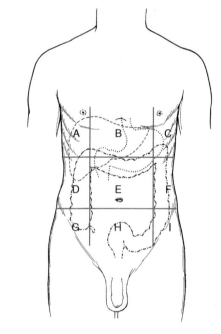

Fig. 2.4 Anatomic divisions of the nine regions of the abdomen.

24. Identify the body habitus illustrated in Figs. 2.5 to 2.8.

   a. Fig. 2.5: _____

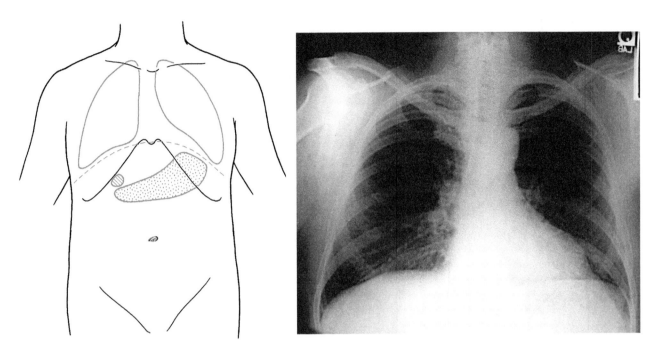

Fig. 2.5 Body habitus diagram and radiograph.

   b. Fig. 2.6: _____

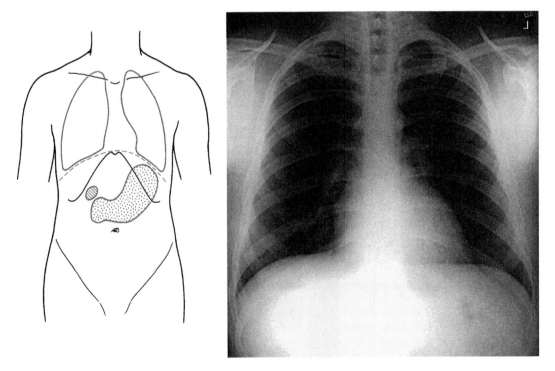

Fig. 2.6 Body habitus diagram and radiograph.

17

c. Fig. 2.7: _____

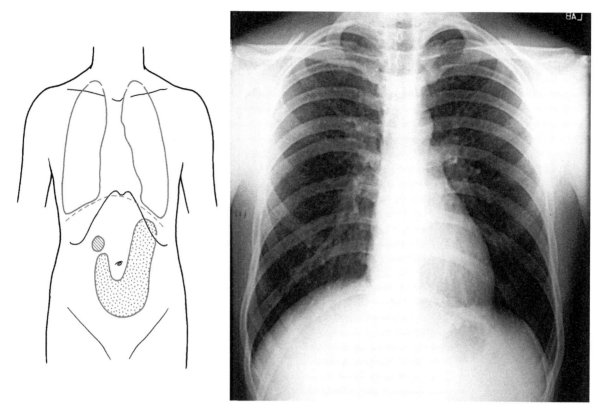

Fig. 2.7 Body habitus diagram and radiograph.

d. Fig. 2.8: _____

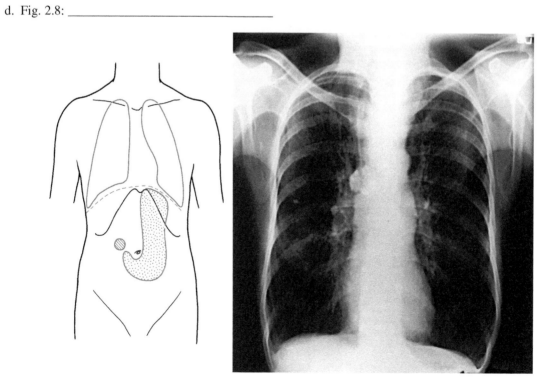

Fig. 2.8 Body habitus diagram and radiograph.

Exercise 2: Osteology

This exercise assists in your understanding of bone types, development, bone and skeletal classifications, and bony landmarks used for radiographic positioning. Identify structures, fill in missing words, or provide a short answer for each question.

For Questions 1 to 12, match the vertebrae (Column A) with the appropriate external landmark present at the same body level (Column B).

Column A

_____ 1. C1

_____ 2. C3, C4

_____ 3. C5

_____ 4. C7, T1

_____ 5. T2, T3

_____ 6. T4, T5

_____ 7. T7

_____ 8. T9, T10

_____ 9. L2, L3

_____ 10. L4, L5

_____ 11. S1, S2

_____ 12. Coccyx

Column B

a. Gonion

b. Mastoid tip

c. Hyoid bone

d. Thyroid cartilage

e. Vertebra prominens

f. Inferior costal margin

g. Level of sternal angle

h. Level of jugular notch

i. Level of xiphoid process

j. Level of inferior angles of scapulae

k. Level of anterior superior iliac spines

l. Level of superior most aspect of iliac crests

m. Level of pubic symphysis and greater trochanters

n. Approximately 2 inches (5 cm) above level of jugular notch

13. Identify the surface landmarks of the head and neck shown in Fig. 2.9.

A. _____

B. _____

C. _____

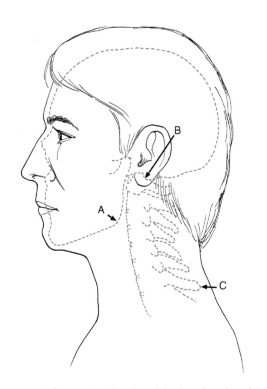

Fig. 2.9 Surface landmarks of the head and neck.

14. Identify the vertebral level or surface landmark (or both) for each marked location shown in Fig. 2.10.

A. _____

B. _____

C. _____

D. _____

E. _____

F. _____

G. _____

H. _____

I. _____

J. _____

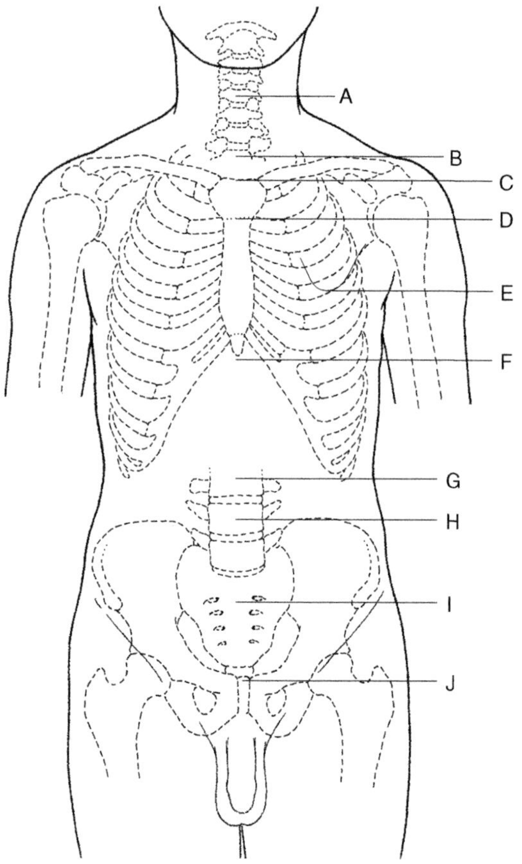

Fig. 2.10 Radiographic landmarks of the torso.

15. How many bones comprise the typical adult skeleton?

16. List the two main skeletal divisions that make up the bony framework of the body.

17. From the following list, circle the four main parts of the appendicular skeleton.
    a. Ribs
    b. Pelvic girdle
    c. Shoulder girdle
    d. Vertebral column
    e. Upper limbs (extremities)
    f. Lower limbs (extremities)

18. From the following list, circle the four main parts of the axial skeleton.
    a. Neck
    b. Skull
    c. Thorax
    d. Vertebral column
    e. Upper limbs (extremities)
    f. Lower limbs (extremities)

For Questions 19 to 22, match the definitions in Column A with the terms in Column B.

Column A	Column B
_____ 19. Outer layer of bony tissue	a. Periosteum
_____ 20. Inner trabeculated portion of the bone	b. Spongy bone
_____ 21. Central cylindric canal of long bones	c. Compact bone
_____ 22. Tough, fibrous membrane that covers the bone (except where bone is covered by articular cartilage)	d. Medullary cavity

23. From the following list, circle the five classifications (by shape) of bones.
    a. Flat
    b. Long
    c. Short
    d. Small
    e. Cranial
    f. Irregular
    g. Appendicular
    h. Sesamoid

For Questions 24 to 30, match the bones in Column A with the classifications in Column B.

Column A	Column B
_____ 24. Tibia	a. Flat
_____ 25. Lunate	b. Long
_____ 26. Radius	c. Short
_____ 27. Patella	d. Irregular
_____ 28. Scapula	e. Sesamoid
_____ 29. Maxilla	
_____ 30. Vertebrae	

31. Define the following bone classifications:

a. Long: _____

_____

b. Short: _____

_____

c. Flat: _____

_____

d. Irregular: _____

_____

e. Sesamoid: _____

_____

Exercise 3: Arthrology

This exercise reviews the classifications and definition of the joints of the human body. Items require a short answer or matching columns.

1. List the two classifications of joints. Which is the more widely used classification?

2. List the three structural classifications of articulations.

For Questions 3 to 5, match the classifications of articulations in Column A with the types of movements in Column B.

Column A	Column B
_____ 3. Synovial	a. Immovable
_____ 4. Fibrous	b. Freely movable
_____ 5. Cartilaginous	c. Limited or slight movement

6. Identify the following articulations according to their functional and structural classifications:

	Functional Classification	Structural Classification
a. Knee:	_____	_____
b. Cranial sutures:	_____	_____
c. Pubic symphysis:	_____	_____

For Questions 7 to 12, match the definitions in Column A with the articulation terms in Column B.

Column A	Column B
_____ 7. Fibrous envelope that encloses a synovial joint	a. Bursae
_____ 8. Joint in which two bones are joined by hyaline cartilage	b. Meniscus
_____ 9. Lubricant and nutrient compound found within synovial joints	c. Symphysis
_____ 10. Joining together of two midline bones in the body by a plate of fibrocartilage	d. Synovial fluid
_____ 11. Fluid-containing sacs that are interposed between sliding surfaces to reduce friction	e. Synchondrosis
_____ 12. Fibrocartilaginous disk pad located between the ends of bones in some synovial joints	f. Articular capsule

For Questions 13 to 18, match each type of synovial joint in Column A with the kinds of movement that are applicable from Column B. Some synovial joints may have more than one selection from Column B. Some selections from Column B may be used more than once.

Column A

_____ 13. Gliding (plane)

_____ 14. Hinge (ginglymus)

_____ 15. Pivot (trochoid)

_____ 16. Ellipsoid (condyloid)

_____ 17. Saddle (sellar)

_____ 18. Ball and socket (spheroid)

Column B

a. Sliding

b. Gliding

c. Flexion

d. Extension

e. Rotation

f. Abduction

g. Adduction

h. Circumduction

For Questions 19 to 28, match the articulations in Column A with the corresponding synovial-type joint in Column B.

Column A

_____ 19. Hip

_____ 20. Knee

_____ 21. Elbow

_____ 22. Wrist

_____ 23. Shoulder

_____ 24. C1 and C2

_____ 25. Intertarsal

_____ 26. Interphalangeal

_____ 27. Metacarpophalangeal

_____ 28. Carpometacarpal joint of the thumb

Column B

a. Saddle (sellar)

b. Gliding (plane)

c. Pivot (trochoid)

d. Hinge (ginglymus)

e. Ellipsoid (condyloid)

f. Ball and socket (spheroid)

Exercise 4: Bony Markings and Features

This exercise provides a review of the markings and features of bones. Items require you to match terms with definitions and work a crossword puzzle.

For Questions 1 to 15, match the process or projection terms in Column A with the definitions in Column B.

Column A

_____ 1. Head

_____ 2. Horn

_____ 3. Crest

_____ 4. Facet

_____ 5. Spine

_____ 6. Styloid

_____ 7. Tubercle

_____ 8. Condyle

_____ 9. Hamulus

_____ 10. Coracoid

_____ 11. Malleolus

_____ 12. Trochanter

_____ 13. Tuberosity

_____ 14. Epicondyle

_____ 15. Protuberance

Column B

a. Sharp process

b. Bony projection

c. Beaklike process

d. Ridgelike process

e. Club-shaped process

f. Hook-shaped process

g. Long, pointed process

h. Projection above a condyle

i. Hornlike process on a bone

j. Expanded end of a long bone

k. Small, rounded, elevated process

l. Large, rounded, elevated process

m. Rounded process at an articular extremity

n. Small, smooth-surfaced process for articulation

o. Large, rounded, elevated process located at the junction of the neck and shaft of the femur

For Questions 16 to 21, match the terms for depressions in Column A with the definitions in Column B.

Column A

_____ 16. Fossa

_____ 17. Sinus

_____ 18. Sulcus

_____ 19. Groove

_____ 20. Fissure

_____ 21. Foramen

Column B

a. Cleft or groove

b. Pit, fovea, or hollow

c. Shallow, linear depression

d. Recess, groove, cavity, or hollow space

e. Furrow, trench, or fissurelike depression

f. Hole in a bone for transmission of blood vessels and nerves

22. Use the following clues to complete the crossword puzzle. All answers refer to anatomic terms for processes or depressions.

Across

3. Hook-shaped process
6. Furrow, trench, or fissurelike depression
8. Long, pointed process
9. Large process located at junction of neck and shaft of femur
11. Rounded process at an articular extremity
12. Large, rounded, elevated process
17. Expanded end of long bone
18. Hole in bone for the transmission of blood vessels and nerves
20. Ridgelike process
21. Shallow, linear depression
22. Cleft or groove
23. Projection above a condyle

Down

1. Pit, fovea, or hollow
2. Club-shaped process
4. Sharp process
5. Bony projection
7. Small, smooth-surfaced process for articulation
10. Indentation into the border of a bone
13. Small, rounded, elevated process
14. Beaklike process
15. Less prominent ridge than a crest
16. Tubelike passageway
19. Recess, groove, cavity, or hollow space

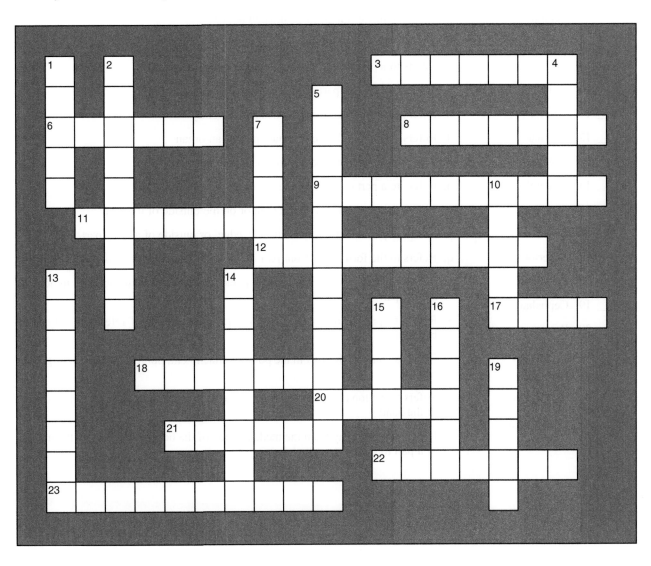

Chapter **2** **General Anatomy and Radiographic Positioning Terminology**

Exercise 5: Body Relationship Terms

This exercise reviews the terminology used to describe locations and relationships of the body and its parts. Items require you to match terms and definitions and complete a crossword puzzle.

For Questions 1 to 24, match the body parts in Column A with the definitions in Column B. Some definitions may be used more than once.

Column A

_____ 1. Deep

_____ 2. Distal

_____ 3. Lateral

_____ 4. Dorsal

_____ 5. Medial

_____ 6. Central

_____ 7. Ventral

_____ 8. Caudad

_____ 9. Palmar

_____ 10. Plantar

_____ 11. Inferior

_____ 12. Internal

_____ 13. Dorsum

_____ 14. Visceral

_____ 15. Anterior

_____ 16. External

_____ 17. Superior

_____ 18. Proximal

_____ 19. Cephalad

_____ 20. Posterior

_____ 21. Ipsilateral

_____ 22. Peripheral

_____ 23. Superficial

_____ 24. Contralateral

Column B

a. Refers to the sole of the foot

b. Refers to the palm of the hand

c. Refers to the covering of an organ

d. Refers to parts far from the surface

e. Refers to a part near the skin or surface

f. Refers to nearer the feet or situated below

g. Refers to nearer the head or situated above

h. Refers to parts toward the head of the body

i. Refers to a part on the same side of the body

j. Refers to the back part of the body or an organ

k. Refers to parts away from the head of the body

l. Refers to the middle area or main part of an organ

m. Refers to a part within or on the inside of an organ

n. Refers to a part or parts on the opposite side of the body

o. Refers to a part outside of an organ or on the outside of the body

p. Refers to parts at or near the surface, edge, or outside of a body part

q. Refers to the forward or front part of the body or to the forward part of an organ

r. Refers to parts toward the median plane of the body or toward the middle of a body part

s. Refers to parts nearest the point of attachment, point of reference, origin, or beginning

t. Refers to parts farthest from the point of attachment, point of reference, origin, or beginning

u. Refers to the top or anterior surface of the foot or to the back or posterior surface of the hand

v. Refers to parts away from the median plane of the body or away from the middle of a part to the right or the left

25. Use the following clues to complete the crossword puzzle. All answers refer to body part terminology.

Across

1. Away from the head of the body
5. Near the skin or surface
7. Sole of the foot
9. Toward the head of the body
10. Within or on the inside of an organ
11. Nearest the point of attachment or origin
14. Away from the median plane to the right or left
15. Outside an organ or the body
16. Pertaining to caudad
17. Opposite of superior

Down

2. Posterior side
3. Opposite of lateral
4. Far from the surface
5. Opposite of inferior
6. Farthest from the point of reference or origin
7. At or near the edge of a body part
8. Front part of the body
9. On the opposite side of the body
10. On the same side of the body
12. Back part of the body or an organ
13. Middle or main part of an organ

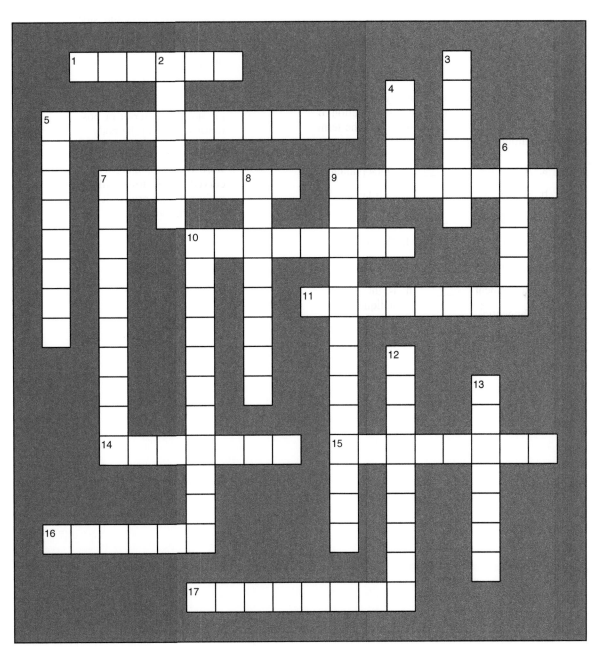

Chapter **2** **General Anatomy and Radiographic Positioning Terminology**

This exercise reviews the terms used in radiographic positioning. Items require a short answer, identification of diagrams, and matching terms to definitions.

1. Define the following radiographic positioning terms:

    a. Projection: _____

    _____

    b. Position: _____

    _____

    c. View: _____

    _____

    d. Method: _____

    _____

2. Classify each of the following terms by writing P in the space provided if the term refers to a projection, *B* if the term refers to a body position, or *R* if the term refers to a radiographic position.

    _____ a. AP   _____ i. Dorsoplantar

    _____ b. Supine   _____ j. Left lateral

    _____ c. Upright   _____ k. Transthoracic

    _____ d. AP axial   _____ l. Trendelenburg

    _____ e. Lordotic   _____ m. Parietoacanthial

    _____ f. Recumbent   _____ n. Right anterior oblique

    _____ g. Tangential   _____ o. Right lateral decubitus

    _____ h. AP oblique

For Questions 3 to 8, match the descriptions in Column A with the projection terms in Column B.

Column A

_____ 3. Central ray is angled longitudinally with the long axis of the body.

_____ 4. Central ray enters the anterior body surface and exits the posterior body surface.

_____ 5. Central ray enters the posterior body surface and exits the anterior body surface.

_____ 6. Central ray enters the side or lateral aspect of the body or body part and exits the other side.

_____ 7. Central ray enters the body or body part from a side angle into the anterior or posterior surface of the body.

_____ 8. Central ray is directed toward the outer margin of a curved body to profile a body part and project it free of superimposition.

Column B

a. AP

b. PA

c. Axial

d. Lateral

e. Oblique

f. Tangential

For Questions 9 to 14, identify the projections illustrated in Figs. 2.11 to 2.16.

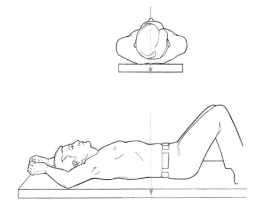

Fig. 2.11 Diagram showing the path of an x-ray beam.

9. Fig. 2.11: _____

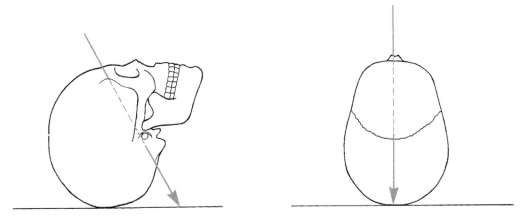

Fig. 2.12 Diagram showing the path of an x-ray beam.

10. Fig. 2.12: _____

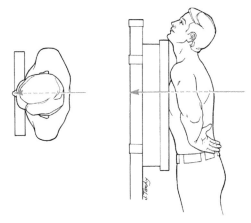

Fig. 2.13 Diagram showing the path of an x-ray beam.

11. Fig. 2.13: _____

29

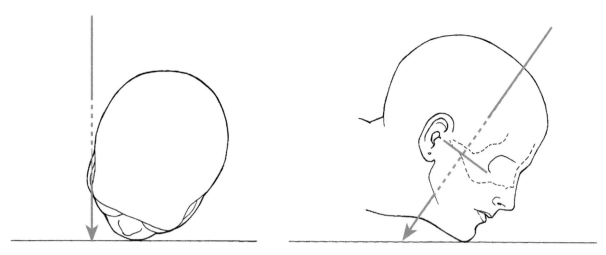

Fig. 2.14 Diagram showing the path of an x-ray beam.

12. Fig. 2.14: _____

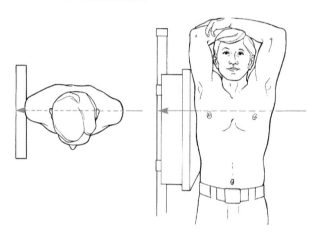

Fig. 2.15 Diagram showing the path of an x-ray beam.

13. Fig. 2.15: _____

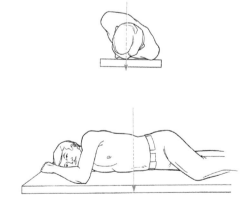

Fig. 2.16 Diagram showing the path of an x-ray beam.

14. Fig. 2.16: _____

For Questions 15 to 20, match the position descriptions in Column A with the terms in Column B.

Column A

_____ 15. Lying face down

_____ 16. Lying on the back

_____ 17. Lying down in any position

_____ 18. Erect or marked by a vertical position

_____ 19. Lying supine with the head lower than the feet

_____ 20. Lying supine with the head higher than the feet

Column B

a. Upright position

b. Fowler position

c. Recumbent position

d. Trendelenburg position

e. Prone (ventral recumbent) position

f. Supine (dorsal recumbent) position

For Questions 21 to 23, identify the body positions illustrated in Figs. 2.17 to 2.19.

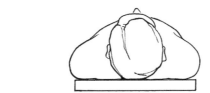

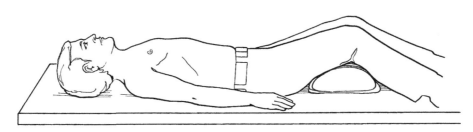

Fig. 2.17 A body position.

21. Fig. 2.17: _____

Chapter **2** **General Anatomy and Radiographic Positioning Terminology**

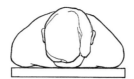

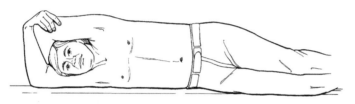

Fig. 2.18 A body position.

22. Fig. 2.18: _____

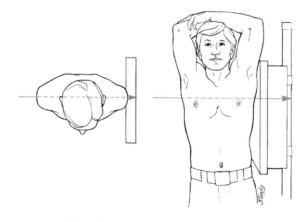

Fig. 2.19 A body position.

23. Fig. 2.19: _____

For Questions 24 to 32, identify the radiographic positions illustrated in Figs. 2.20 to 2.28.

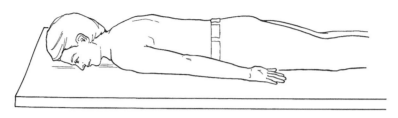

Fig. 2.20 A radiographic position.

24. Fig. 2.20: _____

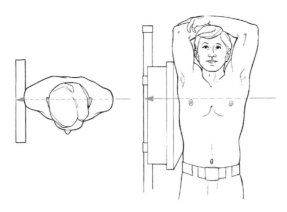

Fig. 2.21 A radiographic position.

25. Fig. 2.21: _____

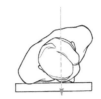

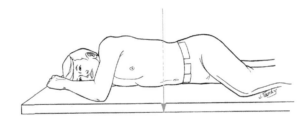

Fig. 2.22 A radiographic position.

26. Fig. 2.22: _____

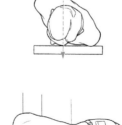

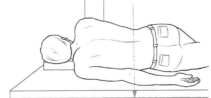

Fig. 2.23 A radiographic position.

27. Fig. 2.23: _____

Chapter **2 General Anatomy and Radiographic Positioning Terminology**

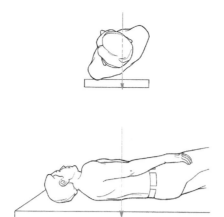

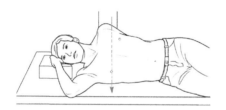

Fig. 2.24 A radiographic position.

28. Fig. 2.24: _____

Fig. 2.25 A radiographic position.

29. Fig. 2.25: _____

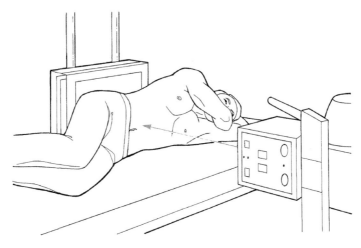

Fig. 2.26 A radiographic position.

30. Fig. 2.26: _____

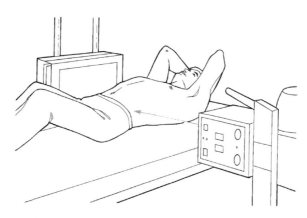

Fig. 2.27 A radiographic position.

31. Fig. 2.27: _____

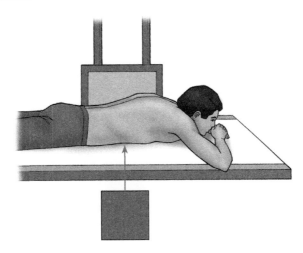

Fig. 2.28 A radiographic position.

32. Fig. 2.28: _____

Chapter **2** **General Anatomy and Radiographic Positioning Terminology**

Exercise 7: Body Movement

Terminology and Chapter 1 Abbreviations. This exercise reviews the terms used to describe the movements of the body and its parts. Items require you to match terms and definitions, write short answers, and identify movements by examining diagrams.

For Questions 1 to 15, match the body movements in Column A with the definitions in Column B.

Column A

_____ 1. Tilt

_____ 2. Rotate

_____ 3. Flexion

_____ 4. Pronate

_____ 5. Eversion

_____ 6. Supinate

_____ 7. Deviation

_____ 8. Extension

_____ 9. Inversion

_____ 10. Abduction

_____ 11. Adduction

_____ 12. Hyperflexion

_____ 13. Circumduction

_____ 14. Hyperextension

_____ 15. Dorsiflexion

Column B

a. To turn around an axis

b. Straightening of a joint

c. Circular movement of a limb

d. Forced or excessive straightening of a joint

e. Forced or excessive flexion of a joint or part

f. Flexion of the foot toward the leg

g. A turning away from the regular standard or course

h. To turn the forearm so that the palm of the hand faces forward

i. To turn the forearm so that the palm of the hand faces backward

j. Movement of a part toward the central axis of a body or body part

k. Movement of the foot when it is turned inward at the ankle joint

l. Movement of the foot when it is turned outward at the ankle joint

m. Movement of a part away from the central axis of a body or body part

n. Bending movement of a joint whereby the angle between contiguous bones is diminished

o. Movement of a part so that the sagittal (longitudinal) plane is angled so that it is not parallel with the long axis of the body

For Questions 16 to 22, identify the body movements illustrated in Figs. 2.29 to 2.35.

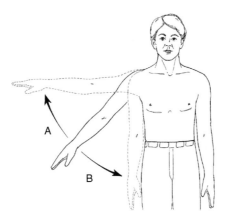

Fig. 2.29 Two types of body movements.

16. Fig. 2.29: A. _____

               B. _____

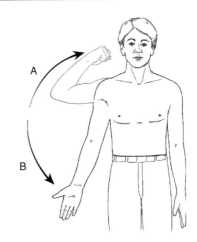

Fig. 2.30 Two types of body movements.

17. Fig. 2.30: A. _____

               B. _____

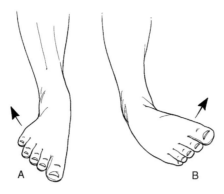

Fig. 2.31 Two types of body movements.

18. Fig. 2.31: A. _____

               B. _____

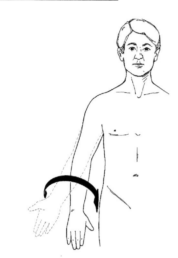

Fig. 2.32 One type of body movement.

19. Fig. 2.32: _____

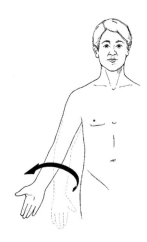

Fig. 2.33 One type of body movement.

20. Fig. 2.33: _____

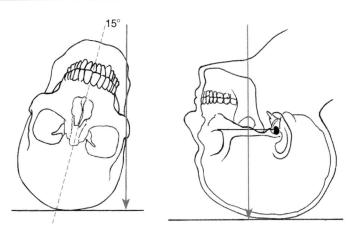

Fig. 2.34 One type of body movement.

21. Fig. 2.34: _____

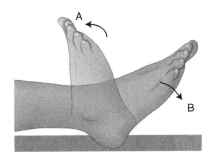

Fig. 2.35 Two types of body movements.

22. Fig. 2.35: A. _____

                B. _____

Chapter **2 General Anatomy and Radiographic Positioning Terminology**

23. Provide the plural form for each of the following medical terms:

a. Ala: _____

b. Alveolus: _____

c. Appendix: _____

d. Calculus: _____

e. Diagnosis: _____

f. Diverticulum: _____

g. Ganglion: _____

h. Ilium: _____

i. Lamina: _____

j. Metastasis: _____

24. Define the following abbreviations:

a. ARRT: _____

b. ASIS: _____

c. RAO: _____

d. LPO: _____

e. US: _____

f. LUQ: _____

g. CT: _____

CHAPTER 2: SELF-TEST: GENERAL ANATOMY AND RADIOGRAPHIC POSITIONING TERMINOLOGY

Answer the following questions by selecting the best choice.

1. Which term refers to the study of the function of the body organs?
   a. Anatomy
   b. Osteology
   c. Physiology

2. Which are the four fundamental body planes?
   a. Sagittal, coronal, horizontal, and oblique
   b. Sagittal, coronal, midaxillary, and transverse
   c. Midsagittal, midcoronal, horizontal, and oblique
   d. Midsagittal, midcoronal, midaxillary, and transverse

3. Which plane divides the body into equal right and left halves?
   a. Oblique
   b. Horizontal
   c. Midsagittal
   d. Midcoronal

4. Which are the two great cavities of the torso?
   a. Pelvic and pleural
   b. Pelvic and abdominal
   c. Thoracic and pleural
   d. Thoracic and abdominal

5. Which body structure is located within the thoracic cavity?
   a. Liver
   b. Heart
   c. Gallbladder
   d. Urinary bladder

6. In which quadrant of the abdomen is the appendix located?
   a. Right upper quadrant
   b. Right lower quadrant
   c. Left upper quadrant
   d. Left lower quadrant

7. Which region of the abdomen is located below the umbilical region?
   a. Epigastrium
   b. Hypogastrium
   c. Left hypochondrium
   d. Right hypochondrium

8. Which vertebra is located at the level of the xiphoid process?
   a. C7
   b. T7
   c. T10
   d. L3

9. Which body habitus represents a person of large, massive stature in whom the stomach is located high and nearly horizontal within the abdomen?
   a. Sthenic
   b. Asthenic
   c. Hyposthenic
   d. Hypersthenic

10. Excluding small sesamoid and accessory bones in the skull, how many bones comprise the skeleton?
    a. 202
    b. 206
    c. 210
    d. 215

11. Which structure belongs to the axial skeleton?
    a. Skull
    b. Lower limb
    c. Upper limb
    d. Pelvic girdle

12. Which bone has a medullary cavity?
    a. Tibia
    b. Sacrum
    c. Parietal
    d. Sternum

13. Bones are classified according to their:
    a. size.
    b. shape.
    c. function.
    d. origin.

14. Which bone classifications are vertebrae?
    a. Flat
    b. Long
    c. Short
    d. Irregular

15. Which bone classification is the trapezium?
    a. Flat
    b. Long
    c. Short
    d. Irregular

16. Which bone classification consists largely of compact cortex tissue in the form of two plates that enclose a layer of diploë?
    a. Flat
    b. Long
    c. Short
    d. Irregular

17. Which term specifically refers to the study of the joints?
    a. Anatomy
    b. Osteology
    c. Arthrology
    d. Physiology

18. Which structural classification of articulations refers to joints that have only limited or slight movement?
    a. Synovial
    b. Fibrous
    c. Cartilaginous
    d. Ellipsoid

19. Which functional classification of articulations are synovial joints?
    a. Diarthroses
    b. Synarthroses
    c. Amphiarthroses
    d. Synchondrosis

20. Which structural classification of articulations are cranial sutures?
    a. Fibrous
    b. Synovial
    c. Cartilaginous
    d. Syndesmosis

21. Which type of movement occurs in a hinge joint?
    a. Rotational
    b. Gliding or sliding
    c. Flexion and extension
    d. Abduction and adduction

22. Which of the following joints is an example of an ellipsoid joint?
    a. Hip
    b. Intercarpal
    c. Interphalangeal
    d. Metacarpophalangeal

23. Which term refers to a long, pointed process?
    a. Crest
    b. Styloid
    c. Condyle
    d. Tuberosity

24. Which term for a depression refers to a hole in a bone through which blood vessels and nerves pass?
    a. Sinus
    b. Sulcus
    c. Groove
    d. Foramen

25. Which term refers to a fracture in which a broken bone projects though the skin?
    a. Open
    b. Closed
    c. Displaced
    d. Nondisplaced

26. Which term refers to a body part on the opposite side of the body?
    a. Lateral
    b. Posterior
    c. Ipsilateral
    d. Contralateral

27. Which term refers to the path of the central x-ray?
    a. View
    b. Method
    c. Position
    d. Projection

28. Which term refers to a general body position?
    a. Axial
    b. Recumbent
    c. Tangential
    d. Left anterior oblique

29. Which term refers to the movement of a body part away from the central axis of the body?
    a. Flexion
    b. Inversion
    c. Abduction
    d. Adduction

30. Which term is the plural form for diagnosis?
    a. Diagnosix
    b. Diagnoses
    c. Diagnosae
    d. Diagnosum

31. Which body position describes the patient lying face down on the radiographic table?
    a. Supine
    b. Dorsal
    c. Prone
    d. Anterior

32. Which plane is positioned at a right angle to the sagittal and coronal planes?
    a. Oblique
    b. Horizontal
    c. Midsagittal
    d. Midcoronal

33. Which vertebra is located at the level of the inferior angles of scapulae?
    a. C7
    b. T7
    c. T10
    d. L3

34. Which vertebra is located at the level of the iliac crest?
    a. T10
    b. L2
    c. L4
    d. S1

35. Which body habitus represents a person with organs and characteristics that are intermediate between sthenic and asthenic body habitus types and is the most difficult to classify?
    a. Sthenic
    b. Asthenic
    c. Hyposthenic
    d. Hypersthenic

3 Thoracic Viscera: Chest and Upper Airway

ANATOMY OF THE NECK AND CHEST

Section 1: Exercise 1

This exercise pertains to the neck, chest, and thoracic viscera. Identify each lettered structure for each illustration.

1. Identify each lettered structure shown in Fig. 3.1.

A. _____

B. _____

C. _____

D. _____

E. _____

F. _____

G. _____

H. _____

I. _____

J. _____

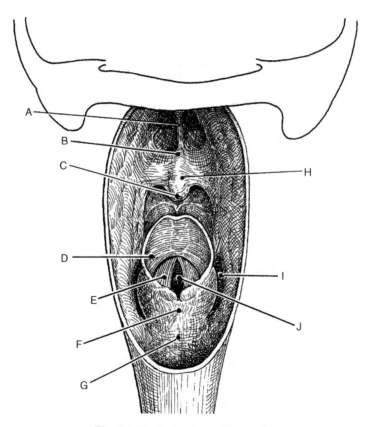

Fig. 3.1 Posterior view of the neck.

2. Identify each lettered structure shown in Fig. 3.2.

A. _____

B. _____

C. _____

D. _____

E. _____

F. _____

G. _____

H. _____

I. _____

J. _____

K. _____

L. _____

M. _____

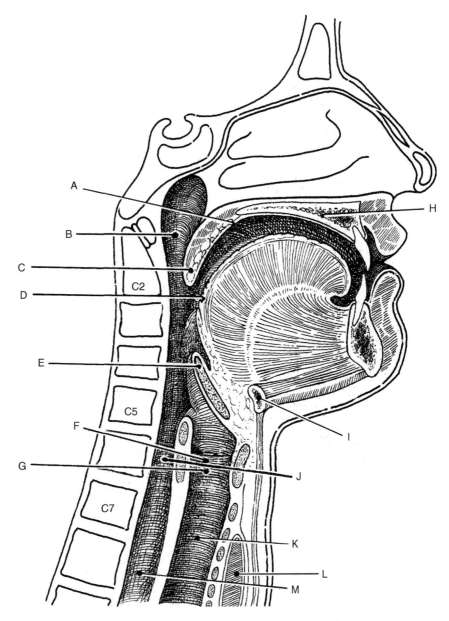

Fig. 3.2 Sagittal section of the face and neck.

3. Identify each lettered structure shown in Fig. 3.3.

A. _____

B. _____

C. _____

D. _____

E. _____

F. _____

G. _____

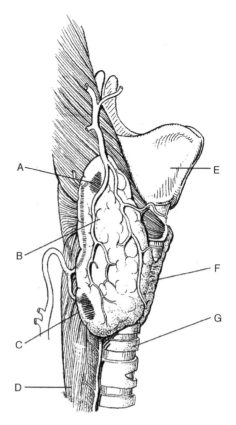

Fig. 3.3 Lateral aspect of the laryngeal area.

4. Identify each lettered structure shown in Fig. 3.4.

A. _____

B. _____

C. _____

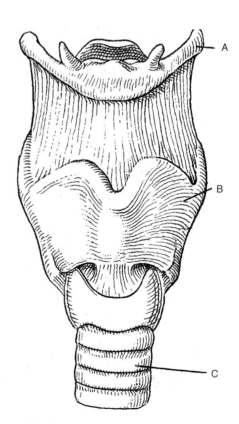

Fig. 3.4 Anterior aspect of the larynx.

5. Identify each lettered structure shown in Fig. 3.5.

A. _____

B. _____

C. _____

D. _____

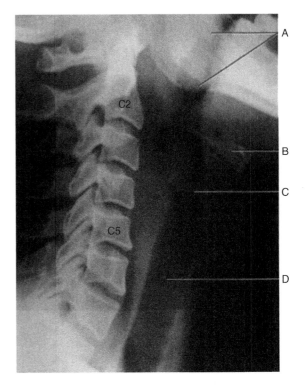

Fig. 3.5 Lateral pharynx and larynx (Valsalva maneuver).

6. Identify each lettered structure shown in Fig. 3.6.

A. _____

B. _____

C. _____

D. _____

E. _____

F. _____

G. _____

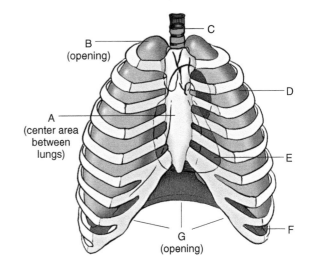

Fig. 3.6 Thoracic cavity.

7. Identify each lettered structure shown in Fig. 3.7.

A. _____

B. _____

C. _____

D. _____

E. _____

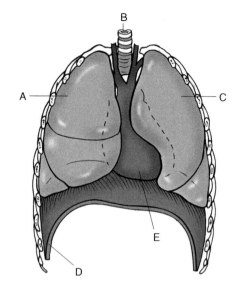

Fig. 3.7 Thoracic cavity with anterior ribs removed.

8. Identify each lettered structure shown in Fig. 3.8.

A. _____

B. _____

C. _____

D. _____

E. _____

F. _____

G. _____

H. _____

I. _____

J. _____

K. _____

L. _____

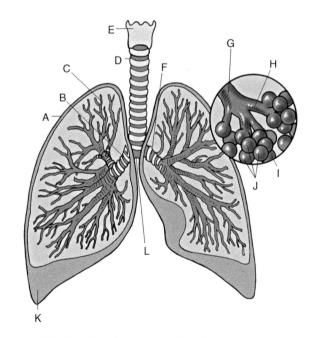

Fig. 3.8 Anterior aspect of respiratory system.

9. Identify each lettered structure shown in Fig. 3.9.

A. _____

B. _____

C. _____

D. _____

E. _____

F. _____

G. _____

H. _____

I. _____

J. _____

K. _____

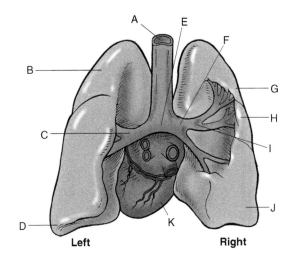

Fig. 3.9 Posterior aspect of heart, lungs, trachea, and bronchial trees.

Chapter **3 Thoracic Viscera: Chest and Upper Airway**

10. Identify each lettered structure in Fig. 3.10.

A. _____

B. _____

C. _____

D. _____

E. _____

F. _____

G. _____

H. _____

I. _____

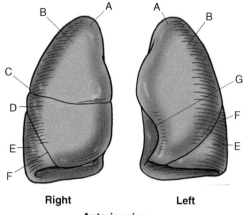

Right   Left

Anterior view

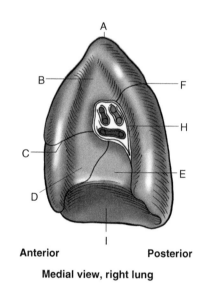

Anterior   Posterior

Medial view, right lung

Lateral view
Right lung

Lateral view
Left lung

Fig. 3.10 Three views of the lungs.

Section 1: Exercise 2

Use the following clues to complete the crossword puzzle. All answers refer to the lungs and thoracic cavity.

Across

1. Found in each lobe
3. Where vessels enter a lung
4. Superior portion of a lung
5. Inferior border of thoracic cavity
7. Respiratory organ
10. Major airway tube
13. Body type
14. Number of lobes in the right lung
16. Side of lung where vessels enter
17. Double-walled, serous membrane sac
18. Respiratory sacs

Down

1. Anterior bony wall of the mediastinum
2. Area between the lungs
3. Mediastinal organ
6. Mediastinal blood vessel
7. Major section of a lung
8. This lung has two lobes
9. Inferior part of a lung
11. Pertaining to the chest cavity
12. These branch from the trachea
15. Separates a lung into lobes

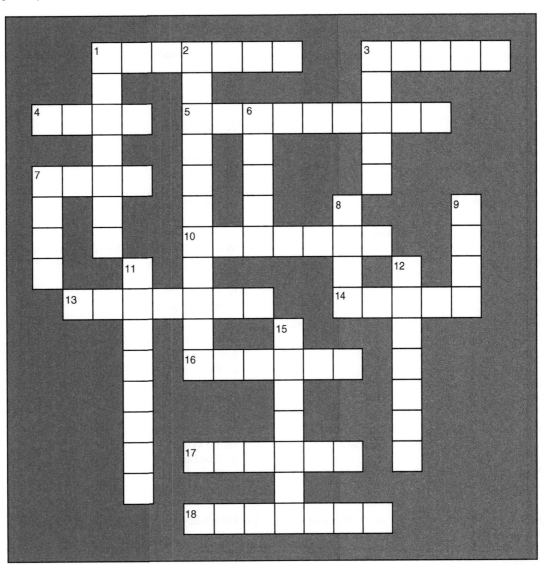

Chapter **3** **Thoracic Viscera: Chest and Upper Airway**

Section 1: Exercise 3

This exercise pertains to the anatomic structures found in the neck and chest. Provide a short answer or select the correct answer from a list for each question.

1. For radiographic purposes, the neck is divided into _____ and _____ portions.

2. Circle the structures located in the anterior neck.
   a. Thyroid gland
   b. Cervical vertebrae
   c. Trachea
   d. Esophagus

3. The structure of the upper neck that serves as a passage for both food and air and is common to the respiratory and digestive systems is the _____.

4. The portion of the pharynx located above the soft palate is the _____.

5. The portion of the pharynx located from the soft palate to the hyoid bone is the _____.

6. The organ of voice is the _____.

7. Which cavity contains the heart and lungs?
   a. Thoracic
   b. Abdominal
   c. Mediastinum
   d. Pelvic

8. Which structure separates the thoracic cavity from the abdominal cavity?
   a. Liver
   b. Heart
   c. Trachea
   d. Diaphragm

9. Which part of the thoracic cavity contains all thoracic organs except the lungs and pleurae?
   a. Mediastinum
   b. Pleural cavity
   c. Abdominal cavity

10. Which bony structure forms the anterior border of the mediastinum?
    a. Sternum
    b. Scapulae
    c. Thoracic vertebral column

11. What mediastinal structure consists of C-shaped cartilaginous rings?
    a. Trachea
    b. Diaphragm
    c. Esophagus

12. What area of the trachea divides into two lesser tubes?
    a. Carina
    b. Larynx
    c. Pharynx

13. Which structures branch from the distal end of the trachea?
    a. Tertiary bronchi
    b. Primary bronchi
    c. Secondary bronchi

14. Which primary bronchus is shorter and wider than the other?
    a. Left
    b. Right
    c. Inferior
    d. Superior

15. What thoracic structures are the organs of respiration?
    a. Lungs
    b. Bronchi
    c. Bronchiole

16. What is the name of the medial aspect of each lung in which the primary bronchus enters?
    a. Apex
    b. Hilum
    c. Pleural space

17. What is the name of the superior portion of each lung?
    a. Base
    b. Apex
    c. Hilum

18. Which structures are at the terminal end of the respiratory system?
    a. Alveoli
    b. Bronchi
    c. Bronchioles

19. How many lobes are found in the right lung? The left lung?

20. Which lung (right or left) is shorter and broader than the other? Explain why.

21. Name the three portions of the pleura.

a. Inner layer: _____

b. Outer layer: _____

c. Space between layers: _____

Section 1: Exercise 4

Match the pathology terms in Column A with the appropriate definition in Column B. Not all choices from Column B should be selected.

Column A	Column B
_____ 1. Atelectasis	a. A collapse of all or part of a lung
_____ 2. Sarcoidosis	b. Collection of fluid in the pleural cavity
_____ 3. Emphysema	c. Pneumonia caused by aspiration of foreign particles
_____ 4. Tuberculosa	
_____ 5. Pneumothorax	d. Underaeration of the lungs caused by a lack of surfactant
_____ 6. Pleural effusion	e. Chronic infection of the lung caused by the tubercle bacillus
_____ 7. Pulmonary edema	
_____ 8. Lobar (bacterial pneumonia)	f. Condition of the lung marked by formation of granuloma
_____ 9. Lobular (bronchopneumonia)	g. Replacement of air with fluid in the lung interstitium and alveoli
_____ 10. Hyaline membrane (respiratory syndrome)	h. Pneumonia involving the bronchi and scattered distress throughout the lung
	i. Condition of unknown origin often associated with pulmonary fibrosis
	j. Accumulation of air in the pleural cavity resulting in collapse of the lung
	k. Pneumonia involving the alveoli of an entire lobe without involving the bronchi
	l. Destructive and obstructive airway changes leading to an increased volume of air in the lungs

POSITIONING OF THE UPPER AIRWAY SOFT TISSUE NECK

Section 2: Exercise 1: Anteroposterior and Lateral Projections

1. List pathologic conditions in which radiography of the soft tissue neck is performed.

2. Radiographs are most commonly made of the upper airway, from the _____ to the _____.

3. When performing the anteroposterior (AP) projection of the soft tissue neck, at what level do you direct the central ray for the upper airway?

4. When performing the AP projection of the soft tissue neck, at what level do you direct the central ray for the larynx and superior mediastinum?

5. Describe the breathing instructions when performing the AP and lateral projections of the soft tissue neck.

6. What are the collimation light field parameters when performing AP and lateral projections of the soft tissue neck?

7. When performing the lateral projection of the soft tissue neck, direct the central ray _____ through the _____ plane at the level of the _____ for the upper airway.

8. When performing the lateral projection of the soft tissue neck, direct the central ray at the level of the _____ through a point midway between the _____ and the _____ plane for trachea and superior mediastinum.

POSITIONING OF THE CHEST

Section 3: Exercise 1: Posteroanterior and Lateral Projections

Various projections are used to obtain views of the heart and lungs. In most cases, two essential projections of the chest are routinely performed to demonstrate thoracic viscera. This exercise pertains to those two projections. Identify structures, provide a short answer, or choose true or false (explaining any statement you believe to be false) for each item.

1. List the two essential projections for the heart and lungs that are routinely used for chest examinations, and describe the positioning steps used for each, as follows:

   Essential projection: _____
   - Size of collimated field:

   - Key patient/part positioning points:

   - Anatomic landmarks and relation to IR:

   - CR orientation and entrance point:

   Essential projection: _____
   - Size of collimated field:

   - Key patient/part positioning points:

   - Anatomic landmarks and relation to IR:

   - CR orientation and entrance point:

Items 2 to 17 pertain to the posteroanterior (PA) projection. Examine Fig. 3.11 as you answer the following questions.

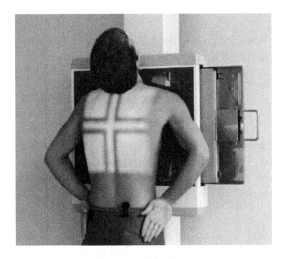

Fig. 3.11 PA chest.

2. What is the recommended source-to-image receptor distance (SID)? Explain why.

3. Why is it preferable to have the patient upright?

4. Which body plane should be perpendicular and centered to the midline of the IR?

55

5. How should the patient's hands be positioned? Explain why.

6. With reference to the patient, where should the upper border of the IR/collimated field be placed?
   a. At the level of the clavicles
   b. At the level of the acromion processes
   c. About 1½ to 2 inches (3.8 to 5 cm) above the top of the shoulders

7. What is the purpose of depressing the shoulders?
   a. To move the scapulae laterally
   b. To keep the clavicles below the apices
   c. To place the midsagittal plane in a vertical position

8. Why should the shoulders be rotated forward?
   a. To keep the clavicles below the apices
   b. To place the diaphragm at its lowest point
   c. To move the scapulae laterally away from the lung fields

9. What special positioning instructions may be given to a woman with large, pendulous breasts to avoid superimposing the lower part of the lung fields?
   a. Instruct the patient to cross both arms above the head.
   b. Instruct the patient to pull her breasts upward and laterally.
   c. Instruct the patient to press her breasts directly in front of her against the vertical IR holder.

10. If a patient were to remove one shoulder from contact with the grid device before the exposure, which of the following image effects would occur?
    a. The clavicles would appear above the apices.
    b. The sternum would superimpose the vertebral column.
    c. The sternoclavicular joints would appear symmetric.
    d. The sternal ends of the clavicles would no longer be equidistant from the vertebral column.

11. What breathing instructions should be given to the patient? Explain why.

12. List two reasons why exposures can be made after both inspiration and expiration.

13. To demonstrate the heart, why should the exposure be made after normal inspiration rather than deep inspiration?

14. Figs. 3.12 and 3.13 are PA projection images of the same patient, but with one difference in positioning. Examine the images and answer the questions that follow.

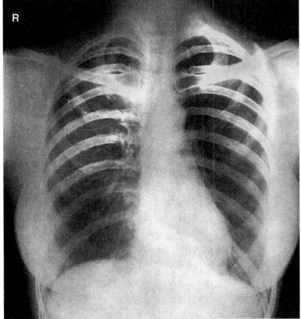

Fig. 3.12 PA chest.

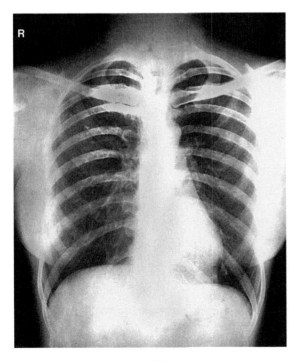

Fig. 3.13 PA chest.

a. Which image was produced with the patient lifting and pulling her breasts laterally before the exposure?

b. Which aspect of the image helped you to determine that answer?

15. Figs. 3.14 and 3.15 are PA projection images for which different breathing instructions were given to the patients. Examine the images and answer the questions that follow.

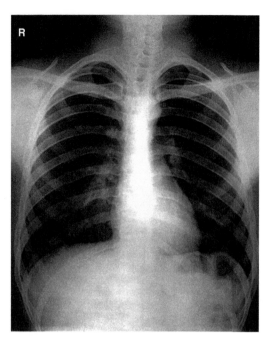

Fig. 3.14 PA chest.

Fig. 3.15 PA chest.

a. Which image was exposed with the patient suspending respiration on full inspiration?

b. Which aspect of the image helped you to determine that answer?

c. How many posterior ribs should be demonstrated above the diaphragm with proper full inspiration?

16. From the following list, circle eight evaluation criteria that indicate a patient was properly positioned for a PA chest projection.
    a. The trachea should be visible in the midline.
    b. The heart and diaphragm should show sharp outlines.
    c. The clavicles should be located superior to the apices.
    d. Ten posterior ribs should be seen above the diaphragm.
    e. The scapulae should be projected outside the lung fields.
    f. The exposure should clearly demonstrate the lung fields.
    g. The ribs should be superimposed posterior to the vertebral column.
    h. The hilum should be seen in the approximate center of the image.
    i. The entire lung fields from the apices to the costophrenic angles should be seen.
    j. No rotation; the sternal ends of the clavicles should be equidistant from the vertebral column.
    k. The clavicles should be lying horizontal with their sternal ends overlapping the first or second ribs.
    l. A faint shadow of the ribs and superior thoracic vertebrae should be seen through the heart shadow.

17. Identify each lettered structure shown in Fig. 3.16.

    A. _____

    B. _____

    C. _____

    D. _____

    E. _____

    F. _____

    G. _____

    H. _____

    I. _____

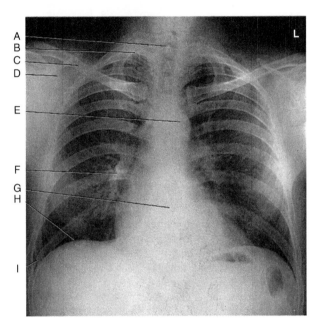

Fig. 3.16 PA chest.

Items 18 to 27 pertain to the lateral projection. Examine Fig. 3.17 as you answer the following questions.

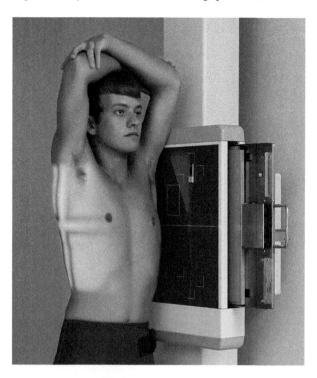

Fig. 3.17 Lateral chest.

18. Which thoracic structures are of primary interest with the left lateral projection?
    a. Heart and left lung
    b. Heart and right lung
    c. Trachea and diaphragm
    d. Trachea and esophagus

19. Which thoracic structure is of primary interest when performing a right lateral projection?
    a. Heart
    b. Trachea
    c. Left lung
    d. Right lung

20. What body plane should be perpendicular and centered to the midline of the IR?

21. Describe how the patient's arms should be positioned.

22. What purpose might an IV medication stand serve when the patient is positioned?

23. What breathing instructions should be given to the patient?

24. True or false. A lateral projection image of the chest should be viewed so that the side of the patient where the central ray entered is nearer the viewer.

25. True or false. The patient's heart will appear larger in the right lateral projection image than in the left lateral projection image.

26. From the following list, circle the nine evaluation criteria that indicate the patient was properly positioned for a lateral projection.
    a. The heart and diaphragm should be seen in sharp outline.
    b. The sternum should be seen in lateral view without rotation.
    c. Penetration of lung fields and heart should be clearly seen.
    d. The ribs should be superimposed posterior to the vertebral column.
    e. Neither the arm nor its soft tissues overlaps the superior lung field.
    f. The hilum should be seen in the approximate center of the image.
    g. The sternal ends of clavicles should be superimposed with the vertebral column.
    h. The sternal ends of clavicles should be seen equidistant from the vertebral column.
    i. The thoracic intervertebral spaces should be open (except in patients with scoliosis).
    j. The costophrenic angles and lower apices of lungs should be clearly demonstrated.
    k. A small amount of the heart should be seen on the right side of the vertebral column.
    l. The long axis of lung fields should be demonstrated in the vertical position without forward-backward leaning.

27. Identify each lettered structure shown in Fig. 3.18.

A. _____

B. _____

C. _____

D. _____

E. _____

F. _____

G. _____

H. _____

I. _____

J. _____

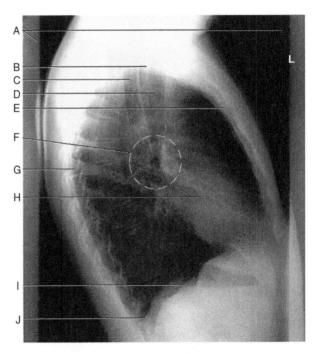

Fig. 3.18 Lateral chest.

Section 3: Exercise 2: Posteroanterior Oblique Projections—Right Anterior Oblique and Left Anterior Oblique Positions

PA oblique projections are sometimes used to supplement the standard PA and lateral views. This exercise pertains to PA oblique projections. Identify structures, provide a short answer, or choose true or false (explaining any statement you believe to be false) for each item.

Examine Figs. 3.19 and 3.20 as you answer the following questions.

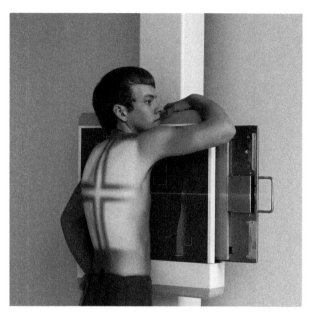

Fig. 3.19 PA oblique chest, LAO position.

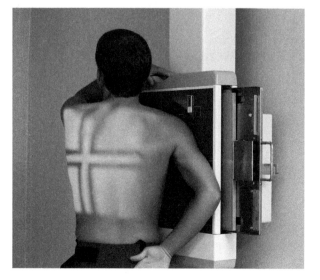

Fig. 3.20 PA oblique chest, RAO position.

1. Which side (the one closer to or farther from the IR) is generally the side of interest?

2. Which side of the chest (right or left) is of primary interest with the PA oblique projection, RAO position?

3. With reference to the patient, where should the upper border of the IR be placed?

4. When performing the PA oblique projection, RAO position, how many degrees should the patient be rotated?

5. What determines how many degrees the patient should be rotated for the PA oblique projection, LAO position?

6. When performing the PA oblique projection, LAO position, to demonstrate lungs, how many degrees should the patient be rotated?

7. When performing the PA oblique projection, LAO position, to demonstrate the heart and great vessels, how many degrees should the patient be rotated?

8. With reference to patient respiration, when should the exposure be made?

9. To what level of the patient should the central ray be directed?

10. Which PA oblique projection provides the best view of the left atrium and the entire left branch of the bronchial tree?

11. True or false. When viewing PA oblique chest images, the patient's left side should be toward the viewer's right side.

12. True or false. When viewing PA oblique chest images (LAO position), the left lung should be partially superimposed by the spine.

13. True or false. The heart and mediastinal structures should be clearly demonstrated within the lung field of the elevated side in oblique images of 45 degrees of body rotation.

63

14. Figs. 3.21 and 3.22 are PA oblique projection images. Examine the images and answer the questions that follow.

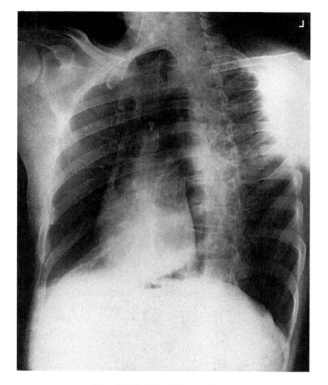

Fig. 3.21 PA oblique chest.

a. Which image represents the RAO position?

b. Which image represents the LAO position?

c. Which image demonstrates the maximum area of the left lung?

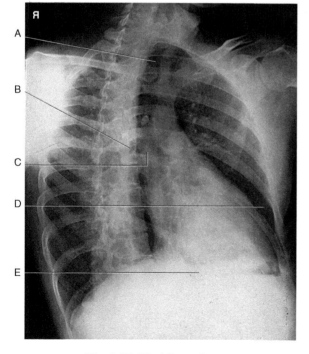

Fig. 3.22 PA oblique chest.

15. Identify each lettered structure shown in Fig. 3.22.

A. _____

B. _____

C. _____

D. _____

E. _____

Section 3: Exercise 3: Anteroposterior Oblique Projections—Right Posterior Oblique and Left Posterior Oblique Positions

AP oblique projections are sometimes used when supplementary positions are needed and the patient is unable to turn for the PA projection. This exercise pertains to AP oblique projections. Identify structures, select the correct choice, or provide a short answer for each item.

Examine Figs. 3.23 and 3.24 as you answer the following questions.

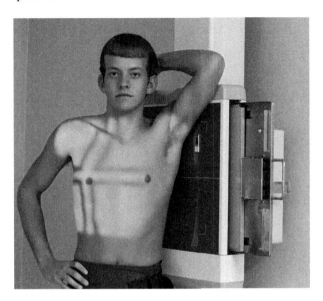

Fig. 3.23 Upright AP oblique chest, LPO position.

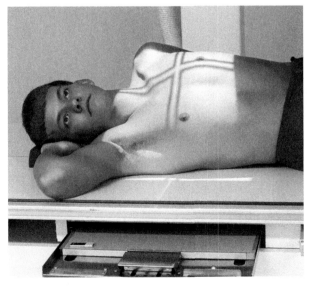

Fig. 3.24 Recumbent AP oblique chest, RPO position.

1. Which side (the one closer to or the one farther from the IR) is generally the side of interest?

2. Which AP oblique image (RPO position or LPO position) demonstrates the maximum area of the left lung?

3. What is the minimum recommended SID?

4. Which AP oblique projection produces an image very similar to that produced by the PA oblique projection, RAO position?
   a. AP oblique projection, LPO position
   b. AP oblique projection, RPO position

5. How many degrees should the patient be rotated?
   a. 25 degrees
   b. 35 degrees
   c. 45 degrees
   d. 55 degrees

6. How far above the top of the shoulders should the upper border of the IR be placed?

7. What breathing instructions should be given to the patient?

8. To what level of the patient should the central ray be directed?

9. Identify each lettered structure shown in Fig. 3.25.

A. _____

B. _____

C. _____

D. _____

E. _____

10. Examine Fig. 3.25 and answer the questions.
   a. In which radiographic position is the patient?

   b. Which side of the patient is closer to the film?

   c. Which lung should be seen in its maximum extent?

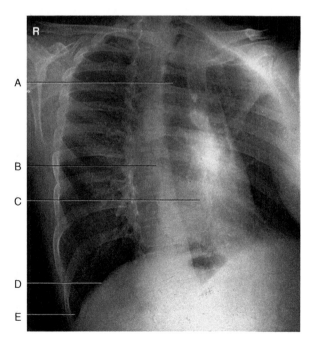

Fig. 3.25 AP oblique chest.

Section 3: Exercise 4: Anteroposterior Projection

The AP projection is used when the patient is too ill to turn to the prone position or to sit for a PA projection; it is often used for bedridden patients. This exercise pertains to the AP projection. Identify structures, select choices from a list, and provide a short answer for each question.

Examine Fig. 3.26 as you answer the following questions.

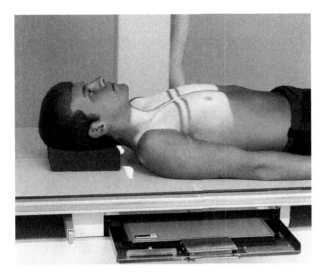

Fig. 3.26 AP chest.

1. What is the recommended SID?

2. What body plane should be centered to the midline of the IR?

3. With reference to the patient, where should the IR be placed?

4. If the patient's condition permits, how should the arms and shoulders be positioned? Explain why.

5. What breathing instructions should be given to the patient?

6. Why should the patient perform the recommended breathing instructions?

7. To what level of the patient should the central ray be directed?

8. Describe how the following structures appear in the AP projection image compared with how they appear in the PA projection image.

   a. Heart and great vessels: _____

   b. Lungs: _____

   c. Clavicles: _____

   d. Ribs: _____

67

9. From the following list, circle the six evaluation criteria that indicate the patient was properly positioned for an AP projection.
   a. The trachea should be seen in the midline.
   b. The sternum should be lateral without rotation.
   c. The ribs should be superimposed posterior to the vertebral column.
   d. The hilum should be seen in the approximate center of the image.
   e. The lung fields should be seen from the apices to the costophrenic angles.
   f. The sternal ends of the clavicles should be equidistant from the vertebral column.
   g. A faint image of the ribs and thoracic vertebrae should be seen through the heart shadow.
   h. The clavicles will lie more horizontal and will obscure more of the apices than in PA projections.
   i. The distance from the vertebral column to the lateral border of the ribs should be equidistant on both sides.
   j. Approximately twice as much distance should be seen between the vertebral column and the outer margin of the ribs on the dependent side compared with the remote side.
   k. Pulmonary vascular markings should be visible from the hilar regions to the periphery of the lungs.

10. Identify each thoracic structure shown in Fig. 3.27.

    A. _____

    B. _____

    C. _____

    D. _____

    E. _____

    F. _____

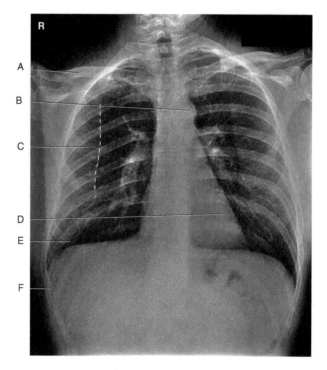

Fig. 3.27 AP chest.

Section 3: Exercise 5: Anteroposterior Axial Projection (Lindblom Method), Lordotic Position

The AP axial projection is used to demonstrate the apices of the lungs. Provide a short answer or select the correct choice from a list for each item to review the AP axial projection.

Examine Fig. 3.28 and answer the following questions.

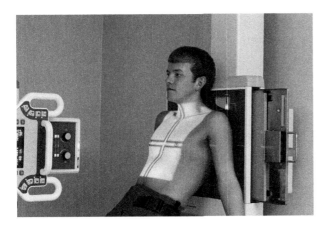

Fig. 3.28 AP axial projection (Lindblom), lordotic position.

1. Which portion of the lung is generally the area of primary interest?
   a. Base
   b. Apex
   c. Hilum

2. Describe how the patient should be positioned.

3. What breathing instructions should be given to the patient?

4. Where should the central ray enter the patient?

5. From the following list, circle the five evaluation criteria that indicate the patient was properly positioned for an AP axial projection (lordotic position).
   a. The clavicles should lie superior to the apices.
   b. The sternum should be lateral without rotation.
   c. The apices and lungs should be included in their entirety.
   d. The ribs should be superimposed posterior to the vertebral column.
   e. Approximately 2 inches of lung apex should be seen above the clavicles.
   f. The sternal ends of the clavicles should be equidistant from the vertebral column.
   g. The ribs should appear distorted with their anterior and posterior portions somewhat superimposed.
   h. The clavicles should be lying horizontal, with their sternal ends overlapping only the first or second ribs.

Chapter **3** **Thoracic Viscera: Chest and Upper Airway**

Section 3: Exercise 6: Lateral Decubitus Positions

This exercise pertains to lateral decubitus positions of the chest. Fill in missing words, provide a short answer, select from a list, or choose true or false (explaining any statement you believe to be false) for each item.

Examine Fig. 3.29 and answer the following questions.

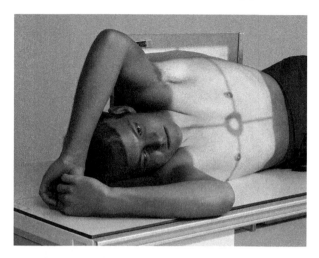

Fig. 3.29 AP projection, right lateral decubitus position.

1. List the essential projections for the lungs and pleurae, and describe the positioning steps used for each, as follows:

   Essential projection: _____

   (_____ position)

   ■ Size of collimated field:

   ■ Key patient/part positioning points:

   ■ Anatomic landmarks and relation to IR:

   ■ CR orientation and entrance point:

2. What is the general purpose for using a lateral decubitus position?

3. True or false. The patient can be positioned upright in a lateral decubitus position.

4. True or false. The IR must be placed vertically against a patient.

5. True or false. The central ray must be directed horizontally.

6. True or false. The affected side should be up to demonstrate a fluid level.

7. True or false. Both sides should be seen in their entirety.

8. To demonstrate fluid in the right thorax, the patient must be positioned in a:
   a. left lateral decubitus position.
   b. right lateral decubitus position.

9. Which side of the thorax (right or left) best demonstrates free air when the patient is in the left lateral decubitus position?

10. To demonstrate free air in the thorax with a lateral decubitus position, why is it preferable to position the patient with the affected side up instead of with the affected side down?

11. To demonstrate a fluid level in the thorax with a lateral decubitus position, why is it preferable to position the patient with the affected side down instead of with the affected side up?

12. What breathing instructions should be given to the patient?

13. Fig. 3.30 is an image of the right lateral decubitus position. Examine the image and answer the following questions.

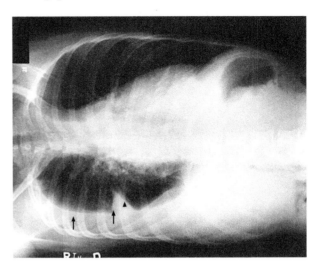

Fig. 3.30 AP projection, right lateral decubitus position.

   a. This position should be used to demonstrate an air level in the _____ side of the thorax.

   b. This position should be used to demonstrate a fluid level in the _____ side of the thorax.

   c. Which level (air or fluid) are the arrows pointing to in the image?

14. Fig. 3.31 is an image of the left lateral decubitus position. Examine the image and complete the statements that follow.

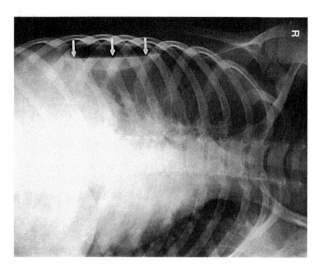

Fig. 3.31 AP projection, left lateral decubitus position.

   a. The arrows in the image are pointing to a(n)

      _____ (air or fluid) level in the

      _____ (right or left) side of the thorax.

   b. In this image, the affected side is _____ (up or down).

15. From the following list, circle the five evaluation criteria that indicate a patient is properly positioned for a lateral decubitus position projection.
   a. The apices should be included.
   b. The clavicles should lie superior to the apices.
   c. The affected side should be included in its entirety.
   d. The patient should not be rotated from a true frontal position.
   e. The patient's arms should be removed from the field of interest.
   f. The ribs should be superimposed posterior to the vertebral column.
   g. Proper identification should be visible to indicate that the decubitus position was used.
   h. The clavicles should be lying horizontal with their sternal ends overlapping only the first or second ribs.

Section 3: Exercise 7: Ventral and Dorsal Decubitus Positions

Sometimes it is necessary to demonstrate an air or fluid level while the patient is in the supine or prone position. This is accomplished through lateral projections using the ventral and dorsal decubitus positions. This exercise pertains to those two positions. Fill in missing words, select from a list, or provide a short answer for each item.

Examine Fig. 3.32 and answer the following questions.

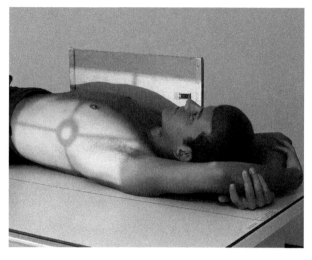

Fig. 3.32 Lateral projection, dorsal decubitus position.

1. For the dorsal decubitus position projection, the patient must be placed in the _____ position.

2. For the ventral decubitus position projection, the patient must be placed in the _____ position.

3. In addition to being perpendicular to the IR, the central ray must also be directed _____.

4. How much should the thorax be elevated?

5. How long should a patient remain in position? Why?

6. Describe how the patient's arms should be positioned.

7. With reference to the patient, how and where should the IR/collimated field be placed?

8. Concerning respiration, when should the exposure be made?

9. Where should the central ray enter the patient?

10. From the following list, circle the four evaluation criteria that indicate the patient was properly positioned for the dorsal decubitus or ventral decubitus position.
    a. The arms should not obscure the upper lung field.
    b. The thorax should not be rotated from a true lateral position.
    c. The sternal ends of the clavicles should be equidistant from the vertebral column.
    d. A small amount of the heart should be seen on the right side of the vertebral column.
    e. Proper identification should be visible to indicate that the decubitus position was used.
    f. The entire lung fields, including the anterior and posterior surfaces, should be demonstrated.
    g. The distance from the vertebral column to the lateral border of the ribs should be equidistant on both sides.
    h. T7 should be in the center of the IR.

Section 3: Exercise 8: Evaluating Images of the Chest

This exercise consists of using images of the chest to give you practice evaluating chest positioning. These images are not from Merrill's Atlas. Each image shows at least one positioning error. Examine each image and answer the questions that follow by providing a short answer.

1. Fig. 3.33 shows a PA projection image that does not meet all evaluation criteria for this type of projection. Examine the image and identify the evaluation criterion that this image does not meet.

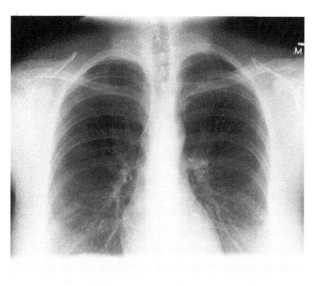

Fig. 3.33 PA chest showing improper positioning.

2. Fig. 3.34 shows a lateral projection image with the patient incorrectly positioned. Examine the image and list the three evaluation criteria that it does not meet.

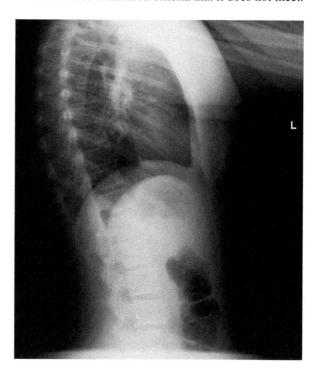

Fig. 3.34 Lateral chest showing improper positioning.

a. _____

b. _____

c. _____

Examine Fig. 3.35 and answer the following questions.

Examine Fig. 3.36 and answer the following question.

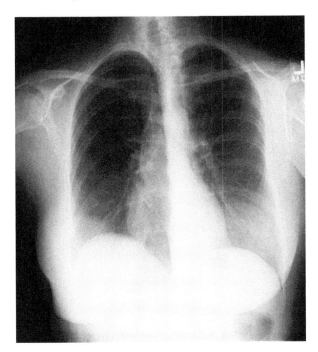

Fig. 3.35 AP chest showing improper positioning.

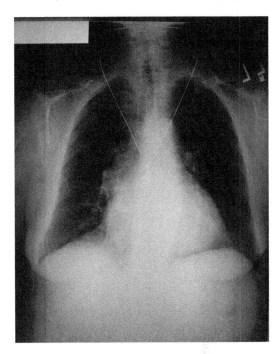

Fig. 3.36 PA chest with error.

3. State the major positioning error that necessitates repetition of the examination.

5. What error is evident in Fig. 3.36?

4. Describe how patient positioning should be adjusted to produce a more acceptable image with a subsequent projection.

Chapter **3 Thoracic Viscera: Chest and Upper Airway**

Examine Fig. 3.37 and answer the following questions.

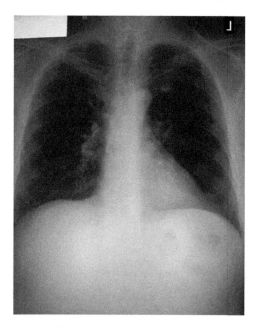

Fig. 3.37 PA chest with errors.

6. What positioning errors are evident in Fig. 3.37?

7. Describe how patient positioning should be adjusted to produce a more acceptable image with a subsequent projection.

Examine Fig. 3.38 and answer the following questions.

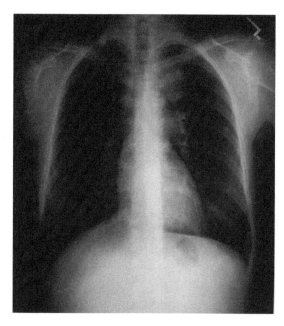

Fig. 3.38 PA chest with error.

8. What positioning error is evident, and which of the evaluation criteria has not been met in Fig. 3.38?

9. What caused the positioning error noted?

10. Describe how the patient positioning should be adjusted to produce a more acceptable image with a subsequent projection.

CHAPTER 3: SELF-TEST: ANATOMY AND POSITIONING OF THE CHEST AND UPPER AIRWAY

Answer the following questions by selecting the best choice.

1. What is the musculomembranous tubular structure located in front of the vertebrae and behind the nose, the mouth, and the larynx?
   a. Glottis
   b. Trachea
   c. Pharynx
   d. Esophagus

2. Which structure of the neck is approximately 1½ inches (3.8 cm) in length and is situated below the root of the tongue and in front of the laryngeal pharynx?
   a. Larynx
   b. Trachea
   c. Esophagus
   d. Oropharynx

3. Which structure forms the laryngeal prominence?
   a. Epiglottis
   b. True vocal cord
   c. Cricoid cartilage
   d. Thyroid cartilage

4. Which structure prevents leakage into the larynx during swallowing?
   a. Pharynx
   b. Epiglottis
   c. Cricoid cartilage
   d. Thyroid cartilage

5. What is the most superiorly located structure of the neck?
   a. Larynx
   b. Glottis
   c. Pharynx
   d. Epiglottis

6. What is the name of the area between the two pleural cavities?
   a. Hilum
   b. Mediastinum
   c. Pleural space
   d. Thoracic cavity

7. Which structure is not demonstrated within the mediastinum in PA projections of the chest?
   a. Heart
   b. Trachea
   c. Diaphragm
   d. Esophagus

8. When performing the AP projection of the soft tissue neck, at what level do you direct the central ray for the upper airway?
   a. Jugular notch
   b. Laryngeal prominence
   c. Manubrium
   d. Xiphoid process

9. When performing the AP projection of the soft tissue neck, at what level do you direct the central ray for the larynx and superior mediastinum?
   a. Jugular notch
   b. Laryngeal prominence
   c. Manubrium
   d. Xiphoid process

10. What is the collimation light field parameters when performing AP and lateral projections of the soft tissue neck?
    a. 10 inches (25 cm) crosswise and 1 inch (2.5 cm) beyond the skin line of the anterior and posterior surfaces
    b. 10 inches (25 cm) lengthwise and 1 inch (2.5 cm) beyond the skin line of the anterior and posterior surfaces
    c. 12 inches (30 cm) crosswise and 1 inch (2.5 cm) beyond the skin line of the anterior and posterior surfaces
    d. 12 inches (30 cm) lengthwise and 1 inch (2.5 cm) beyond the skin line of the anterior and posterior surfaces

11. Identify the breathing instructions when performing the AP and lateral projections of the soft tissue neck.
    a. Hold breath
    b. Expiration
    c. Fast inspiration
    d. Slow inspiration

12. Which pathologic condition of the lung involves the replacement of air with fluid in the lung interstitium and alveoli?
    a. Atelectasis
    b. Tuberculosis
    c. Pneumothorax
    d. Pulmonary edema

13. Why should chest images be performed with a 72-inch (183-cm) SID?
    a. To blur involuntary heart motion
    b. To minimize magnification of the heart
    c. To maximize magnification of the heart
    d. To project the clavicles above the apices

77

14. Why should chest images be performed after the patient has suspended respiration after the second inspiration?
    a. To blur rib markings
    b. To expand the lungs better
    c. To demonstrate a collapsed lung
    d. To calm the heart and reduce cardiac motion

15. With reference to the IR, how are the midsagittal plane and the midcoronal plane positioned for the PA projection of the chest?
    a. Midsagittal: parallel; midcoronal: parallel
    b. Midsagittal: parallel; midcoronal: perpendicular
    c. Midsagittal: perpendicular; midcoronal: parallel
    d. Midsagittal: perpendicular; midcoronal: perpendicular

16. For the PA projection of the chest, which positioning maneuver should be performed for the best removal of the scapulae from lung fields?
    a. Place the hands on the hips.
    b. Rotate the shoulders forward.
    c. Cross both arms over the head.
    d. Place the hands behind the back.

17. Why would the chest most likely be demonstrated using two PA projections (in which the patient is seen in suspended inspiration and suspended expiration)?
    a. To demonstrate pneumothorax
    b. To evaluate the heart and great vessels
    c. To measure the width of the mediastinum
    d. To demonstrate movement of the diaphragm

18. Which of the following is an effective way to detect rotation of the patient with the PA projection image of the chest?
    a. The number of ribs demonstrated above the diaphragm
    b. The asymmetric appearance of the sternoclavicular joints
    c. The amount of apical area demonstrated above the clavicles
    d. The appearance of the lateral border of the scapulae outside the lung fields

19. For which projection of the chest should the midsagittal plane be parallel with the IR?
    a. Lateral projection
    b. AP projection, left lateral decubitus position
    c. AP axial projection, lordotic position (Lindblom method)
    d. PA projection

20. With reference to the IR, how are the midcoronal plane and the midsagittal plane positioned for the lateral projection of the chest?
    a. Midcoronal: parallel; midsagittal: parallel
    b. Midcoronal: parallel; midsagittal: perpendicular
    c. Midcoronal: perpendicular; midsagittal: parallel
    d. Midcoronal: perpendicular; midsagittal: perpendicular

21. Which projection of the chest best demonstrates lung apices free from superimposition with the clavicles?
    a. PA projection
    b. Left lateral projection
    c. AP projection, left lateral decubitus position
    d. AP axial projection, lordotic position (Lindblom method)

22. Which PA oblique projection of the chest may be used to evaluate the heart and great vessels when performing a cardiac series?
    a. 45-degree RAO
    b. 45-degree LAO
    c. 55- to 60-degree LAO
    d. 10- to 20-degree RAO and LAO

23. How many degrees should the patient be rotated for PA oblique projections of the chest to evaluate the lungs?
    a. RAO: 45 degrees; LAO: 45 degrees
    b. RAO: 45 degrees; LAO: 55 to 60 degrees
    c. RAO: 55 to 60 degrees; LAO: 45 degrees
    d. RAO: 55 to 60 degrees; LAO: 55 to 60 degrees

24. Using a lateral decubitus position for patients who are unable to stand upright best demonstrates which of the following pathologic conditions of the chest?
    a. Rib fractures
    b. Cardiomegaly
    c. Collapsed lung
    d. Air or fluid levels

25. With reference to the IR, how are the midsagittal plane and the midcoronal plane positioned for the AP chest, left lateral decubitus position?
    a. Midsagittal: parallel; midcoronal: parallel
    b. Midsagittal: parallel; midcoronal: perpendicular
    c. Midsagittal: perpendicular; midcoronal: parallel
    d. Midsagittal: perpendicular; midcoronal: perpendicular

26. Which pathologic condition of the lungs is best demonstrated with the AP chest, left lateral decubitus position?
    a. Free air in both sides of the chest
    b. Fluid levels in both sides of the chest
    c. Free air in the left side or fluid levels in the right side of the chest
    d. Fluid levels in the left side or free air in the right side of the chest

27. Which pathologic condition of the lungs is best demonstrated with the AP chest, right lateral decubitus position?
    a. Free air in both sides of the chest
    b. Fluid levels in both sides of the chest
    c. Free air in the left side or fluid levels in the right side of the chest
    d. Fluid levels in the left side or free air in the right side of the chest

28. Which radiographic position requires that the patient be placed supine with the IR placed vertically against the patient's right side and a horizontal central ray directed to the center of the IR?
    a. Ventral decubitus
    b. Dorsal decubitus
    c. Right lateral decubitus
    d. Left lateral decubitus

29. Which radiographic position requires that the patient be placed prone?
    a. Left lateral decubitus
    b. Right lateral decubitus
    c. Dorsal decubitus
    d. Ventral decubitus

30. Which evaluation criterion pertains to the PA projection image of the chest?
    a. The ribs should appear distorted.
    b. The sternum should be lateral, not rotated.
    c. Ten posterior ribs should be visible above the diaphragm.
    d. The ribs posterior to the vertebral column should be superimposed.

31. Which evaluation criterion pertains to the PA projection image of the chest?
    a. The ribs should appear distorted.
    b. The clavicles should lie superior to the apices.
    c. The scapulae should be projected outside the lung fields.
    d. The ribs posterior to the vertebral column should be superimposed.

32. Which evaluation criterion pertains to the lateral projection image of the chest?
    a. A small amount of the heart should be seen on the right side.
    b. The ribs posterior to the vertebral column should be superimposed.
    c. A faint shadow of superior thoracic vertebrae should be seen through the heart shadow.
    d. The distance from the vertebral column to the lateral border of the ribs should be equidistant on both sides.

33. Which evaluation criterion pertains to the AP axial projection, lordotic position image of the chest?
    a. The ribs should appear distorted.
    b. The clavicles should lie below the apices.
    c. The sternum should be lateral, not rotated.
    d. The thoracic intervertebral disk spaces should be open.

34. Which evaluation criterion pertains to the AP axial projection, lordotic position image of the chest?
    a. The clavicles should lie superior to the apices.
    b. The thoracic intervertebral disk spaces should be open.
    c. The ribs posterior to the vertebral column should be superimposed.
    d. There should be 2 inches (5 cm) of lung apices visible above the clavicles.

35. When performing the AP axial projection, lordotic position image of the chest, at what level do you direct the central ray?
    a. Jugular notch
    b. Manubrium
    c. Midsternum
    d. Xiphoid process

4 Abdomen

ANATOMY OF THE ABDOMINOPELVIC CAVITY

Section 1: Exercise 1

This exercise pertains to the contents of the abdomino-pelvic cavity. Identify each lettered structure for each illustration.

1. Identify each lettered structure shown in Fig. 4.1.

A. _____

B. _____

C. _____

D. _____

E. _____

F. _____

G. _____

H. _____

I. _____

J. _____

K. _____

L. _____

M. _____

N. _____

O. _____

P. _____

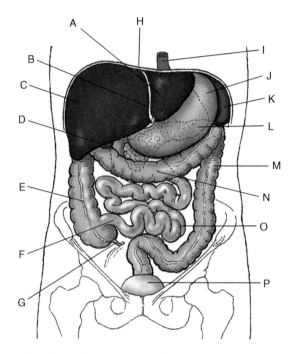

Fig. 4.1 Anterior aspect of the abdominal viscera.

2. Identify each lettered structure shown in Fig. 4.2.

A. _____

B. _____

C. _____

D. _____

E. _____

F. _____

G. _____

H. _____

I. _____

J. _____

K. _____

L. _____

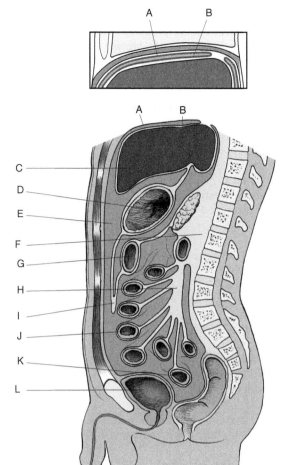

Fig. 4.2 Lateral view of abdomen demonstrating the peritoneal sac and its components.

3. Identify each lettered structure shown in Fig. 4.3.

A. _____

B. _____

C. _____

D. _____

E. _____

F. _____

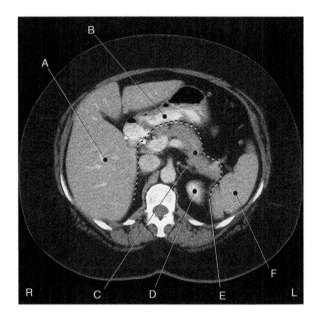

Fig. 4.3 Axial CT scan of upper abdomen showing relationship of abdominal organs.

81

Section 1: Exercise 2

This exercise reviews the anatomy of the abdominopelvic cavity. Fill in missing words, provide a short answer, or choose true or false (explaining any statement you believe to be false) for each item.

1. Circle the organs located in the abdominal cavity.
   a. Spleen
   b. Pancreas
   c. Uterus
   d. Gallbladder
   e. Stomach
   f. Small intestines
   g. Urinary bladder
   h. Kidneys

2. Circle the organs located in the pelvic cavity.
   a. Spleen
   b. Pancreas
   c. Uterus
   d. Rectum
   e. Gallbladder
   f. Stomach
   g. Small intestines
   h. Urinary bladder
   i. Kidneys

3. The name of the double-walled seromembranous sac that lines the abdominal cavity is the

   _____.

4. The two layers of the peritoneum are the

   _____ layer and the

   _____ layer.

5. The outer layer of the peritoneum that contacts the underside of the diaphragm is called the

   _____ layer.

6. The inner layer of the peritoneum that contacts various organs is called the _____

   layer.

7. The retroperitoneum is the _____.

8. List two organs located in the retroperitoneum.

9. List the two folds in the peritoneum.

10. What is the function of these two folds?

Section 1: Exercise 3

Use the following clues to complete the crossword puzzle. All answers refer to anatomy and pathology of the abdomen.

Across

2. Outer layer of the peritoneum
5. Cavity that contains reproductive organs, urinary bladder, and rectum
6. Double-walled seromembranous sac that encloses the abdominopelvic cavity
11. Pathologic condition defined as a blockage of the bowel lumen
12. Pathologic condition that is a localized dilatation of the abdominal aorta

Down

1. Presence of air in the peritoneal cavity
3. Cavity that contains organs such as the stomach, spleen, pancreas, and liver
4. Pathologic condition of the abdomen that is defined as the failure of bowel peristalsis
7. One of the folds of the peritoneum that serves to support the viscera
8. Inner layer of the peritoneum
9. One of the folds of the peritoneum that serves to support the viscera
10. Abdominal organs located in the retroperitoneum

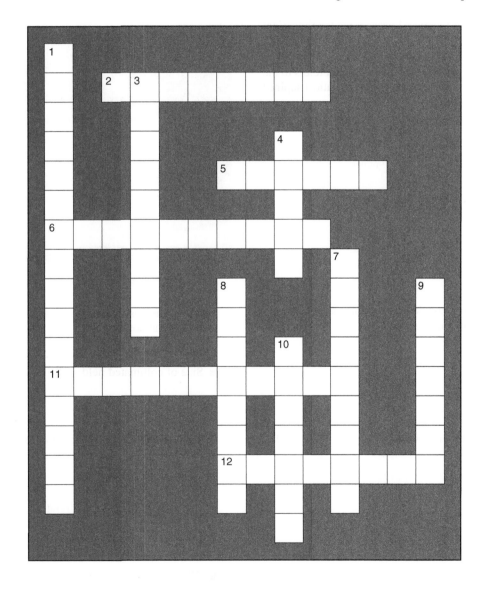

Chapter **4** **Abdomen**

POSITIONING OF THE ABDOMEN

Section 2: Exercise 1: Positioning for the Abdomen

Various radiographic procedures are used to demonstrate the abdomen and its contents. A patient is usually first examined with plain radiography before specialized studies are performed using contrast media. This exercise reviews the positions and projections commonly used to produce images of the abdomen without the introduction of a contrast medium. Fill in missing words, provide a short answer, select answers from a list, or choose true or false (explaining any statement you believe to be false) for each item.

Items 1 to 5 pertain to general procedures for abdominal radiography.

1. What is the commonly used acronym that refers to the AP projection of the abdomen with the patient supine?

2. What is the meaning of this acronym?

3. What three projections usually comprise the three-way or acute abdomen series?

4. Why is an upright chest image included as part of the acute abdomen series?

5. In the acute abdomen series, what image should be substituted for the upright abdomen radiograph when the patient is unable to stand?

Items 6 to 14 pertain to *anteroposterior* (AP) and *posteroanterior* (PA) projections. Examine Fig. 4.4 and answer the following questions.

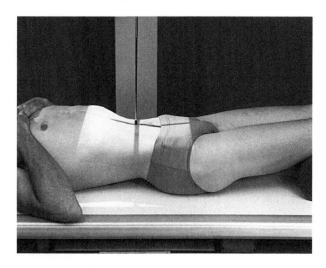

Fig. 4.4 AP abdomen, supine.

6. Describe the positioning steps used for the AP projection of the abdomen.

   Essential projection:_____

   ■ Size of collimated field:

   ■ Key patient/part positioning points:

   ■ Anatomic landmarks and relation to IR:

   ■ CR orientation and entrance point

7. Which plane of the body should be positioned perpendicular to the IR? Parallel with the IR?

8. For the AP projection with the patient supine, which structure should be seen at the bottom of the image?

9. What structure of the upper abdomen should be seen on the abdomen image when the patient is upright? Explain why.

10. What breathing instructions should be given to the patient?

11. What is the advantage of exposing abdominal images at the suspension of the recommended phase of respiration compared with the other respiration phase?

12. What two identification markers should be seen on the image when the patient is upright?

13. With reference to radiation protection, what is the advantage of the PA projection over the AP projection?

14. Circle the three evaluation criteria that indicate the patient was properly positioned without rotation for a KUB image.
   a. Intervertebral foramina should be open.
   b. Alae or wings of the ilia should be symmetric.
   c. Lumbar vertebrae pedicles should be superimposed.
   d. If seen, ischial spines of the pelvis should be symmetric.
   e. Spinous processes should be in the center of the lumbar vertebrae.

15. Examine Fig. 4.5 and identify the labeled structures.

A. _____

B. _____

C. _____

D. _____

E. _____

F. _____

G. _____

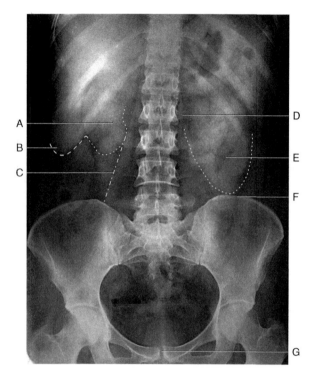

Fig. 4.5 AP projection of the abdomen (KUB).

Items 16 to 24 pertain to the *AP projection, left lateral decubitus position*. Examine Fig. 4.6 and answer the following questions.

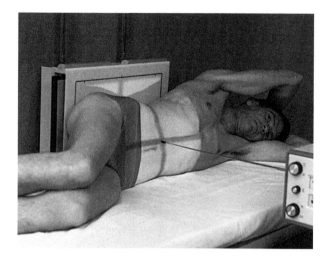

Fig. 4.6 AP abdomen, left lateral decubitus position.

16. Describe the positioning steps used for the AP projection, left lateral decubitus position of the abdomen.

Essential projection: _____,

_____

position

- Size of collimated field:

- Key patient/part positioning points:

- Anatomic landmarks and relation to IR:

- CR orientation and entrance point:

17. What is the advantage of the left lateral decubitus position compared with the supine position in AP projection of the abdomen?

18. Why is the left lateral decubitus position preferred over the right lateral decubitus position when the patient is unable to stand?

19. Why is it advisable to let the patient remain in the lateral recumbent position for several minutes before making the exposure?

20. What breathing instructions should be given to the patient?

21. Which side of the abdomen (the "up" side or the "down" side) should be demonstrated if only one side can be imaged and the patient is suspected to have fluid levels within the abdominal cavity?

22. Which side of the abdomen (the "up" side or the "down" side) should be demonstrated if only one side can be imaged and the patient is suspected to have free air in the abdomen?

23. What structure of the upper abdomen should be demonstrated on the image?

24. What identification markers should be seen on the image?

Items 25 to 30 pertain to the *lateral projection*. Examine Fig. 4.7 and answer the following questions.

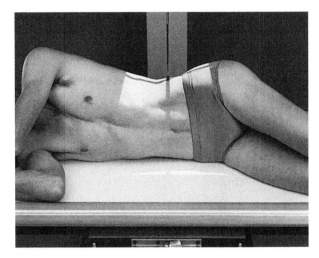

Fig. 4.7 Right lateral abdomen.

25. Describe the positioning steps used for the lateral projection of the abdomen:

Essential projection: _____
- Size of collimated field:

- Key patient/part positioning points:

- Anatomic landmarks and relation to IR:

- CR orientation and entrance point:

26. True or false. A lateral projection of the abdomen can be performed with the patient placed in either the right lateral recumbent position or the left lateral recumbent position.

27. True or false. The midsagittal plane should be perpendicular and centered to the IR.

28. True or false. The exposure should be made after the patient has suspended respiration after full inspiration.

29. Which body plane is perpendicular to IR?

30. What two areas of the image can be closely examined to determine if the patient was rotated?

Items 31 to 38 pertain to the *lateral projection, dorsal decubitus position*. Examine Fig. 4.8 and answer the following questions.

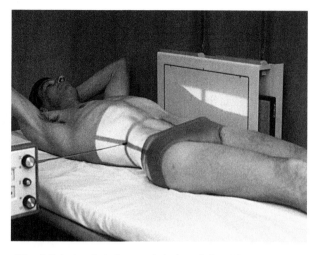

Fig. 4.8 Lateral abdomen, left dorsal decubitus position.

31. Describe the positioning steps used for the lateral projection, dorsal decubitus position of the abdomen:

Essential projection: _____,

_____ position

■ Size of collimated field:

■ Key patient/part positioning points:

■ Anatomic landmarks and relation to IR:

■ CR orientation and entrance point:

32. What is the name of the radiographic position that produces a lateral image of the abdomen with the patient in the supine position?

33. What purpose is served by having the patient slightly flex his or her knees?

34. To what level of the patient should the long axis of the IR be centered?

35. How far above the level of the iliac crests should the central ray enter the patient?

36. True or false. Anatomists define the "true pelvis" as the portion of the abdominopelvic cavity inferior to a plane passing through the sacral promontory posteriorly and the superior surface of the pubic bones anteriorly.

37. True or false. The central ray should be directed horizontally and perpendicular relative to the center of the IR.

38. Circle the three evaluation criteria that indicate the patient was correctly positioned for a lateral projection while placed in the dorsal decubitus position.
   a. The wings of the ilia should be symmetric.
   b. The ilia should be superimposed.
   c. The lumbar vetebrae pedicles should be superimposed and intervertebral foramina should be open.
   d. As much of the remaining abdomen as possible when the diaphragm
   e. The spinous processes should be seen in the center of the lumbar vertebrae.
   f. The ribs and pelvis should be equidistant to the edge of the IR on both sides.

CHAPTER 4: SELF-TEST: ABDOMEN

Answer the following questions by selecting the best choice.

1. The abdomen is divided into two cavities. The inferior cavity is the:
   a. abdominal cavity.
   b. pelvic cavity.
   c. gonadal cavity.
   d. retroperitoneal cavity.

2. The liver, stomach, and pancreas are located in the:
   a. abdominal cavity.
   b. pelvic cavity.
   c. digestive cavity.
   d. retroperitoneal cavity.

3. The portions of the peritoneum that function to support the viscera of the abdomen in position are the:
   a. retroperitoneal viscera and omentery.
   b. diaphragm and visceral folds.
   c. abdominal aorta and diaphragm.
   d. mesentery and omenta folds.

4. Which structure forms the mesentery and omenta folds?
   a. Liver
   b. Pancreas
   c. Gallbladder
   d. Peritoneum

5. Which three projections usually comprise the acute abdomen series for ambulatory patients?
   a. Supine KUB, AP upright abdomen, and upright PA chest
   b. Supine KUB, right lateral decubitus abdomen, and upright PA chest
   c. Left lateral decubitus abdomen, dorsal decubitus abdomen, and upright PA chest
   d. Right lateral decubitus abdomen, left lateral decubitus abdomen, and dorsal decubitus abdomen

6. To which level of the patient should the central ray be centered for the KUB when the patient is supine?
   a. T10 vertebral body
   b. L3 vertebral body
   c. 2 inches (5 cm) above the iliac crests
   d. Iliac crests

7. For the AP upright abdomen image of an adult of average size, why should the centering be slightly higher than the centering level used for the supine KUB image?
   a. To include the bladder
   b. To include the diaphragm
   c. To visualize gallstones
   d. To visualize kidney stones

8. For the KUB image, when should respiration be suspended, and what effect will that have on the patient?
   a. On full expiration; elevate the diaphragm
   b. On full expiration; depress the diaphragm
   c. On full inspiration; elevate the diaphragm
   d. On full inspiration; depress the diaphragm

9. Why is it desirable to include the diaphragm in the upright abdomen image?
   a. To demonstrate free air in the abdomen
   b. To demonstrate fluid levels in the thorax
   c. To demonstrate fluid levels in the abdomen
   d. To demonstrate calculi in the gallbladder and kidneys

10. Which projection should be used to demonstrate free air within the abdominal cavity when the patient is unable to stand for an upright abdomen image?
    a. AP projection with the patient supine
    b. Lateral projection, dorsal decubitus position
    c. AP projection, left lateral decubitus position
    d. AP projection, right lateral decubitus position

11. Which projection does not demonstrate free air levels within the abdomen?
    a. AP projection with the patient supine
    b. AP projection with the patient upright
    c. Lateral projection, dorsal decubitus position
    d. AP projection, left lateral decubitus position

12. What is the major advantage of the PA projection of the abdomen over the AP projection of the abdomen?
    a. The PA projection reduces the exposure dose to the gonads.
    b. The PA projection magnifies gallstones for better visualization.
    c. The PA projection demonstrates the pubic rami below the urinary bladder.
    d. The PA projection reduces the object-to-image receptor distance of the kidneys.

13. Which radiographic position of the abdomen requires that the patient be placed in the lateral recumbent position on his or her left side and that the horizontal central ray be directed along the midsagittal plane, entering the anterior surface of the patient's abdomen at the level of the iliac crests?
    a. Dorsal decubitus
    b. Ventral decubitus
    c. Left lateral decubitus
    d. Right lateral decubitus

14. Which radiographic position of the abdomen requires that the patient be supine and that the central ray be directed to a lateral side of the patient, entering slightly anterior to the midcoronal plane?
    a. Dorsal decubitus
    b. Ventral decubitus
    c. Left lateral decubitus
    d. Right lateral decubitus

15. Which radiographic position of the abdomen requires that the patient be placed in the lateral recumbent position on his or her left side, that the IR be placed under the patient and centered to the abdomen at the level of the iliac crests, and that the central ray be directed to enter the right side of the patient slightly anterior to the midcoronal plane?
    a. Left lateral
    b. Right lateral
    c. Left lateral decubitus
    d. Right lateral decubitus

16. The lateral projection with the patient placed in the dorsal decubitus position, the left lateral projection, and the left lateral decubitus position of the abdomen all require which of the following?
    a. The central ray should enter the left side of the patient.
    b. The patient should suspend respiration after expiration.
    c. The patient should suspend respiration after inspiration.
    d. The central ray should enter the anterior side of the abdomen.

17. For the lateral projection with the patient placed in the dorsal decubitus position, where should the central ray enter the patient?
    a. 2 inches (5 cm) anterior to the midcoronal plane at the level of the iliac crests
    b. 2 inches (5 cm) anterior to the midcoronal plane and 2 inches (5 cm) above the level of the iliac crests
    c. 2 inches (5 cm) posterior to the midcoronal plane at the level of the iliac crests
    d. 2 inches (5 cm) posterior to the midcoronal plane and 2 inches (5 cm) above the level of the iliac crests

18. For the lateral projection with the patient placed in the dorsal decubitus position, which procedure should be performed to ensure that the entire abdomen is included on the image?
    a. Use support cushions to elevate the patient.
    b. Center the IR to the level of the xiphoid process.
    c. Center the IR to the anterior surface of the abdomen.
    d. Direct the central ray to a point 2 inches (5 cm) below the iliac crests.

19. Which structures should be examined to see whether the patient was rotated for a lateral projection of the abdomen?
    a. Pelvis and lumbar vertebrae
    b. Pelvis and thoracic vertebrae
    c. Diaphragm and lumbar vertebrae
    d. Diaphragm and thoracic vertebrae

20. How is proper patient alignment evaluated on an AP projection, supine position (KUB) image of the abdomen?
    a. The spinous processes are seen in the midline of the lumbar vertebrae.
    b. The transverse processes of the lumbar vertebrae are visible.
    c. The vertebral column is centered in the collimated field.
    d. The psoas muscles are clearly demonstrated on each side of the lumbar spine.

21. Which of the following is evaluated to check for rotation on an AP projection, supine position image of the abdomen?
    a. The vertebral column is centered in the collimated field.
    b. The ala of the ilia are symmetric.
    c. The transverse processes of the lumbar vertebrae are visible.
    d. Ribs, pelvis, and hips are equidistant to the edge of the image on both sides.

22. Which side must be demonstrated on an AP abdomen with the patient positioned left lateral decubitus when a pneumoperitoneum is suspected?
    a. Anterior
    b. Posterior
    c. Right
    d. Left

23. Which side must be demonstrated on an AP abdomen with the patient positioned left lateral decubitus when fluid accumulation is being evaluated?
    a. Anterior
    b. Posterior
    c. Right
    d. Left

91

24. The exposure factors for an AP projection image of the abdomen must be sufficient to demonstrate the soft tissues of the:
    1. lower border of the liver
    2. kidneys
    3. psoas muscles

    a. 1 and 2 only
    b. 2 and 3 only
    c. 1 and 3 only
    d. 1, 2, and 3

25. An acute abdominal series may be ordered for all of the following reasons *except to*:
    a. check for a pneumoperitoneum.
    b. evaluate the presence of free fluid in the abdominopelvic cavity.
    c. use as a preliminary examination before contrast agent administration.
    d. rule out bowel obstruction or infection.

26. What is the recommended sequence for performing an acute abdomen series when the patient cannot stand?
    1. Seated upright chest
    2. Supine AP abdomen
    3. Upright AP abdomen
    4. Left lateral decubitus abdomen

    a. 1, 3, 4
    b. 2, 3, 1
    c. 4, 2, 1
    d. 4, 1, 2

27. To which level of the patient should the central ray be centered for the KUB when the patient is upright and the diaphragm is of interest?
    a. T10 vertebral body
    b. L3 vertebral body
    c. 2 inches (5 cm) above the iliac crests
    d. Iliac crests

28. To which level of the patient should the central ray be centered for the KUB when the patient is upright and the bladder is of interest?
    a. T10 vertebral body
    b. L3 vertebral body
    c. 2 inches (5 cm) above the iliac crests
    d. Iliac crests

29. What is the recommended exposure field or CR plate size when performing a KUB?
    a. 10 × 12 inches (25.4 × 30.5 cm) lengthwise
    b. 10 × 12 inches (25.4 × 30.5 cm) crosswise
    c. 14 × 17 inches (35.6 × 43.2 cm) lengthwise
    d. 14 × 17 inches (35.6 × 43.2 cm) crosswise

30. If free intraperitoneal air is suspected when performing a left lateral decubitus abdomen, how long should the patient lie on their side before exposure?
    a. 0 minutes
    b. 2 minutes
    c. 5 minutes
    d. 25 minutes

OSTEOLOGY AND ARTHROLOGY OF THE UPPER EXTREMITY

Section 1: Exercise 1

1. Label the diagram of the hand shown in Fig. 5.1 by writing D on each distal phalanx, M on each middle phalanx, and P on each proximal phalanx. Label each metacarpal by writing its identification number (1 through 5) on the appropriate bone.

2. Identify each lettered bone or articulation shown in Fig. 5.1.

   A. _____

   B. _____

   C. _____

   D. _____

   E. _____

   F. _____

   G. _____

   H. _____

   I. _____

   J. _____

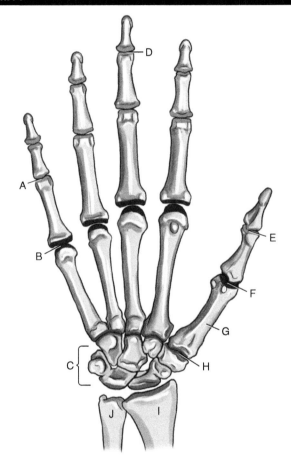

Fig. 5.1 Anterior aspect of hand and wrist.

Section 1: Exercise 2

Identify each lettered carpal bone shown in Fig. 5.2.

A. _____

B. _____

C. _____

D. _____

E. _____

F. _____

G. _____

H. _____

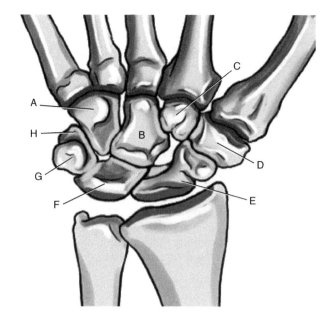

Fig. 5.2 Anterior aspect of wrist.

Section 1: Exercise 3

Identify each lettered bone shown in Fig. 5.3.

A. _____

B. _____

C. _____

D. _____

E. _____

F. _____

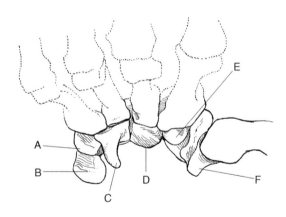

Fig. 5.3 Inferosuperior aspect of the carpal sulcus.

Section 1: Exercise 4

Identify each lettered structure shown in Fig. 5.4.

A. _____

B. _____

C. _____

D. _____

E. _____

F. _____

G. _____

H. _____

I. _____

J. _____

K. _____

L. _____

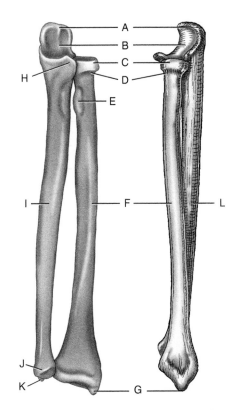

Fig. 5.4 Anterior and lateral aspects of the forearm.

Section 1: Exercise 5

This exercise allows you to apply what you have learned about anatomy. This diagram cannot be found in Merrill's Atlas, but the articulations are discussed in the textbook. Identify each lettered articulation shown in Fig. 5.5.

A. _____

B. _____

C. _____

D. _____

E. _____

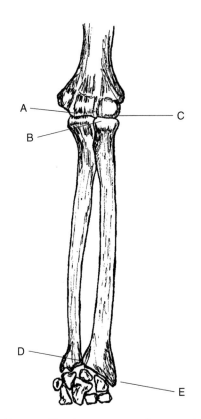

Fig. 5.5 The forearm—anterior aspect.

Section 1: Exercise 6

Identify each lettered structure shown in Fig. 5.6.

A. _____

B. _____

C. _____

D. _____

E. _____

F. _____

G. _____

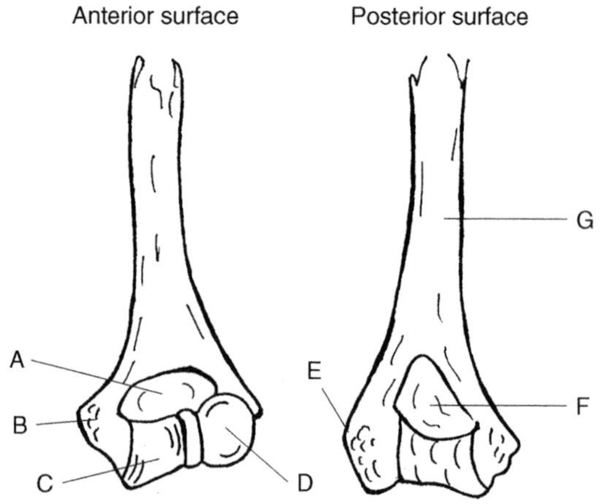

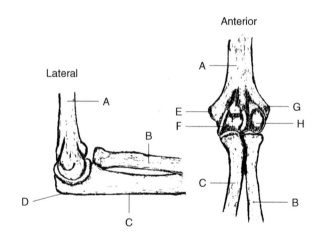

Fig. 5.6 Distal end of the humerus.

Section 1: Exercise 7

Identify each lettered structure shown in Fig. 5.7.

A. _____

B. _____

C. _____

D. _____

E. _____

F. _____

G. _____

H. _____

Fig. 5.7 Two views of the elbow.

Chapter **5** **Upper Extremity**

Section 1: Exercise 8

Identify each lettered structure illustrated in Fig. 5.8.

A. _____

B. _____

C. _____

D. _____

E. _____

F. _____

G. _____

H. _____

I. _____

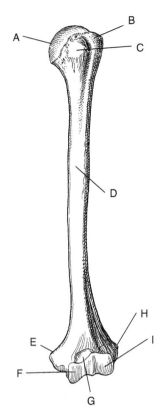

Fig. 5.8 Anterior aspect of the humerus.

Section 1: Exercise 9

Match the structures located on the distal portion of the humerus in Column A with the descriptions in Column B. Not all descriptions may apply to the listed structures.

Column A

_____ 1. Trochlea

_____ 2. Capitulum

_____ 3. Coronoid fossa

_____ 4. Olecranon fossa

_____ 5. Medial epicondyle

Column B

a. A round, marblelike structure

b. Bony prominence; easily palpated

c. A spool-like structure

d. Depression; located on the anterior surface

e. Depression; located on the posterior surface

f. Lateral to the humeral head

Section 1: Exercise 10

Structures found on the radius, ulna, or humerus are listed. In the space provided, write P if the structure is proximal or D if the structure is distal on the bone.

_____ 1. Trochlea

_____ 2. Capitulum

_____ 3. Ulnar head

_____ 4. Radial head

_____ 5. Humeral head

_____ 6. Radial tubercle

_____ 7. Coronoid fossa

_____ 8. Trochlear notch

_____ 9. Greater tubercle

_____ 10. Olecranon fossa

_____ 11. Coronoid process

_____ 12. Olecranon process

_____ 13. Medial epicondyle

_____ 14. Ulnar styloid process

_____ 15. Radial styloid process

Section 1: Exercise 11

Structures found on the radius, ulna, or humerus are listed. In the space provided, write R for radius, U for ulna, or H for humerus to indicate on which bone the part is located. Some structures may be found on more than one bone.

_____ 1. Head

_____ 2. Trochlea

_____ 3. Capitulum

_____ 4. Radial notch

_____ 5. Radial fossa

_____ 6. Coronoid fossa

_____ 7. Styloid process

_____ 8. Olecranon fossa

_____ 9. Trochlear notch

_____ 10. Greater tubercle

_____ 11. Radial tuberosity

_____ 12. Coronoid process

_____ 13. Olecranon process

_____ 14. Medial epicondyle

_____ 15. Lateral epicondyle

Section 1: Exercise 12

Match the articulations in Column A with the types of movement listed in Column B. More than one choice from Column B may be used for some articulations.

Column A

_____ 1. Intercarpal

_____ 2. Radiocarpal

_____ 3. Interphalangeal

_____ 4. Metacarpophalangeal

_____ 5. Distal radioulnar

_____ 6. Proximal radioulnar

_____ 7. Elbow joint (humeroulnar and humeroradial)

Column B

a. Gliding

b. Flexion

c. Extension

d. Abduction

e. Adduction

f. Circumduction

g. Rotational (around a single axis)

Section 1: Exercise 13

Match the pathology terms in Column A with the appropriate definition in Column B. Not all choices from Column B should be selected.

Column A

_____ 1. Gout

_____ 2. Fracture

_____ 3. Bone cyst

_____ 4. Dislocation

_____ 5. Joint effusion

_____ 6. Osteomyelitis

_____ 7. Osteoarthritis

_____ 8. Enchondroma

_____ 9. Osteosarcoma

_____ 10. Ewing sarcoma

_____ 11. Colles fracture

_____ 12. Smith fracture

_____ 13. Boxer's fracture

_____ 14. Bennett fracture

_____ 15. Torus or buckle fracture

Column B

a. Loss of bone density

b. Disruption in the continuity of bone

c. Benign tumor consisting of cartilage

d. Fracture at the base of the first metacarpal

e. Fracture at the neck of the fifth metacarpal

f. Displacement of a bone from the joint space

g. Malignant tumor arising from cartilage cells

h. Fluid-filled cyst with a wall of fibrous tissue

i. Impacted fracture with bulging of the periosteum

j. Inflammation of bone resulting from a pyogenic infection

k. Chronic, systemic, inflammatory collagen disease

l. Malignant tumor of bone arising in medullary tissue

m. Hereditary form of arthritis in which uric acid is deposited in joints

n. Malignant, primary tumor of bone with bone or cartilage formation

o. Fracture of the distal radius and ulnar styloid with anterior displacement

p. Fracture of the distal radius and ulnar styloid with posterior displacement

q. Accumulation of fluid in the joint associated with an underlying condition

r. Form of arthritis marked by progressive cartilage deterioration in synovial joints and vertebrae

Section 1: Exercise 14: Common Abbreviations of the Upper Extremity

Abbreviations are often used to save time when speaking or writing. Students must master the language and abbreviations used by radiographers. This exercise is provided to help familiarize the student with common abbreviations used in the imaging profession. Write the correct term beside its abbreviation.

1. PIP joint: _____

2. MCP joint: _____

3. DIP joint: _____

4. IP: _____ (anatomy)

5. IP: _____ (equipment)

Section 1: Exercise 15

This exercise is a comprehensive review of the osteology and arthrology of the upper extremity. Provide a short answer or select the correct answer for each question.

1. List the names of the three groups of bones that comprise the hand and wrist, and indicate the quantity of bones in that group in each upper extremity.

2. Which bone classification are the metacarpals?
   a. Flat
   b. Long
   c. Short
   d. Irregular

3. Which bone classification are the carpal bones?
   a. Flat
   b. Long
   c. Short
   d. Irregular

4. Which bones articulate with the heads of the metacarpal bones?
   a. Carpals
   b. Distal phalanges
   c. Proximal phalanges
   d. Tarsals

5. What group of bones articulates with the bases of metacarpal bones?

6. What part of a metacarpal bone (base or head) forms part of each metacarpophalangeal joint?

7. Which of the following types of upper extremity joints are formed in part by the bases of the metacarpals?
   a. Interphalangeal
   b. Carpometacarpal
   c. Metacarpophalangeal

8. How are the metacarpals identified?
   a. Letters A to E from medial (little finger side) to lateral (thumb side)
   b. Letters A to E from lateral (thumb side) to medial (little finger side)
   c. Numbered 1 through 5 from lateral (thumb side) to medial (little finger side)
   d. Numbered 1 through 5 from medial (little finger side) to lateral (thumb side)

9. What is the most distal portion of each metacarpal?
   a. Head
   b. Base
   c. Tubercle

10. How many proximal, middle, and distal phalanges are found in one hand?

    a. Proximal: _____

    b. Middle: _____

    c. Distal: _____

11. Which kinds of movements do the interphalangeal joints allow?
    a. Gliding and sliding
    b. Flexion and extension
    c. Rotational movements around a single axis

12. Which joint is the most distal joint in the upper extremity?
    a. Carpometacarpal
    b. Distal interphalangeal
    c. Metacarpophalangeal
    d. Proximal interphalangeal

13. Identify each carpal bone by listing its name first, followed by any additional names it may have. Indicate whether each bone is proximal or distal by writing P for proximal or D for distal in the parentheses found after each blank.

    a. _____ ( )
    b. _____ ( )
    c. _____ ( )
    d. _____ ( )
    e. _____ ( )
    f. _____ ( )
    g. _____ ( )
    h. _____ ( )

14. What other name refers to the radiocarpal joint?

15. List the names of the two bones that comprise the forearm, and indicate which bone is lateral and which bone is medial.

16. On which end of the radius (proximal or distal) is the styloid process located?

17. On which end of the radius (proximal or distal) is the radial head located?

18. On which end of the ulna (proximal or distal) is the styloid process located?

19. On which end of the ulna (proximal or distal) is the olecranon process located?

20. Which two bony processes are located on the proximal end of the ulna?
    a. Ulnar head and styloid process
    b. Ulnar head and coronoid process
    c. Olecranon process and styloid process
    d. Olecranon process and coronoid process

21. Which of the following is located on the proximal ulna?
    a. Ulnar notch
    b. Humeral notch
    c. Trochlear notch

22. On which bone is the trochlear notch located?
    a. Ulna
    b. Radius
    c. Humerus

23. Which joint do the radial notch of the ulna and the head of the radius form?
    a. Humeroulnar
    b. Humeroradial
    c. Distal radioulnar
    d. Proximal radioulnar

24. Which joint do the head of the ulna and the ulnar notch of the radius form?
    a. Humeroulnar
    b. Humeroradial
    c. Distal radioulnar
    d. Proximal radioulnar

25. With which of the following structures of the distal humerus does the radial head articulate?
    a. Trochlea
    b. Capitulum
    c. Lateral epicondyle
    d. Medial epicondyle

26. With which of the following structures of the distal humerus does the trochlear notch articulate?
    a. Trochlea
    b. Capitulum
    c. Lateral epicondyle
    d. Medial epicondyle

27. From the following list, circle the three articulations that form the complete elbow joint.
    a. Radiocarpal
    b. Humeroulnar
    c. Humeroradial
    d. Scapulohumeral
    e. Distal radioulnar
    f. Proximal radioulnar

28. With reference to the capitulum, where is the trochlea located?
    a. Lateral
    b. Medial
    c. Distal
    d. Proximal

29. Write the name of each articulation of the humerus.

30. Write the name of each fossa found on the distal humerus, and indicate on which surface each is located.

103

Section 1: Exercise 16: Upper Extremity Anatomy Crossword Puzzle

Use the following clues to fill in the crossword puzzle.

Across

1. Prominence on anterior surface of distal, medial humerus
4. End of bone on which radial head is located
5. Depression on posterior surface of distal humerus, olecranon
8. Medial to trapezium
10. Carpal between scaphoid and triquetrum
12. Finger bones
15. Portion of distal humerus that articulates with radial head
18. Raised process on proximal, lateral humerus
19. Prominent process on proximal ulna
20. End of bone on which ulnar head is located

Down

2. Carpal that articulates with third metacarpal
3. Distal process on radius and ulna
6. Bones in the wrist
7. Carpal bone with hooklike process
9. IP portion of DIP abbreviation
11. Lateral bone of forearm
13. Palpable landmarks on each side of distal humerus
14. Bones in the palm of the hand
16. Process located on anterior, proximal ulna
17. Upper arm bone

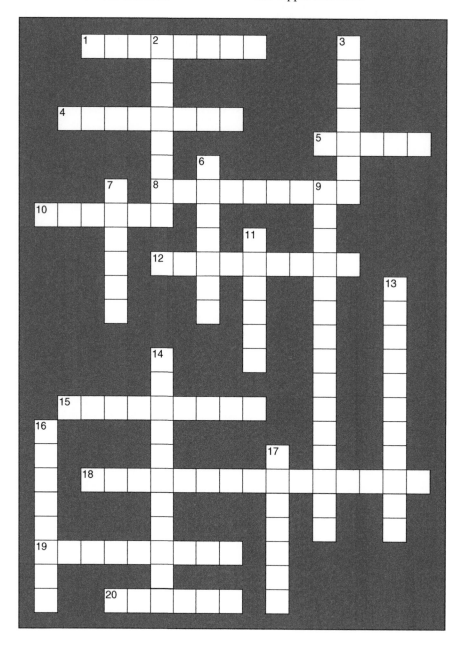

POSITIONING OF THE UPPER EXTREMITY

Section 2: Exercise 1: Positioning for the Fingers

This exercise pertains to the essential projections of the fingers, as identified in your Merrill's Atlas textbook. Identify structures, fill in missing words, or provide a short answer for each question.

1. List each essential projection for digits 2 through 5, and describe the positioning steps used for each as follows:

   Essential projection: _____
   - Size of collimated field:

   - Key patient/part positioning points:

   - Anatomic landmarks and relation to IR:

   - CR orientation and entrance point:

   Essential projection: _____
   - Size of collimated field:

   - Key patient/part positioning points:

   - Anatomic landmarks and relation to IR:

   - CR orientation and entrance point:

   Essential projection: _____
   - Size of collimated field:

   - Key patient/part positioning points:

   - Anatomic landmarks and relation to IR:

   - CR orientation and entrance point:

2. Identify each lettered bone or joint shown in Fig. 5.9.

A. _____

B. _____

C. _____

D. _____

E. _____

F. _____

G. _____

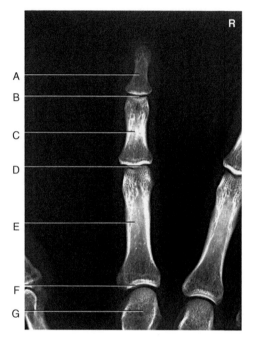

Fig. 5.9 Second digit (index finger).

3. What projection is demonstrated in Fig. 5.9?

4. Fig. 5.10 demonstrates the _____ projection of the second digit.

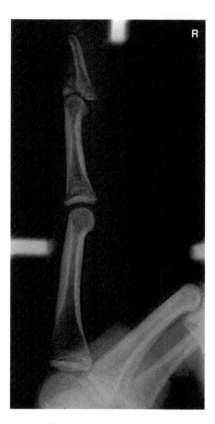

Fig. 5.10 Second digit.

5. Compare Fig. 5.9 with Fig. 5.10. Describe how the patient's position, as shown in Fig. 5.9, was adjusted to produce the image shown in Fig. 5.10.

6. On which hand surface should the hand be rested when performing the lateral projection image of the fourth or fifth digit?
   a. Medial (ulnar)
   b. Lateral (radial)
   c. Anterior (palmar)
   d. Posterior (ventral)

7. For lateral projections of the third or fourth digits, why should the affected digit be positioned so that its long axis is parallel with the IR?

8. How many degrees from the PA position should a finger be rotated for PA oblique projection?

9. For the PA oblique projection of the second digit, what is the advantage of rotating the second digit medially compared with the advantage of rotating the digit laterally?

10. For the PA oblique projection of the third digit, what is the advantage of placing the patient's fingers on a 45-degree foam wedge?

Section 2: Exercise 2: Positioning for the First Digit (Thumb)

This exercise pertains to projections of the first digit, or thumb. Identify structures, fill in missing words, choose the correct answer, or provide a short answer for each question.

1. List the essential projections for the first digit (thumb), and describe the positioning steps used for each, as follows:

   Essential projection: _____
   ■ Size of collimated field:

   ■ Key patient/part positioning points:

   ■ Anatomic landmarks and relation to IR:

   ■ CR orientation and entrance point:

   Essential projection: _____
   ■ Size of collimated field:

   ■ Key patient/part positioning points:

   ■ Anatomic landmarks and relation to IR:

   ■ CR orientation and entrance point:

Essential projection: _____
- Size of collimated field:

- Key patient/part positioning points:

- Anatomic landmarks and relation to IR:

- CR orientation and entrance point:

2. What projection of the thumb may be substituted if the patient is unable to maintain the required position for the AP projection?

3. What is the disadvantage of using the substitute projection mentioned above?

4. All thumb images should include the _____ carpal within the collimated field.

5. Identify each lettered structure or joint shown in Fig. 5.11.

A.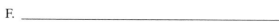

B. _____

C. _____

D. _____

E. _____

F. _____

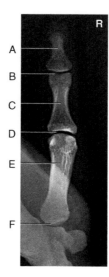

Fig. 5.11 AP thumb.

Section 2: Exercise 3: Positioning for the Hand

This exercise pertains to the essential radiographic positions for the hand. Identify structures, fill in missing words, provide a short answer, or choose an answer from a list for each question.

1. List the essential projections for the hand, and describe the positioning steps used for each, as follows:

   Essential projection: _____
   - Size of collimated field:

   - Key patient/part positioning points:

   - Anatomic landmarks and relation to IR:

   - CR orientation and entrance point:

   Essential projection: _____
   - Size of collimated field:

   - Key patient/part positioning points:

   - Anatomic landmarks and relation to IR:

   - CR orientation and entrance point:

   Essential projection: _____
   - Size of collimated field:

   - Key patient/part positioning points:

   - Anatomic landmarks and relation to IR:

   - CR orientation and entrance point:

2. Which two groups of joints of the hand and digits should be demonstrated open on the image of the PA projection of the hand?
   a. Intercarpal and interphalangeal
   b. Intercarpal and carpophalangeal
   c. Metacarpophalangeal and interphalangeal
   d. Metacarpophalangeal and carpophalangeal

3. Identify each lettered bone or joint shown in Fig. 5.12.

A. _____

B. _____

C. _____

D. _____

E. _____

F. _____

G. _____

H. _____

I. _____

J. _____

K. _____

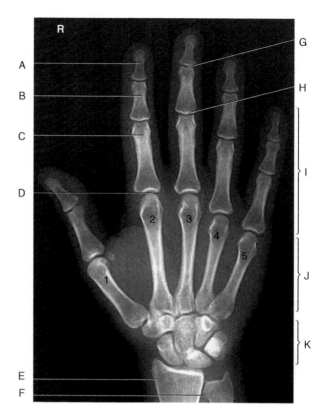

Fig. 5.12 PA hand.

4. Figs. 5.13 and 5.14 illustrate two different ways to position the hand for PA oblique projections. Which figure represents the position that best demonstrates interphalangeal joints? Explain why.

5. Examine the images shown in Figs. 5.15 and 5.16. What difference in positioning most likely caused the difference in appearance of these two images?

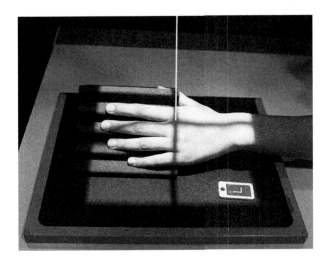

Fig. 5.13 PA oblique hand.

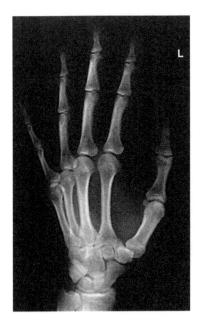

Fig. 5.15 PA oblique hand.

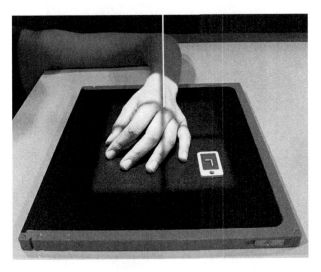

Fig. 5.14 PA oblique hand.

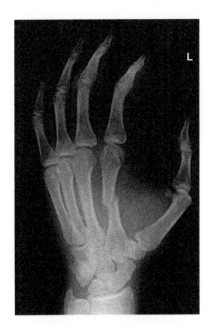

Fig. 5.16 PA oblique wrist.

6. Figs. 5.17 and 5.18 represent two lateral projections of the hand. Identify the position used for each image.

   Fig. 5.17 position: _____

   Fig. 5.18 position: _____

7. Which projection of the hand should demonstrate superimposed phalanges?
   a. PA oblique
   b. Lateral, in fan lateral position
   c. Lateral, in extension

8. Fig. 5.17 shows a lateral projection image of the hand. In this image, which group of bones is of primary interest?
   a. Carpals
   b. Phalanges
   c. Metacarpals

9. The projection demonstrated in Fig. 5.18 is best used to demonstrate:
   1. foreign bodies.
   2. displacement of fractures in the metacarpals.
   3. the phalanges.

   a. 1 and 2 only
   b. 1 and 3 only
   c. 2 and 3 only
   d. 1, 2, and 3

10. Identify each lettered individual bone or group of bones shown in Fig. 5.18.

    A. _____

    B. _____

    C. _____

    D. _____

    E. _____

    F. _____

    G. _____

    H. _____

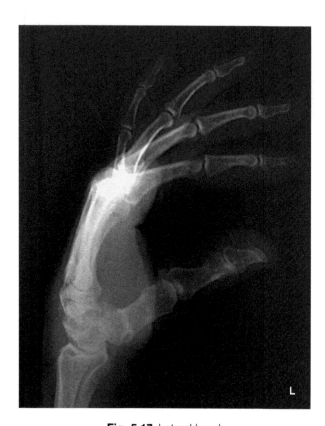

Fig. 5.17 Lateral hand.

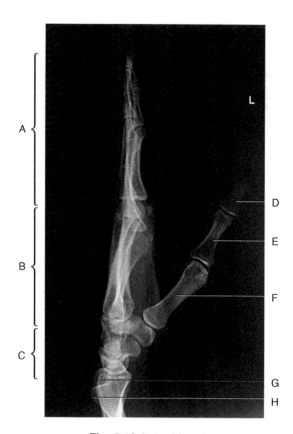

Fig. 5.18 Lateral hand.

Section 2: Exercise 4: Positioning for the Wrist and Scaphoid

This exercise pertains to the essential radiographic positions for the wrist and scaphoid. Identify structures, fill in missing words, provide a short answer, or select answers from a list for each question.

1. List the essential projections for the wrist and scaphoid carpal, and describe the positioning steps used for each, as follows:

   Essential projection: _____
   - Size of collimated field:

   - Key patient/part positioning points:

   - Anatomic landmarks and relation to IR:

   - CR orientation and entrance point:

   Essential projection: _____
   - Size of collimated field:

   - Key patient/part positioning points:

   - Anatomic landmarks and relation to IR:

   - CR orientation and entrance point:

   Essential projection: _____
   - Size of collimated field:

   - Key patient/part positioning points:

   - Anatomic landmarks and relation to IR:

   - CR orientation and entrance point:

   Essential projection: _____
   - Size of collimated field:

   - Key patient/part positioning points:

   - Anatomic landmarks and relation to IR:

   - CR orientation and entrance point:

   Essential projection: _____
   - Size of collimated field:

   - Key patient/part positioning points:

   - Anatomic landmarks and relation to IR:

   - CR orientation and entrance point:

2. Flexing the fingers for the PA projection of the wrist decreases _____ and increases _____.

3. Identify each lettered carpal bone shown in Fig. 5.19.

A. _____

B. _____

C. _____

D. _____

E. _____

F. _____

G. _____

H. _____

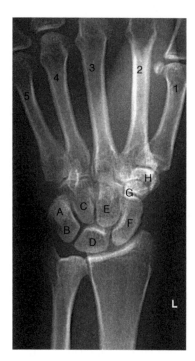

Fig. 5.19 PA wrist.

4. For the lateral projection of the wrist, how should the elbow be positioned?
   a. Fully extended
   b. Flexed 45 degrees
   c. Flexed 90 degrees

5. For the lateral projection of the wrist, which surface of the wrist should be in contact with the IR?
   a. Medial
   b. Lateral
   c. Anterior
   d. Posterior

6. Identify each lettered structure shown in Fig. 5.20.

A. _____

B. _____

C. _____

D. _____

E. _____

F. _____

G. _____

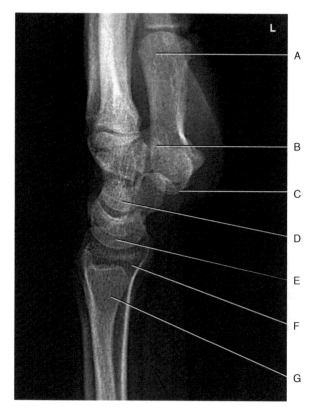

Fig. 5.20 Lateral wrist.

7. Referring again to Fig. 5.20, what other bones in addition to the metacarpals and the carpals should be superimposed for this projection?

8. How much should the wrist be rotated for the PA oblique projection?
   a. 25 degrees
   b. 35 degrees
   c. 45 degrees

114

9. For the PA oblique projection when the scaphoid is of primary interest, the scaphoid can sometimes be better demonstrated if the patient deviates the hand and wrist toward the _____.

10. Identify each lettered structure shown in Fig. 5.21.

A. _____

B. _____

C. _____

D. _____

E. _____

F. _____

G. _____

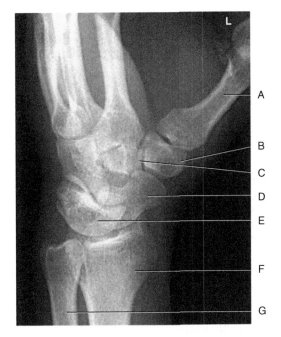

Fig. 5.21 PA oblique wrist.

Questions 11 to 13 pertain to Fig. 5.22.

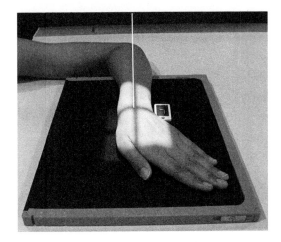

Fig. 5.22 An essential wrist projection.

11. Fig. 5.22 demonstrates the _____ projection of the wrist in _____ position.

12. Which bone is of primary interest with this projection?
    a. Ulna
    b. Lunate
    c. Radius
    d. Scaphoid

13. To delineate a fracture line better with a PA projection of the wrist in ulnar deviation, how many degrees and in which direction may the central ray be directed?
    a. 10 to 15 degrees medially or laterally
    b. 20 to 25 degrees medially or laterally
    c. 10 to 15 degrees proximally or distally
    d. 20 to 25 degrees proximally or distally

Questions 14 to 18 pertain to Fig. 5.23.

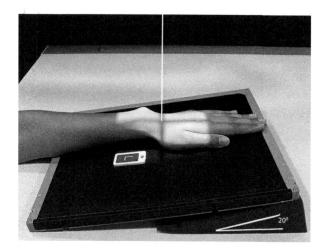

Fig. 5.23 An essential wrist projection.

14. Fig. 5.23 demonstrates the _____

    projection (_____ method).

15. Which carpal bone is of primary interest with this position?
    a. Lunate
    b. Capitate
    c. Scaphoid

16. How far from horizontal should the IR be inclined toward the elbow?
    a. 10 degrees
    b. 20 degrees
    c. 30 degrees

17. When using a wedge to elevate the IR (as seen in Fig. 5.23), how should the central ray be directed toward the wrist?
    a. Perpendicularly
    b. At a 10-degree angle toward the elbow
    c. At a 20-degree angle toward the elbow
    d. At a 30-degree angle toward the elbow

18. If no wedge is used to angle the IR, how should the central ray be directed toward the wrist?
    a. Perpendicularly
    b. At a 10-degree angle toward the elbow
    c. At a 20-degree angle toward the elbow
    d. At a 30-degree angle toward the elbow

Section 2: Exercise 5: Positioning for the Carpal Canal

This exercise pertains to the essential projection for the carpal canal. Identify structures, provide a short answer, or select the answer from a list for each question.

1. List the essential projections for the carpal canal, and describe the positioning steps used for each, as follows:

    Essential projection: _____

    (_____ method).
    ■ Size of collimated field:

    ■ Key patient/part positioning points:

    ■ Anatomic landmarks and relation to IR:

    ■ CR orientation and entrance point:

2. With reference to the plane of the IR, how should the long axis of the hand be positioned?
    a. Angled
    b. Vertical
    c. Parallel

3. With reference to the long axis of the hand, how much should the central ray be angled?
    a. 5 to 10 degrees
    b. 15 to 20 degrees
    c. 25 to 30 degrees

4. Identify each lettered structure shown in Fig. 5.24.

A. _____

B. _____

C. _____

D. _____

E. _____

F. _____

G. _____

H. _____

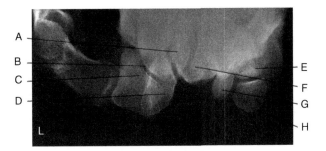

Fig. 5.24 Tangential (inferosuperior) carpal canal.

Section 2: Exercise 6: Positioning for the Forearm

This exercise pertains to the essential projections for the forearm. Identify structures, provide a short answer, select the answer from a list, or choose true or false (explaining any statement you believe to be false) for each question.

1. List the essential projections for the forearm and describe the positioning steps used for each, as follows:

   Essential projection: _____
   - Size of collimated field:

   - Key patient/part positioning points:

   - Anatomic landmarks and relation to IR:

   - CR orientation and entrance point:

   Essential projection: _____
   - Size of collimated field:

   - Key patient/part positioning points:

   - Anatomic landmarks and relation to IR:

   - CR orientation and entrance point:

2. For the AP projection of the forearm, how should the elbow be positioned?
   a. Fully extended
   b. Flexed 45 degrees
   c. Flexed 90 degrees

3. If the hand is pronated for the AP projection of the forearm, what will the image demonstrate?

4. Identify each lettered structure shown in Fig. 5.25.

A. _____

B. _____

C. _____

D. _____

E. _____

F. _____

G. _____

H. _____

I. _____

5. For the lateral projection of the forearm, how should the elbow be positioned?
   a. Fully extended
   b. Flexed 45 degrees
   c. Flexed 90 degrees
   d. Rotated medially 45 degrees

6. True or false. The hand should be pronated for the lateral projection.

7. Identify each lettered structure shown in Fig. 5.26.

A. _____

B. _____

C. _____

D. _____

E. _____

F. _____

G. _____

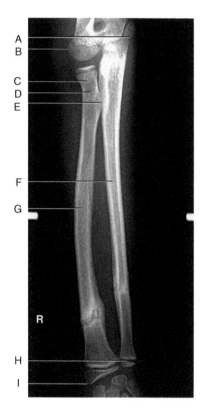

Fig. 5.25 AP forearm.

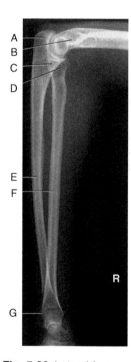

Fig. 5.26 Lateral forearm.

Section 2: Exercise 7: Positioning for the Elbow

This exercise pertains to the essential projections for the elbow. Identify structures, provide a short answer, match columns, or select answers from a list for each question.

1. List the essential projections for the elbow, and describe the positioning steps used for each, as follows:

   Essential projection: _____
   - Size of collimated field:

   - Key patient/part positioning points:

   - Anatomic landmarks and relation to IR:

   - CR orientation and entrance point:

   Essential projection: _____
   - Size of collimated field:

   - Key patient/part positioning points:

   - Anatomic landmarks and relation to IR:

   - CR orientation and entrance point:

   Essential projection: _____
   - Size of collimated field:

   - Key patient/part positioning points:

   - Anatomic landmarks and relation to IR:

   - CR orientation and entrance point:

   Essential projection: _____
   - Size of collimated field:

   - Key patient/part positioning points:

   - Anatomic landmarks and relation to IR:

   - CR orientation and entrance point:

   Essential projection: _____
   - Size of collimated field:

   - Key patient/part positioning points:

   - Anatomic landmarks and relation to IR:

   - CR orientation and entrance point:

Essential projection: _____
- Size of collimated field:

- Key patient/part positioning points:

- Anatomic landmarks and relation to IR:

- CR orientation and entrance point:

Essential projection: _____

(_____ method).
- Size of collimated field:

- Key patient/part positioning points:

- Anatomic landmarks and relation to IR:

- CR orientation and entrance point:

2. For the AP projection of the elbow, why should the hand be positioned with the palm facing up?

3. Identify each lettered structure shown in the AP projection of an elbow in Fig. 5.27.

A. _____

B. _____

C. _____

D. _____

E. _____

F. _____

G. _____

H. _____ (tuberosity)

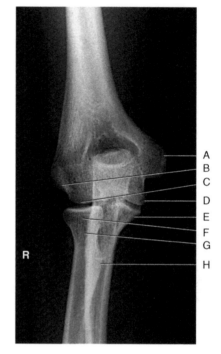

Fig. 5.27 AP elbow.

4. For the lateral projection of the elbow, how should the hand be adjusted?
   a. Pronated
   b. Supinated
   c. Lateral with the thumb side up
   d. Lateral with the thumb side down

5. How many degrees of flexion of the elbow are necessary for the lateral projection?

6. How should the humeral epicondyles appear in the image of the lateral projection of the elbow?

7. Identify each lettered structure shown in Fig. 5.28.

A. _____

B. _____

C. _____

D. _____

E. _____

F. _____

G. _____

H. _____

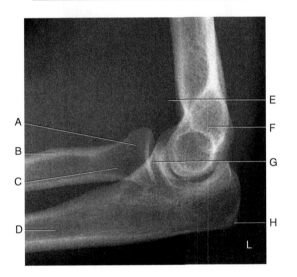

Fig. 5.28 Lateral elbow.

8. How much medial rotation of the elbow is needed to position it for AP oblique projections?
   a. 25 degrees
   b. 35 degrees
   c. 45 degrees
   d. 55 degrees

9. Which AP oblique projection positioning movement (medial rotation or lateral rotation) requires the hand to be pronated?

10. Identify each lettered structure shown in Fig. 5.29.

A. _____

B. _____

C. _____

D. _____

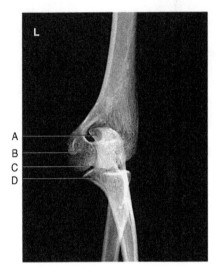

Fig. 5.29 AP oblique elbow (medial rotation).

11. Identify each lettered structure shown in Fig. 5.30.

A. _____

B. _____

C. _____

D. _____

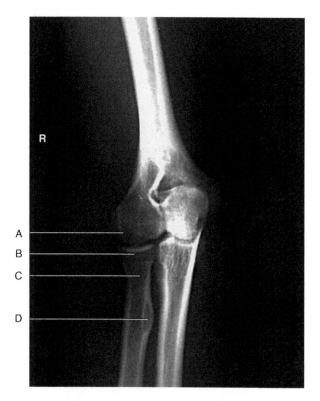

Fig. 5.30 AP oblique elbow (lateral rotation).

12. Again examining Figs. 5.29 and 5.30, identify which image best demonstrates the following structures.

_____ a. Open elbow joint

_____ b. Coronoid process in profile

_____ c. Radial head projected free of the ulna

_____ d. Elongated medial humeral epicondyle

_____ e. Ulna superimposed by the radial head and neck

Figs. 5.31 and 5.32 are AP projection images of the partially flexed elbow. Examine the images and answer questions 13 to 19.

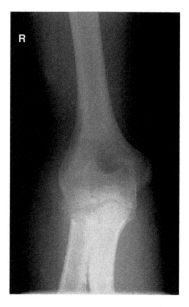

Fig. 5.31 AP elbow, partial flexion.

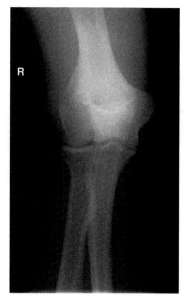

Fig. 5.32 AP elbow, partial flexion.

13. Which image demonstrates an AP projection of the distal humerus?

14. Which image demonstrates an AP projection of the proximal forearm?

15. Which image demonstrates the elbow joint partially opened?

16. For the AP distal humerus projection (partially flexed elbow), what part of the upper extremity should be parallel and in contact with the IR?

17. In the AP distal humerus projection (partially flexed elbow) image, what part of the upper extremity will appear greatly foreshortened in the image?

18. For the AP proximal forearm projection (partially flexed elbow), what part of the upper extremity should be parallel and in contact with the IR?

19. In the AP proximal forearm projection (partially flexed elbow) image, what part of the upper extremity will appear greatly foreshortened in the image?

20. What position is the hand in for the axiolateral projection (Coyle method) of the elbow?

21. What specific anatomy is best demonstrated on the axiolateral projection (Coyle method) of the elbow when the central ray is directed 45 degrees toward the shoulder?

22. What anatomy is best demonstrated in Fig. 5.33?

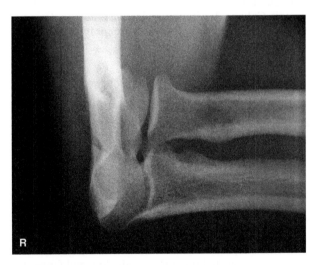

Fig. 5.33 Axiolateral projection (Coyle method).

23. What anatomy is best demonstrated in Fig. 5.34?

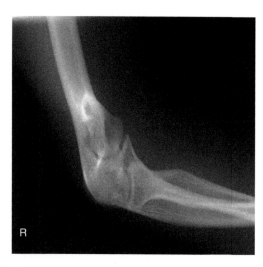

Fig. 5.34 Axiolateral projection (Coyle method).

For Questions 24 to 28, match the projections of the elbow in Column A with the evaluation criteria in Column B. Not all evaluation criteria may apply to the listed projections.

Column A

_____ 24. AP projection

_____ 25. Lateral projection

_____ 26. AP oblique projection, lateral rotation position

_____ 27. AP oblique projection, medial rotation position

_____ 28. AP proximal forearm projection (partially flexed elbow)

Column B

a. Distal humerus will be foreshortened.

b. Coronoid process should be seen in profile.

c. Olecranon process should be seen in profile.

d. Proximal forearm will be greatly foreshortened.

e. Radial head should be projected free of the ulna.

f. Humeral epicondyles should not be rotated or superimposed.

Section 2: Exercise 8: Positioning for the Humerus

This exercise pertains to the essential projections of the humerus. Identify structures, fill in missing words, provide a short answer, or select answers from a list for each question.

1. List the essential projections for the carpal canal, and describe the positioning steps used for each, as follows:

Essential projection: _____
- Size of collimated field:

- Key patient/part positioning points:

- Anatomic landmarks and relation to IR:

- CR orientation and entrance point:

Essential projection: _____
- Size of collimated field:

- Key patient/part positioning points:

- Anatomic landmarks and relation to IR:

- CR orientation and entrance point:

2. The humerus can be examined with the patient in either the _____ or _____ position.

3. How should the hand be placed for the AP projection of the humerus?

4. For the AP projection with the patient supine, why is it sometimes necessary to elevate the unaffected shoulder on a firm support?

5. From the following list, circle the three evaluation criteria that indicate the humerus was correctly positioned for the AP projection.
   a. Epicondyles are superimposed.
   b. Epicondyles are maximally seen and not rotated.
   c. Greater tubercle is superimposed over the humeral head.
   d. Humeral head and greater tubercle are both seen in profile.
   e. Lesser tubercle is seen in profile and toward the glenoid fossa.
   f. Outline of the lesser tubercle is located between the humeral head and the greater tubercle.

6. Identify each lettered structure shown in Fig. 5.35.

   A. _____

   B. _____

   C. _____

   D. _____

   E. _____

   F. _____

   G. _____

   H. _____

   I. _____

   J. _____

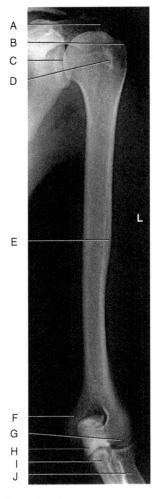

Fig. 5.35 Upright AP humerus.

7. How does the divergence of the beam affect the demonstration of the elbow joint in the lateral projection image?

8. The superimposition of what structures confirms that a true lateral image was produced?

9. For the lateral projection with the patient in the lateral recumbent position and an IR placed between the arm and the thorax, which portion of the humerus is missing from the image?

10. Identify each lettered structure shown in Fig. 5.36.

A. _____

B. _____

C. _____

D. _____

E. _____

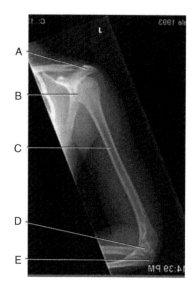

Fig. 5.36 Upright lateral humerus.

Section 2: Exercise 9: Positioning of the Upper Extremity

This exercise is a comprehensive review of the standard projections that demonstrate structures of the upper extremity. Provide a short answer for each question.

1. Where is the centering point for the central ray for the AP projection of the thumb?

2. Which projection of the thumb requires the patient to rotate the hand into extreme internal rotation?

3. Where is the centering point for the central ray for the PA projection of the third digit of the hand?

4. Explain why the hand should be rotated into extreme internal rotation until the lateral surface of the index finger (second digit) is in contact with the IR, rather than positioning that finger with its medial (ulnar) surface toward the IR, for the lateral projection of the index finger.

5. Name the four bones that should be completely seen in the image of the AP projection of the thumb.

6. Excluding the thumb, name the two digits of the hand that should rest directly on the IR for the lateral projection of individual digits.

7. Describe how and where the central ray should be directed for the PA projection of the hand.

8. What surface of the hand should be in contact with the IR for the PA projection of the hand?

9. From the prone position, how many degrees should the hand be rotated for the PA oblique projection? For the lateral projection?

10. For the best demonstration of all digits, how should the thumb and index finger be positioned with respect to the IR for the PA oblique projection of the hand?

11. Which bones of the hand are of primary interest if the fingertips are allowed to rest on the IR for the PA oblique projection of the hand?

12. What group of bones of the hand is best demonstrated with the fan lateral projection of the hand?

13. For the PA projection of the wrist, why should the hand be slightly arched by flexing the fingers?

14. Describe how and where the central ray should be directed for the PA projection of the wrist.

15. In addition to the eight carpal bones, what other bones should be seen in the image of the PA projection of the wrist?

16. How many degrees from the prone position should the wrist be rotated for the PA oblique projection of the wrist?

17. Which projection of the wrist requires the superimposition of the radial and ulnar styloid processes?

18. Which surface of the wrist should be in contact with the IR for the lateral projection of the wrist?

19. In which projection of the wrist should the metacarpals appear superimposed in the image?

20. For the PA oblique projection of the wrist, which side of the wrist should be elevated from the IR?

21. What two carpal bones on the lateral side of the wrist should be clearly demonstrated in the image of the PA oblique projection of the wrist?

22. What carpal bone is best demonstrated with the ulnar deviation position of the wrist?

23. How does the placement of the IR for the PA axial projection of the scaphoid (Stecher method) differ from IR placement for PA projections of the wrist?

24. How does the forearm appear if the hand is pronated when performing the AP projection of the forearm?

25. To prevent radial crossover, how should the hand be positioned for the AP projection of the forearm?

26. What structure on the distal end of the ulna should be seen in the image of the AP projection of the forearm?

27. How should the humeral epicondyles appear in the image of the lateral projection of the forearm?

28. How should the hand be positioned for the lateral projection of the forearm?

29. What would most likely cause the bones of the forearm to appear rotated in the image of the AP projection of the elbow?

30. Why should the patient lean laterally for the AP projection of the elbow?

31. What structures of the proximal radius are seen slightly superimposed over the proximal ulna in the AP projection of the elbow?

32. How should the hand be positioned for the lateral projection of the elbow? Explain why.

33. What projection and position of the elbow best demonstrates the coronoid process in profile?

34. How should the forearm and elbow be rotated for the best demonstration of the radial head free of superimposition from the ulna?

129

35. How many AP projections are necessary for the best demonstration of the elbow without distortion when an injury prevents full extension of the elbow?

36. Explain how the humerus and the forearm are positioned differently for each AP projection of the elbow when the elbow is in partial flexion.

37. What is the CR orientation for the axiolateral projection of the elbow (Coyle method) to demonstrate the coronoid process?

38. What humeral processes should be palpated to ensure proper alignment when the humerus is being positioned?

39. Which projection for the humerus requires the patient's hand to be supinated?

40. Describe best how to position the IR for the lateral projection of the humerus if the AP projection image clearly shows a fracture 2 inches (5 cm) superior to the elbow.

Section 2: Exercise 10: Identifying Projections of the Upper Extremity

This exercise features images of the various projections of the upper extremity. Examine each image, and identify the projection by name and the part of the upper extremity that is demonstrated.

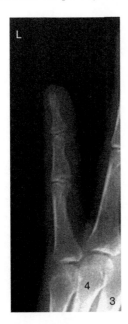

Fig. 5.37

1. Fig. 5.37: _____

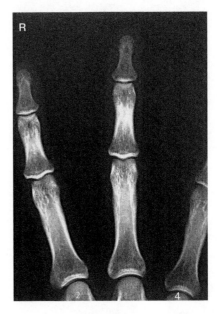

Fig. 5.39

3. Fig. 5.39: _____

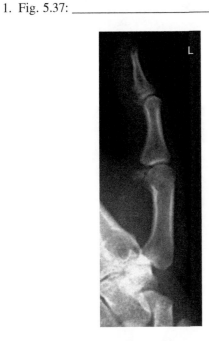

Fig. 5.38

2. Fig. 5.38: _____

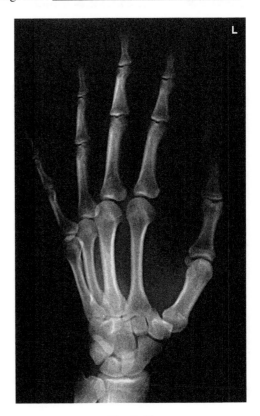

Fig. 5.40

4. Fig. 5.40: _____

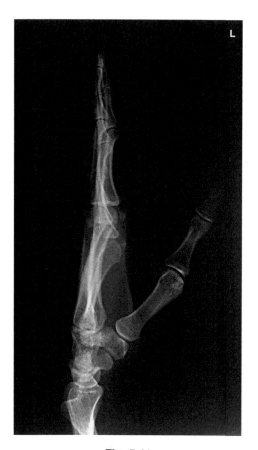

Fig. 5.41

5. Fig. 5.41: _____

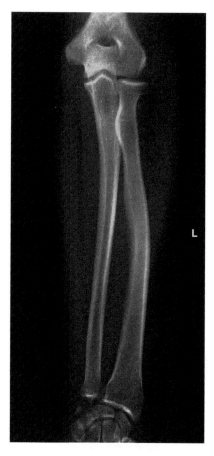

Fig. 5.43

7. Fig. 5.43: _____

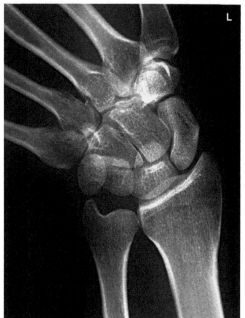

Fig. 5.42

6. Fig. 5.42: _____

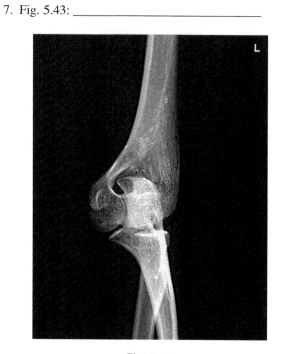

Fig. 5.44

8. Fig. 5.44: _____

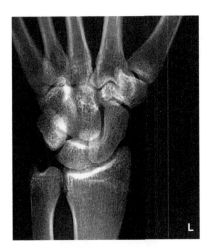

Fig. 5.45

9. Fig. 5.45: _____

    (_____ method)

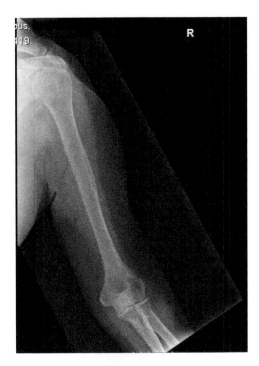

Fig. 5.46

10. Fig. 5.46: _____

Section 2: Exercise 11: Upper Extremity Image Evaluation

This exercise consists of images of the upper extremity to give you practice evaluating extremity positioning. These images are not from Merrill's Atlas. Each image shows at least one positioning error. Examine each image and answer the questions that follow by providing a short answer or choosing the correct answer from a list.

1. Fig. 5.47 shows a PA finger projection of inferior quality. Examine the image and state why it does not meet the evaluation criteria for this projection.

2. Fig. 5.48 shows an AP projection image of the thumb. Examine the image and state why it does not meet the evaluation criteria for this projection.

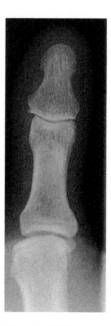

Fig. 5.48 AP thumb with improper positioning.

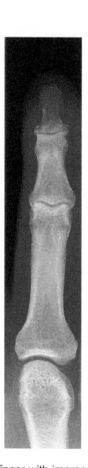

Fig. 5.47 PA finger with improper positioning.

3. Fig. 5.49 shows an AP projection image with the forearm incorrectly positioned. State the positioning error that occurred in this image.

4. Fig. 5.50 shows an attempted lateral projection image with the forearm incorrectly positioned. From the following list, select the positioning error that most likely occurred in this image.
   a. The hand was pronated.
   b. The hand was supinated.
   c. The upper arm was not parallel and in contact with the IR and table.

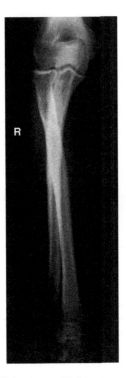

Fig. 5.49 AP forearm with improper positioning.

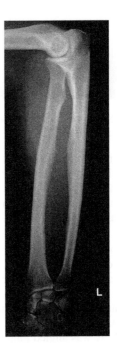

Fig. 5.50 Lateral forearm with improper positioning.

Fig. 5.51 shows a lateral projection image with the elbow incorrectly positioned. Examine the image and answer the questions that follow.

Fig. 5.52 is another lateral projection image with the elbow incorrectly positioned. Examine the image and answer the questions that follow.

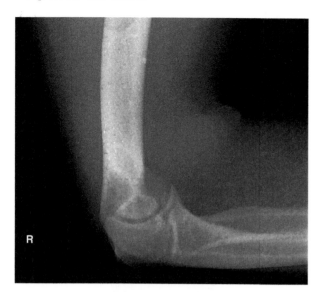

Fig. 5.51 Lateral elbow with improper positioning.

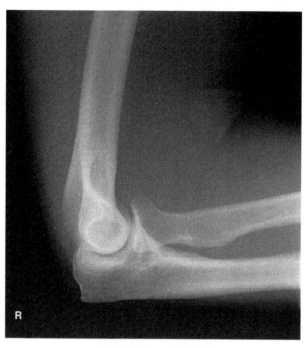

Fig. 5.52 Lateral elbow with improper positioning.

5. Which part of the image indicates that the elbow was incorrectly positioned for this view?
   a. The radial head is seen in profile.
   b. The radial tuberosity is facing anteriorly.
   c. The humeral epicondyles are not superimposed.

6. Which positioning error most likely caused the elbow to appear as it does in this image?
   a. The hand was pronated, causing radial crossover of the ulna.
   b. The upper arm was not parallel and in contact with the IR and table.
   c. The central ray was angled longitudinally with the long axis of the forearm.

7. Which part of the image indicates that the elbow was incorrectly positioned?
   a. The olecranon process is seen in profile.
   b. The radial tuberosity does not face anteriorly.
   c. The humeral epicondyles are not superimposed.

8. Which positioning error most likely caused the elbow to appear as it does in this image?
   a. The hand was supinated.
   b. The hand was medially rotated.
   c. The upper arm was not parallel and in contact with the IR and table.

Fig. 5.53 is a lateral projection of the hand in extension with positioning errors. Examine the image and answer the questions that follow.

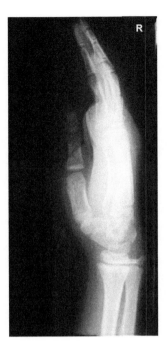

Fig. 5.53 Lateral hand in extension with improper positioning.

Fig. 5.54 is a lateral projection of the forearm with improper positioning. Examine this image and answer the following questions.

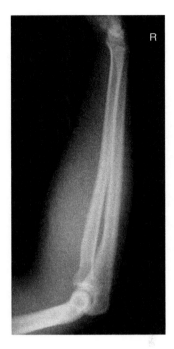

Fig. 5.54 Lateral forearm with improper positioning.

9. Which of the following are errors in Fig. 5.53?
   1. Rotation (not in a true lateral position)
   2. Tip of digit clipped
   3. Thumb not abducted

   a. 1 and 2 only
   b. 1 and 3 only
   c. 2 and 3 only
   d. 1, 2, and 3

10. Describe the positioning methods that would correct the errors in Fig. 5.53.

11. True or false. The wrist is not in a true lateral position.

12. True or false. The elbow is flexed 90 degrees.

Fig. 5.55 is an incorrectly positioned AP oblique projection of the elbow in medial rotation position. Examine this image and answer the questions that follow.

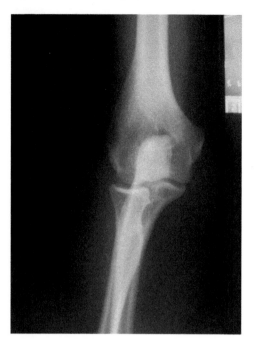

Fig. 5.55 AP oblique elbow in medial rotation with improper positioning.

Fig. 5.56 is an incorrectly positioned AP oblique projection of the elbow in lateral rotation. Examine this image and answer the question that follows.

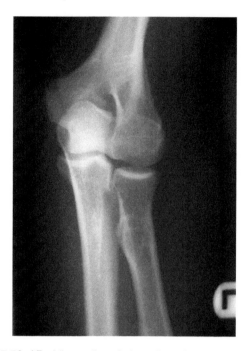

Fig. 5.56 AP oblique elbow in lateral rotation with improper positioning.

13. Explain why this image does not meet the evaluation criteria for this projection.

14. What positioning maneuver would be required to correct the positioning error seen in Fig. 5.55?

CHAPTER 5: SELF-TEST: OSTEOLOGY, ARTHROLOGY, AND POSITIONING OF THE UPPER EXTREMITY

Answer the following questions by selecting the best choice.

1. How many interphalangeal joints are found in one upper extremity?
   a. 8
   b. 9
   c. 10
   d. 14

2. Each proximal phalanx articulates with a:
   a. middle phalanx.
   b. metacarpal bone.
   c. carpal bone.
   d. distal phalanx.

3. Which bones comprise the palm of the hand?
   a. Carpals
   b. Phalanges
   c. Metatarsals
   d. Metacarpals

4. Which joint is formed by the articulation of the proximal end of the middle phalanx with the distal end of the proximal phalanx of the ring finger?
   a. The distal interphalangeal joint of the third digit
   b. The distal interphalangeal joint of the fourth digit
   c. The proximal interphalangeal joint of the third digit
   d. The proximal interphalangeal joint of the fourth digit

5. Which joint is formed by the articulation of the distal end of the middle phalanx with the proximal end of the distal phalanx of the index finger?
   a. The distal interphalangeal joint of the first digit
   b. The distal interphalangeal joint of the second digit
   c. The proximal interphalangeal joint of the first digit
   d. The proximal interphalangeal joint of the second digit

6. Which joint is a hinge-type joint?
   a. Interphalangeal
   b. Scapulohumeral
   c. Carpometacarpal
   d. Metacarpophalangeal

7. How many metacarpal bones are found in one upper extremity?
   a. 2
   b. 5
   c. 8
   d. 14

8. Which of the following articulates with the bases of metacarpal bones?
   a. Carpals
   b. Phalanges
   c. Forearm
   d. Metacarpophalangeal joints

9. Which joint of the hand is formed by the articulation of the head of a metacarpal with a digit?
   a. Carpometacarpal
   b. Metacarpophalangeal
   c. Distal interphalangeal
   d. Proximal interphalangeal

10. Which joints of the hand are formed by the articulation of the bases of the metacarpals with the bones of the wrist?
    a. Radiocarpal
    b. Interphalangeals
    c. Carpometacarpals
    d. Metacarpophalangeals

11. Which joint is an ellipsoidal joint?
    a. Interphalangeal
    b. Scapulohumeral
    c. Carpometacarpal
    d. Metacarpophalangeal

12. Which articulation of the upper extremity is a saddle joint that allows the thumb to oppose the fingers?
    a. Radiocarpal
    b. Distal radioulnar
    c. Proximal radioulnar
    d. First carpometacarpal

13. Which bones are located in the proximal row of the wrist?
    a. Scaphoid, lunate, capitate, and hamate
    b. Scaphoid, lunate, pisiform, and triquetrum
    c. Trapezium, trapezoid, capitate, and hamate
    d. Trapezium, trapezoid, pisiform, and triquetrum

14. Which bones are located in the distal row of the wrist?
    a. Hamate, capitate, lunate, and scaphoid
    b. Hamate, capitate, trapezium, and trapezoid
    c. Pisiform, triquetrum, lunate, and scaphoid
    d. Pisiform, triquetrum, trapezium, and trapezoid

15. Where in the wrist is the scaphoid located?
    a. Medial side of the distal row
    b. Medial side of the proximal row
    c. Lateral side of the distal row
    d. Lateral side of the proximal row

139

16. Where in the wrist is the trapezium located?
    a. Medial side of the distal row
    b. Medial side of the proximal row
    c. Lateral side of the distal row
    d. Lateral side of the proximal row

17. Where in the wrist is the hamate located?
    a. Medial side of the distal row
    b. Medial side of the proximal row
    c. Lateral side of the distal row
    d. Lateral side of the proximal row

18. What other name refers to the carpal bone known as the hamate?
    a. Unciform
    b. Capitatum
    c. Cuneiform
    d. Os magnum

19. What other name refers to the carpal bone known as the capitate?
    a. Pisiform
    b. Unciform
    c. Scaphoid
    d. Os magnum

20. What other name refers to the carpal bone known as the trapezium?
    a. Trapezoid
    b. Semilunar
    c. Lesser multangular
    d. Greater multangular

21. What other name refers to the carpal bone known as the trapezoid?
    a. Pisiform
    b. Unciform
    c. Lesser multangular
    d. Greater multangular

22. Which carpal bone has only one name?
    a. Hamate
    b. Capitate
    c. Pisiform
    d. Scaphoid

23. Which bones are classified as short bones?
    a. Carpals
    b. Vertebrae
    c. Phalanges
    d. Metacarpals

24. Which joint is the most distal articulation of the wrist?
    a. Intercarpal
    b. Radiocarpal
    c. Carpometacarpal
    d. Metacarpophalangeal

25. Which joint is the most proximal articulation of the wrist?
    a. Intercarpal
    b. Radiocarpal
    c. Carpometacarpal
    d. Metacarpophalangeal

26. Which two carpal bones are the most lateral bones of the wrist?
    a. Lunate and trapezoid
    b. Lunate and trapezium
    c. Scaphoid and trapezoid
    d. Scaphoid and trapezium

27. The lunate is situated between the:
    a. trapezoid and scaphoid.
    b. trapezoid and trapezium.
    c. triquetrum and scaphoid.
    d. triquetrum and trapezium.

28. What other name refers to the carpal bone known as the scaphoid?
    a. Unciform
    b. Navicular
    c. Semilunar
    d. Capitatum

29. Which carpal bone does not articulate with the radius?
    a. Lunate
    b. Capitate
    c. Scaphoid
    d. Triquetrum

30. Which bony structures are located on the proximal end of the ulna?
    a. Radial notch, styloid process, and ulnar head
    b. Radial head, olecranon process, and ulnar head
    c. Radial head, styloid process, and coronoid process
    d. Radial notch, olecranon process, and coronoid process

31. Which bony structures are located on the distal end of the ulna?
    a. Ulnar head and styloid process
    b. Ulnar head and olecranon process
    c. Coronoid process and styloid process
    d. Coronoid process and olecranon process

32. Which bony structure is located on the distal end of the radius?
    a. Head
    b. Neck
    c. Tubercle
    d. Styloid process

33. Which bony structures are located on the proximal radius?
    a. Head and tuberosity
    b. Head and styloid process
    c. Olecranon process and tubercle
    d. Olecranon process and styloid process

34. Which bones comprise the forearm?
    a. Radius and ulna
    b. Radius and carpals
    c. Humerus and ulna
    d. Humerus and carpals

35. Which structure is located on the lateral aspect of the distal forearm?
    a. Ulnar head
    b. Radial head
    c. Ulnar styloid process
    d. Radial styloid process

36. Which large bony process is easily located by touching on the posterior aspect of the proximal forearm?
    a. Styloid process
    b. Radial tuberosity
    c. Coronoid process
    d. Olecranon process

37. Which structure is located on the medial side of the distal forearm?
    a. Coronoid process
    b. Olecranon process
    c. Ulnar styloid process
    d. Radial styloid process

38. Where is the trochlear notch located?
    a. Distal ulna
    b. Distal radius
    c. Proximal ulna
    d. Proximal radius

39. Which two structures articulate to form the proximal radioulnar joint?
    a. Head of the ulna and radial notch of the ulna
    b. Head of the ulna and ulnar notch of the radius
    c. Head of the radius and radial notch of the ulna
    d. Head of the radius and ulnar notch of the radius

40. Which two structures articulate to form the distal radioulnar joint?
    a. Head of the ulna and radial notch of the ulna
    b. Head of the ulna and ulnar notch of the radius
    c. Head of the radius and radial notch of the ulna
    d. Head of the radius and ulnar notch of the radius

41. Which articulation do the trochlea and the trochlear notch form?
    a. Humeroulnar
    b. Humeroradial
    c. Distal radioulnar
    d. Proximal radioulnar

42. Which structure articulates with the capitulum?
    a. Ulnar head
    b. Radial head
    c. Glenoid fossa
    d. Humeral head

43. Which structure articulates with the trochlea?
    a. Distal ulna
    b. Distal radius
    c. Proximal ulna
    d. Proximal radius

44. In which joint is the capitulum located?
    a. Hip
    b. Wrist
    c. Elbow
    d. Shoulder

45. In which joint is the trochlea located?
    a. Hip
    b. Wrist
    c. Elbow
    d. Shoulder

46. Which type of joint is the elbow?
    a. Hinge
    b. Gliding
    c. Condyloid
    d. Ball and socket

47. Where is the capitulum located?
    a. Medial side of the distal humerus
    b. Medial side of the proximal humerus
    c. Lateral side of the distal humerus
    d. Lateral side of the proximal humerus

48. With reference from the trochlea, where is the capitulum located?
    a. Distal
    b. Lateral
    c. Medial
    d. Proximal

141

49. What is the roughened process of the humerus superior and lateral to the intertubercular groove?
    a. Lesser tubercle
    b. Greater tubercle
    c. Lateral epicondyle
    d. Medial epicondyle

50. Which bony process is located on the anterior surface of the proximal humerus?
    a. Lesser tubercle
    b. Greater tubercle
    c. Lateral epicondyle
    d. Medial epicondyle

51. Which structure articulates with the ulna to form the humeroulnar joint?
    a. Trochlea
    b. Capitulum
    c. Radial head
    d. Humeral head

52. How many articulations does the humerus have?
    a. 2
    b. 3
    c. 4
    d. 5

53. Which structure articulates with the radius to form the humeroradial joint?
    a. Trochlea
    b. Capitulum
    c. Radial notch
    d. Humeral head

54. Which depression is located on the anterior surface of the distal humerus?
    a. Radial notch
    b. Coronoid fossa
    c. Olecranon fossa
    d. Intertubercular groove

55. Which depression is located on the posterior surface of the distal humerus?
    a. Radial notch
    b. Coronoid fossa
    c. Olecranon fossa
    d. Intertubercular groove

56. Which depression is located between the lesser and greater tubercles of the proximal humerus?
    a. Radial notch
    b. Coronoid fossa
    c. Intertubercular groove
    d. Olecranon fossa

57. What is the appropriate collimated field for the PA projection of the second digit?
    a. 1 inch (2.5 cm) on all sides of the digit, including 1 inch (2.5 cm) proximal to the MCP joint
    b. 1 inch (2.5 cm) on all sides of the digit, including 1 inch (2.5 cm) distal to the MCP joint
    c. 0.5 inch (1.3 cm) on all sides of the digit, including 1 inch (2.5 cm) proximal to the MCP joint
    d. 0.5 inch (1.3 cm) on all sides of the digit, including 1 inch (2.5 cm) distal to the MCP joint

58. Which digit of the hand produces the greatest OID in the lateral projection of that digit?
    a. Third digit
    b. Second digit
    c. First digit
    d. Fifth digit

59. For lateral projections of the second through fifth digits of the hand, through which joint should the central ray be directed?
    a. Carpometacarpal
    b. Metacarpophalangeal
    c. Distal interphalangeal
    d. Proximal interphalangeal

60. From the prone position, how many degrees should a finger be rotated for the PA oblique projection of that finger?
    a. 15
    b. 30
    c. 45
    d. 90

61. Which digit of the hand produces the least OID in the lateral projection of that digit?
    a. Second digit
    b. Third digit
    c. Fourth digit
    d. OID is equal for all lateral projections of the digits.

62. How should the hand be positioned for the PA oblique projection of the hand?
    a. From the prone position, rotate the hand ulnar side up.
    b. From the prone position, rotate the hand radial side up.
    c. From the supine position, rotate the hand ulnar side up.
    d. From the supine position, rotate the hand radial side up.

63. What is the centering point for the central ray for the PA projection of the third finger?
    a. Head of the third metacarpal
    b. Base of the third metacarpal
    c. Distal interphalangeal joint of the third digit
    d. Proximal interphalangeal joint of the third digit

64. What is the centering point for the central ray on the AP projection of the first digit (thumb)?
    a. Head of the first metacarpal
    b. First MCP joint
    c. First CMC joint
    d. First IP joint

65. What is the appropriate collimated field for all projections of the first digit (thumb)?
    a. 0.5 inches (1.3 cm) on all sides of the digit, including 1 inch (2.5 cm) proximal to the MCP joint
    b. 0.5 inches (1.3 cm) on all sides of the digit, including 1 inch (2.5 cm) proximal to the CMC joint
    c. 1 inch (2.5 cm) on all sides of the digit, including 1 inch (2.5 cm) proximal to the MCP joint
    d. 1 inch (2.5 cm) on all sides of the digit, including 1 inch (2.5 cm) proximal to the CMC joint

66. From the prone position, how many degrees should a finger be rotated for the lateral projection of that finger?
    a. 15 degrees
    b. 30 degrees
    c. 45 degrees
    d. 90 degrees

67. What is the appropriate collimated field for the PA projection of the hand?
    a. 0.5 inch (1.3 cm) on all sides of the hand, including 1 inch (2.5 cm) proximal to the ulnar styloid
    b. 0.5 inches (1.3 cm) on all sides of the hand, including 1 inch (2.5 cm) distal to the ulnar styloid
    c. 1 inch (2.5 cm) on all sides of the hand, including 1 inch (2.5 cm) proximal to the ulnar styloid
    d. 1 inch (2.5 cm) on all sides of the hand, including 1 inch (2.5 cm) distal to the ulnar styloid

68. For the PA projection of the hand, where should the central ray be directed?
    a. Midcarpal area
    b. Base of the third metacarpal
    c. Third metacarpophalangeal joint
    d. Proximal interphalangeal joint of the third digit

69. From the prone position, how many degrees should a hand be rotated for the PA oblique projection of that hand?
    a. 15 degrees
    b. 25 degrees
    c. 35 degrees
    d. 45 degrees

70. Which of the following is best to demonstrate a foreign body in the hand?
    a. Lateral in extension
    b. Lateral in fan lateral position
    c. PA oblique projection
    d. AP oblique projection

71. Which wrist-positioning maneuver opens the carpal interspaces on the lateral side of the wrist?
    a. Hyperflexion
    b. Hyperextension
    c. Ulnar deviation
    d. Radial deviation

72. Which wrist projection requires that the IR be inclined toward the elbow at an angle of 20 degrees from horizontal?
    a. PA
    b. PA oblique
    c. PA with ulnar deviation
    d. PA axial (Stecher method)

73. Which projection of the wrist corrects foreshortening of the scaphoid carpal bone?
    a. PA
    b. Lateral
    c. PA with ulnar deviation
    d. PA with radial deviation

74. Which projection of the wrist requires that the radial styloid process be superimposed over the ulnar styloid process?
    a. PA
    b. Lateral
    c. PA oblique
    d. PA axial (Stecher method)

75. What is the appropriate collimated field for the PA projection of the wrist?
    a. 2.5 inches (6 cm) on all sides of the wrist joint
    b. 2.5 inches (6 cm) proximal and distal to the wrist joint and 1 inch (2.5 cm) on the sides
    c. 1 inch (2.5 cm) on all sides of the wrist joint
    d. 3 inches (7.6 cm) proximal and distal to the wrist joint and 2 inches (5 cm) on the sides

76. For the PA projection of the wrist, which positioning maneuver should be used to place the anterior surface of the wrist in contact with the IR?
    a. Ulnar-flex the hand
    b. Radial-flex the hand
    c. Slightly arch the hand
    d. Pronate the hand in full extension

77. How should the hand and wrist be positioned for the PA oblique projection of the wrist?
    a. With the hand pronated, rotate the wrist ulnar side up.
    b. With the hand pronated, rotate the wrist radial side up.
    c. With the hand supinated, rotate the wrist ulnar side up.
    d. With the hand supinated, rotate the wrist radial side up.

78. Which projection of the wrist best demonstrates the scaphoid carpal bone and its related articulations?
    a. Lateromedial projection
    b. Mediolateral projection
    c. PA projection, ulnar deviation position
    d. PA projection, radial deviation position

79. How should the hand be positioned for the AP projection of the forearm?
    a. Supinated
    b. Pronated
    c. Lateral, with medial surface on IR
    d. Lateral, with lateral surface on IR

80. What is the appropriate collimated field for all projections of the forearm?
    a. 2 inches (5 cm) on all sides of the forearm
    b. 2 inches (5 cm) distal to the wrist and proximal to the elbow and 1 inch (2.5 cm) on the sides
    c. 1 inch (2.5 cm) on all sides of the forearm
    d. 1 inch (2.5 cm) distal to the wrist and proximal to the elbow and 0.5 inch (1.3 cm) on the sides

81. Which description best explains how radial crossover occurs when the forearm is demonstrated?
    a. During the AP projection, the hand is pronated.
    b. During the AP projection, the hand is supinated.
    c. During the lateral projection, the arm is fully extended with the hand flexed.
    d. During the lateral projection, the radial and ulnar styloid processes are superimposed with each other.

82. For the AP projection of the forearm, which positioning step should be taken to prevent radial crossover?
    a. Pronate the hand.
    b. Supinate the hand.
    c. Keep the humeral epicondylar coronal plane parallel with the IR.
    d. Keep the humeral epicondylar coronal plane perpendicular with the IR.

83. Which projection of the forearm requires that the elbow be flexed 90 degrees?
    a. AP
    b. Lateral
    c. AP oblique, lateral rotation position
    d. AP oblique, medial rotation position

84. When performing an image of a forearm in a fiberglass cast, approximately which compensation to exposure technique should occur?
    a. Increase mAs 25% or 4 kVp
    b. Increase mAs 50% or 8 kVp
    c. Decrease mAs 25% or 4 kVp
    d. Decrease mAs 50% or 8 kVp

85. How much should the elbow be flexed for the lateral projection of the elbow?
    a. 25 degrees
    b. 45 degrees
    c. 80 degrees
    d. 90 degrees

86. Which projection of the elbow best demonstrates the radial head free of bony superimposition?
    a. AP
    b. Lateral
    c. AP oblique, lateral rotation position
    d. AP oblique, medial rotation position

87. Which of the following should be used to image the radial head on a trauma patient?
    a. Lateral projection without flexion of elbow joint
    b. Axiolateral projection (Coyle method) of elbow joint
    c. AP elbow, partial flexion position
    d. AP oblique projection of the forearm

88. What is the direction and amount of central ray angulation for the axiolateral projection (Coyle method) to demonstrate the radial head and capitulum?
    a. 0 degrees; perpendicular to IR
    b. 10 degrees toward the shoulder
    c. 25 degrees toward the shoulder
    d. 45 degrees toward the shoulder

89. Which projection and position of the upper extremity best demonstrates the coronoid process in profile and free of superimposition?
    a. AP oblique of the wrist in lateral rotation position
    b. PA oblique of the wrist with lateral side elevated 45 degrees from IR
    c. AP oblique of the elbow in lateral rotation position
    d. AP oblique of the elbow in medial rotation position

90. What is the appropriate collimated field for the AP projection of the elbow?
    a. 2 inches (5 cm) on all sides of the elbow joint
    b. 2 inches (5 cm) proximal and distal to the elbow joint and 1 inch (2.5 cm) on the sides
    c. 1 inch (2.5 cm) on all sides of the elbow joint
    d. 3 inches (7.6 cm) proximal and distal to the elbow joint and 1 inch (2.5 cm) on the sides

91. With reference to the plane of the IR, how should the humeral epicondylar coronal plane be positioned for the AP projection of the elbow?
    a. Parallel
    b. Perpendicular
    c. 45 degrees lateral rotation
    d. 45 degrees medial rotation

92. Which projection of the elbow best demonstrates the olecranon process in profile?
    a. AP projection
    b. Lateral projection
    c. AP oblique projection, lateral rotation position
    d. AP oblique projection, medial rotation position

93. For the axiolateral projection (Coyle method) of the elbow to demonstrate the coronoid process, the elbow is:
    a. flexed 80 degrees.
    b. flexed 90 degrees.
    c. in hyperflexion.
    d. in hyperextension.

94. What is the central ray orientation for the axiolateral projection of the elbow (Coyle method) to demonstrate the coronoid process when the patient is seated?
    a. Angled 45 degrees toward the shoulder
    b. Angled 45 degrees away from the shoulder
    c. Angled 45 degrees cephalic
    d. Angled 45 degrees caudal

95. Which positioning characteristic best indicates that the humerus is properly positioned for the AP projection of the humerus?
    a. The hand is pronated on the table.
    b. The hand is true lateral on the table.
    c. The humeral epicondylar coronal plane is parallel with the IR.
    d. The humeral epicondylar coronal plane is perpendicular to the IR.

96. Which evaluation criterion indicates that the humerus was properly positioned for the AP projection?
    a. The epicondyles are superimposed.
    b. The lesser tubercle is seen in profile.
    c. The greater tubercle is superimposed over the humeral head.
    d. The humeral head and greater tubercle are both seen in profile.

97. One way that the lateral image of a humerus, produced with the patient in the lateral decubitus position and the IR placed between the arm and thorax, appears different from the lateral position with the patient standing is that the former demonstrates:
    a. the humeral head in profile.
    b. less than the entire humerus.
    c. the lesser tubercle in profile.
    d. the greater tubercle in profile.

98. With reference to the plane of the IR, how is it determined that the humerus is properly positioned in true lateral position?
    a. The hand is pronated.
    b. The hand is placed true lateral.
    c. The humeral epicondylar coronal plane is parallel.
    d. The humeral epicondylar coronal plane is perpendicular.

99. Which evaluation criterion indicates that the humerus was properly positioned for the lateral projection?
    a. The lesser tubercle is seen in profile.
    b. Beam divergence opens the elbow joint.
    c. The humeral head and greater tubercle are both seen in profile.
    d. Maximum visualization of the epicondyles without rotation is seen.

100. What is the appropriate collimated field for the AP and lateral projection of the humerus?
    a. 2 inches (5 cm) distal to the elbow and superior to the shoulder and 1 inch (2.5 cm) on the sides
    b. 2 inches (5 cm) proximal to the elbow and superior to the shoulder and 1 inch (2.5 cm) on the sides
    c. 2 inches (5 cm) on all sides of the humerus
    d. 3 inches (7.6 cm) on all sides of the humerus

145

6 Shoulder Girdle

OSTEOLOGY AND ARTHROLOGY OF THE SHOULDER GIRDLE

Section 1: Exercise 1

This exercise pertains to the clavicle. Identify structures, fill in missing words, choose the correct answer, or provide a short answer for each question.

1. Identify each lettered structure shown in Fig. 6.1.

   A. _____

   B. _____

   C. _____

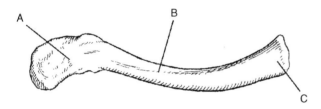

Fig. 6.1 Anterior aspect of the clavicle.

2. What classification of bone is the clavicle?

3. The medial end is also known as the _____ extremity.

4. The lateral end is also known as the _____ extremity.

5. Which end (medial or lateral) articulates with part of the scapula?

6. Which end (medial or lateral) articulates with the manubrium?

7. At what level is the clavicle (with reference to the ribs)?

8. Which classification of joint are sternoclavicular (SC) joints and acromioclavicular (AC) joints?
   a. Synovial
   b. Fibrous
   c. Cartilaginous
   d. Synchondroses

9. Which type of joint are SC joints and AC joints?
   a. Hinge
   b. Gliding
   c. Ball and socket
   d. Pivot

10. Which gender of adults (males or females) has more sharply curved clavicles?

146

Section 1: Exercise 2

Identify each lettered structure shown in Fig. 6.2.

A. _____ (cavity)

B. _____

C. _____ (process)

D. _____ (notch)

E. _____ (border)

F. _____ (angle)

G. _____ (border)

H. _____ (angle)

I. _____ (border)

J. _____ (fossa)

Section 1: Exercise 3

Identify each lettered structure shown in Fig. 6.3.

A. _____ (angle)

B. _____

C. _____ (border)

D. _____ (angle)

E. _____ (fossa)

F. _____ (fossa)

G. _____ (border)

H. _____ (notch)

I. _____ (process)

J. _____

K. _____

L. _____ (cavity)

M. _____ (border)

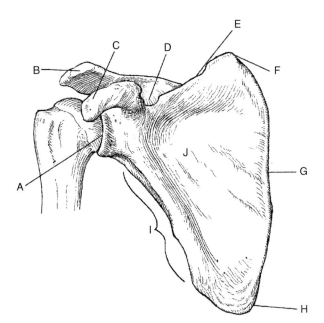

Fig. 6.2 Anterior aspect of the scapula.

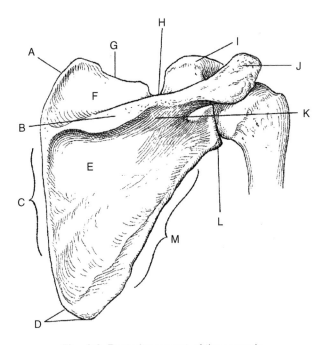

Fig. 6.3 Posterior aspect of the scapula.

Section 1: Exercise 4

Identify each lettered structure shown in Fig. 6.4.

A. _____

B. _____

C. _____ (surface)

D. _____ (border)

E. _____ (angle)

F. _____ (angle)

G. _____ (process)

H. _____ (cavity)

I. _____ (surface)

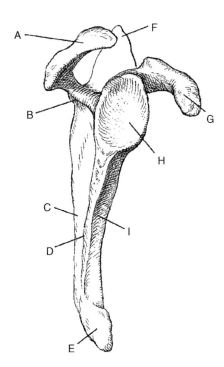

Fig. 6.4 Lateral aspect of the scapula.

Section 1: Exercise 5

Match the structures located on the scapula listed in Column A with the descriptions in Column B. Not all descriptions may apply to the listed structures.

Column A

_____ 1. Spine

_____ 2. Acromion

_____ 3. Medial border

_____ 4. Glenoid cavity

_____ 5. Scapular notch

_____ 6. Costal surface

_____ 7. Inferior angle

_____ 8. Superior angle

_____ 9. Lateral border

_____ 10. Superior border

_____ 11. Coracoid process

_____ 12. Subscapular fossa

_____ 13. Supraspinous fossa

_____ 14. Infraspinous fossa

Column B

a. Anterior aspect of scapula

b. Also known as the sternal surface

c. Deep depression on superior border

d. Large protrusion on dorsal surface

e. Lateral extension of scapular spine

f. Large fossa at lateral angle

g. Extends from superior angle to coracoid process

h. The junction of the medial and superior borders

i. Large depression on the costal surface

j. The junction of the medial and lateral borders

k. Area above the scapular spine on dorsal surface

l. Large, broad area below the spine on dorsal surface

m. Extends from the glenoid cavity to the inferior angle

n. Extends from the superior angle to the inferior angle

o. Slender, finger-like projection extending anteriorly and laterally from near the lateral angle

Section 1: Exercise 6

Identify each lettered structure shown in Fig. 6.5.

A. _____

B. _____

C. _____

D. _____

E. _____

F. _____

G. _____

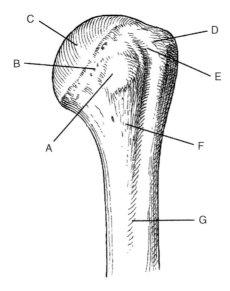

Fig. 6.5 Anterior aspect of proximal humerus.

Section 1: Exercise 7

Match the structures located on the proximal portion of the humerus listed in Column A with the descriptions in Column B. Not all descriptions may apply to the listed structures.

Column A

_____ 1. Head

_____ 2. Surgical neck

_____ 3. Anatomic neck

_____ 4. Lesser tubercle

_____ 5. Greater tubercle

_____ 6. Intertubercular (bicipital) groove

Column B

a. Depression that receives the olecranon process

b. Deep depression that separates the two tubercles

c. Narrow constriction superior to the tubercles

d. Constriction of the shaft inferior to the tubercles

e. Bony process on the lateral surface of the bone

f. Rounded bony process that articulates with the radial head

g. Large, rounded eminence that articulates with the glenoid cavity

h. Bony process on the anterior surface of the shaft, inferior from the anatomic neck

Section 1: Exercise 8

Use the following clues to complete the crossword puzzle. All answers refer to the bones and joints of the shoulder girdle.

Across

1. Most distal angle
3. Scapular spinal process
5. Posterior shoulder girdle bone
6. Articulates with scapula
9. Ball and socket joint
11. Scapula border
13. Scapular spine ridge
14. On superior border
16. Bone classification for humerus
17. Anterior scapular process
18. Anterior scapular fossa
19. Bone classification for scapula

Down

1. Posterior-inferior scapular fossa
2. Anterior part of shoulder girdle
4. Anterior scapular surface
7. Cavity for humeral head
8. Top scapular border
9. Posterior-superior scapular fossa
10. Scapular border
12. Lateral end of clavicle
15. Medial end of clavicle

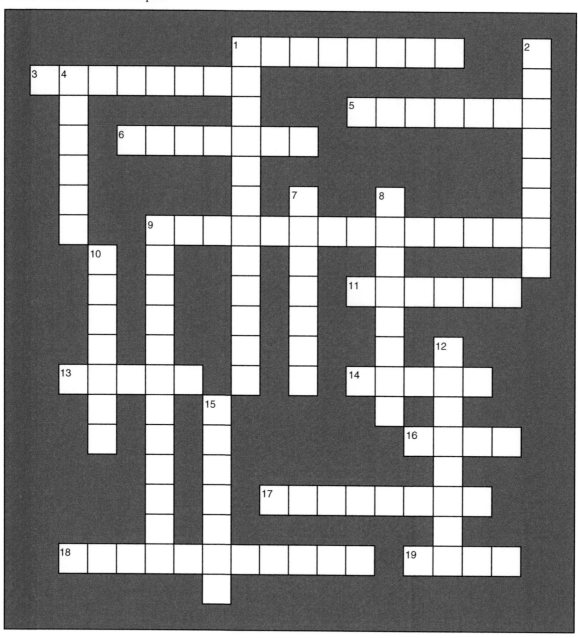

Section 1: Exercise 9

Match the pathology terms in Column A with the appropriate definition in Column B. Not all choices from Column B should be selected.

Column A

_____ 1. Tumor

_____ 2. Bursitis

_____ 3. Fracture

_____ 4. Metastases

_____ 5. Dislocation

_____ 6. Osteoporosis

_____ 7. Osteoarthritis

_____ 8. Osteopetrosis

_____ 9. Chondrosarcoma

_____ 10. Rheumatoid arthritis

Column B

a. Loss of bone density

b. Inflammation of the bursa

c. Disruption in the continuity of bone

d. Benign tumor consisting of cartilage

e. Increased density of atypically soft bone

f. Displacement of a bone from the joint space

g. Malignant tumor arising from cartilage cells

h. Inflammation of bone caused by a pyogenic infection

i. Malignant tumor of bone arising in medullary tissue

j. Chronic, systemic, inflammatory collagen disease

k. Transfer of a cancerous lesion from one area to another

l. New tissue growth where cell proliferation is uncontrolled

m. Form of arthritis marked by progressive cartilage deterioration in synovial joints and vertebrae

Section 1: Exercise 10

This exercise is a comprehensive review of the osteology and arthrology of the shoulder girdle. Fill in missing words or provide a short answer for each question.

1. What bone classification is the scapula?

2. How many surfaces, borders, and angles does a scapula have?

   a. Surfaces: _____

   b. Borders: _____

   c. Angles: _____

3. Which surface (anterior or posterior) of the scapula is the costal surface?

4. Name the two fossae located on the posterior surface of the scapula.

5. What structure separates the two fossae on the posterior surface of the scapula?

6. What is the name of the lateral end of the scapular spine?

7. Where on the scapula is the scapular notch located?

8. What is the most anterior bony projection of the scapula?

9. List the names of the scapular borders.

10. List the names of the scapular angles.

11. What bone forms the anterior part of the shoulder girdle?

12. What muscle covers and attaches to the costal (anterior) surface of the scapula?

13. The portion of the humerus located between the tubercles and the head is called the _____ neck.

14. Small, synovial fluid–filled sacs that relieve pressure and reduce friction in tissue are called _____.

15. How many articulations does the shoulder girdle have?

16. List the names of each shoulder girdle articulation.

17. Identify the joint type for each articulation of the shoulder girdle.

18. What bone articulates with the glenoid cavity?

19. What bone articulates with the medial end of the clavicle?

20. What abbreviation is used to denote the articulation noted in question 19?

21. What structure of the scapula articulates with the lateral end of the clavicle?

22. What abbreviation is used to denote the articulation at the lateral end of the clavicle?

POSITIONING OF THE SHOULDER GIRDLE

Section 2: Exercise 1: Positioning for the Shoulder

This exercise pertains to the essential projections of the shoulder. Identify structures, fill in missing words, provide a short answer, select answers from a list, or choose true or false (explaining any statement you believe to be false) for each question.

1. List the essential projections and positions for the shoulder joint, and describe the positioning steps used for each, as follows:

   Essential projection: _____
   - Size of collimated field:

   - Key patient/part positioning points:

   - Anatomic landmarks and relation to IR:

   - CR orientation and entrance point:

   Essential projection: _____
   - Size of collimated field:

   - Key patient/part positioning points:

   - Anatomic landmarks and relation to IR:

   - CR orientation and entrance point:

   Essential projection: _____
   - Size of collimated field:

   - Key patient/part positioning points:

   - Anatomic landmarks and relation to IR:

   - CR orientation and entrance point:

   Essential projection: _____
   (_____ method)
   - Size of collimated field:

   - Key patient/part positioning points:

   - Anatomic landmarks and relation to IR:

   - CR orientation and entrance point:

   Essential projection: _____
   (_____ method)
   - Size of collimated field:

   - Key patient/part positioning points:

   - Anatomic landmarks and relation to IR:

   - CR orientation and entrance point:

Essential projection: _____

(_____ method)

■ Size of collimated field:

■ Key patient/part positioning points:

■ Anatomic landmarks and relation to IR:

■ CR orientation and entrance point:

Essential projection: _____

(_____)

■ Size of collimated field:

■ Key patient/part positioning points:

■ Anatomic landmarks and relation to IR:

■ CR orientation and entrance point:

Questions 2 to 5 pertain to the AP *projection*.

2. What positioning maneuver should be avoided if the patient possibly has a fractured humerus or dislocation of the scapulohumeral joint?

3. For AP projections, the patient's respiration should be

_____ .

4. Figs. 6.6 to 6.8 are AP projections of the shoulder. Examine the images and answer the questions that follow.

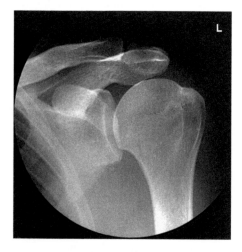

Fig. 6.6 AP shoulder.

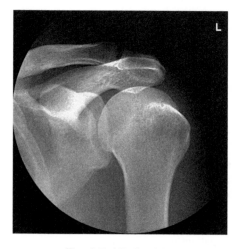

Fig. 6.7 AP shoulder.

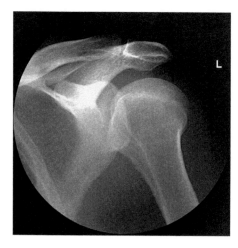

Fig. 6.8 AP shoulder.

a. What positioning maneuver causes the appearance of these three images to be different?

b. Which image shows the humerus in external rotation?

c. Which image shows the humerus in internal rotation?

d. Which image shows the humerus in neutral rotation?

e. Which image was obtained by positioning the humeral epicondyles parallel to the IR?

f. Which image was obtained by positioning the humeral epicondyles at an angle of approximately 45 degrees with the IR?

g. Which image was obtained by positioning the humeral epicondyles perpendicular to the IR?

h. Which image shows the greater tubercle in profile on the lateral aspect of the humerus?

i. Which image shows the lesser tubercle in profile and pointing medially?

j. Which image shows the outline of the lesser tubercle between the humeral head and the greater tubercle?

5. Identify each lettered structure shown in Fig. 6.9.

A. _____

B. _____

C. _____

D. _____

E. _____

F. _____

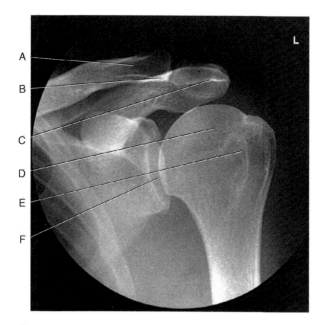

Fig. 6.9 AP shoulder with external rotation of the humerus.

Questions 6 to 10 pertain to the *AP oblique projection (Grashey method)* for the glenoid cavity.

6. What patient position would be required if the patient's right shoulder is to be examined?
   a. 35 to 45 degree RPO
   b. 35 to 45 degree LPO
   c. 45 to 60 degree RAO
   d. 45 to 60 degree LAO

7. The _____ should be parallel with the plane of the IR.

8. What is the proper arm position for the Grashey method?
   a. Abducted in slight internal rotation
   b. Abducted in slight external rotation
   c. Adducted in extreme internal rotation
   d. Adducted in extreme external rotation

9. A properly positioned AP oblique (Grashey method) image will demonstrate the _____ in profile.

10. Identify each lettered structure shown in Fig. 6.10.

A. _____

B. _____

C. _____

D. _____

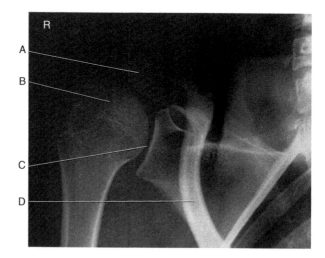

Fig. 6.10 AP oblique glenoid cavity (Grashey method).

Items 11 to 14 pertain to the transthoracic lateral projection (Lawrence method).

11. The transthoracic lateral projection may be performed with the patient positioned upright or:
    a. prone.
    b. supine.
    c. lateral recumbent.

12. To what specific area of the humerus should the IR be centered for the transthoracic lateral projection (Lawrence method)?
    a. Epicondyles
    b. Surgical neck
    c. Distal third of the diaphysis

13. How many degrees and in which direction should the central ray be directed if it cannot be directed perpendicular to the IR because the patient is unable to elevate the unaffected shoulder?
    a. 10 to 15 degrees caudad
    b. 10 to 15 degrees cephalad
    c. 20 to 25 degrees caudad
    d. 20 to 25 degrees cephalad

14. Which change to radiographic exposure factors should be used to aid effectively the blurring of lung detail by the action of the heart when the patient is able to hold his or her breath for a sustained period?
    a. Use a low mA/long exposure time combination with the usual mAs factor.
    b. Use a high mA/short exposure time combination with the usual mAs factor.

15. Identify each lettered structure shown in Fig. 6.11.

    A. _____

    B. _____

    C. _____

    D. _____

    E. _____

    F. _____

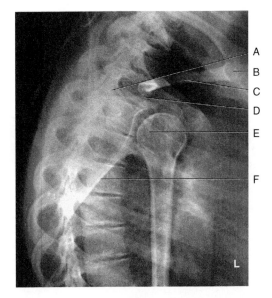

Fig. 6.11 Transthoracic lateral shoulder (Lawrence method).

Questions 16 to 23 pertain to the inferosuperior axial projection (Lawrence method).

16. Identify each lettered structure shown in Fig. 6.12.

A. _____

B. _____

C. _____

D. _____

E. _____

F. _____

G. _____

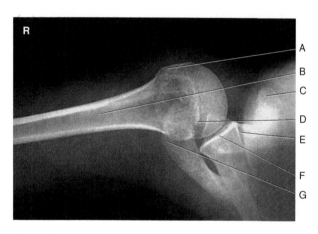

Fig. 6.12 Inferosuperior axial projection (Lawrence method).

17. True or false. When the patient is recumbent, the head and upper torso should be elevated 3 inches (7.6 cm).

18. True or false. When using a horizontally directed central ray, the patient should be placed in the supine body position.

19. With reference to the long axis of the body, how should the affected arm be positioned?

20. Into which rotational position should the humerus be placed?
    a. Neutral
    b. Internal
    c. External

21. Which area of the body should the central ray enter?
    a. Axilla of the affected arm
    b. Top of the affected shoulder
    c. Anterior point of the coracoid process

22. What positioning factor determines how many degrees the central ray should be directed medially?

23. Examine Fig. 6.12, an image of the inferosuperior axial projection (Lawrence method). From the following list, circle four radiographic evaluation criteria indicating that the patient was properly positioned for the inferosuperior axial projection (Lawrence method).
   a. The scapula should be seen in lateral profile.
   b. The coracoid process should be seen pointing anteriorly.
   c. The lesser tubercle should be seen in profile and pointing anteriorly.
   d. The scapulohumeral joint should be seen slightly overlapping.
   e. The scapula, clavicle, and humerus should be seen through the lung field.
   f. The greater tubercle should be seen in profile on the lateral aspect of the humerus.
   g. The AC joint, acromion, and acromial end of the clavicle should be seen through the humeral head.

Questions 24 to 28 pertain to the PA *oblique projection (scapular Y)*.

24. True or false. In an image of a normal shoulder, the humeral head should be directly superimposed over the junction of the scapular Y.

25. What breathing instructions should be given to the patient?

26. What position would be used to examine a patient's injured left shoulder?
   a. 35 to 45 degree RPO
   b. 35 to 45 degree LPO
   c. 45 to 60 degree RAO
   d. 45 to 60 degree LAO

27. With reference from the thorax, where should the scapular body be demonstrated in the image of the PA oblique projection?
   a. Superimposed with the clavicle
   b. Superimposed with ribs and lung
   c. Along the lateral aspect but not superimposed

28. Identify each lettered structure shown in Fig. 6.13.

   A. _____

   B. _____

   C. _____

   D. _____

   E. _____

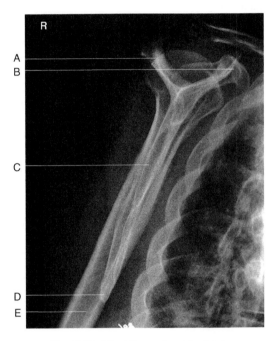

Fig. 6.13 PA oblique shoulder joint.

Questions 29 to 33 pertain to the tangential projection for the intertubercular (bicipital) groove.

29. List the essential projection for the intertubercular (bicipital) groove, and describe the positioning steps used for each, as follows:

   Essential projection: _____

   (_____ modification)
   ■ Size of collimated field:

   ■ Key patient/part positioning points:

■ Anatomic landmarks and relation to IR:

■ CR orientation and entrance point:

30. For the Fisk modification, the IR is supported on the patient's _____.

31. For the Fisk modification, a standing patient should lean forward or backward to place the vertical humerus at an angle of _____ to _____ degrees.

32. For the Fisk modification, how should the central ray be directed?
    a. Angled 10 to 15 degrees anteriorly
    b. Angled 10 to 15 degrees posteriorly
    c. Perpendicular to the IR

33. Identify each lettered structure shown in Fig. 6.14.
    A. _____
    B. _____
    C. _____
    D. _____

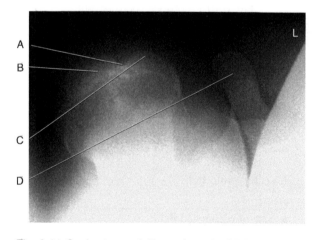

Fig. 6.14 Supine tangential intertubercular (bicipital) groove.

Section 2: Exercise 2: Positioning for the Acromioclavicular Articulations

This exercise pertains to the essential projections for the AC joints. Provide a short answer or choose true or false (explaining any statement you believe to be false) for each question.

1. List the essential projections for the AC joints, and describe the positioning steps used for each, as follows:

   Essential projection: _____

   (_____ method)
   ■ Size of collimated field:

   ■ Key patient/part positioning points:

   ■ Anatomic landmarks and relation to IR:

   ■ CR orientation and entrance point:

2. True or false. The patient may be positioned either upright or supine to demonstrate AC joints.

3. True or false. The central ray should be directed perpendicularly to the affected AC joint for each image.

4. What procedure should be performed to demonstrate both AC joints on a patient who has wide shoulders?

5. What is the purpose of the weight-bearing projections for the AC joints?

6. What is the proper method to attach the weights? Why?

7. The recommended SID for radiography of the AC joints is _____.

Section 2: Exercise 3: Positioning for the Clavicle

This exercise reviews the essential projections of the clavicle. Identify structures, provide a short answer, choose the correct answer, or choose true or false (explaining any statement you believe to be false) for each question.

1. List the essential projections and positions for the shoulder joint, and describe the positioning steps used for each, as follows:

Essential projection: _____
- Size of collimated field:

- Key patient/part positioning points:

- Anatomic landmarks and relation to IR:

- CR orientation and entrance point:

Essential projection: _____
- Size of collimated field:

- Key patient/part positioning points:

- Anatomic landmarks and relation to IR:

- CR orientation and entrance point:

Essential projection: _____
- Size of collimated field:

- Key patient/part positioning points:

- Anatomic landmarks and relation to IR:

- CR orientation and entrance point:

Essential projection: _____
- Size of collimated field:

- Key patient/part positioning points:

■ Anatomic landmarks and relation to IR:

■ CR orientation and entrance point:

Items 2 to 6 pertain to the *AP and PA projections*.

2. What breathing instructions should be given to the patient?

3. The AP and PA projections produce similar images. Identify which projection (AP or PA) produces the best spatial resolution and explain why.

4. True or false. The entire clavicle should be demonstrated with either AP or PA projection.

5. True or false. The AP and PA projections should demonstrate the entire clavicle free from superimposition with other bony structures.

6. Identify each lettered structure shown in Fig. 6.15.

A. _____

B. _____

C. _____

D. _____

E. _____

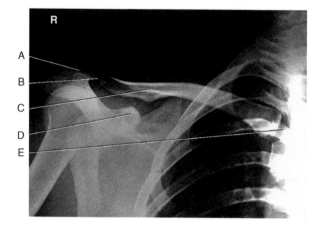

Fig. 6.15 AP clavicle.

Items 7 to 12 pertain to the AP axial and PA axial projections.

7. At how many degrees and in which direction should the central ray be directed for the following projections?

a. AP axial, with the patient supine: _____

_____

b. PA axial, with the patient prone: _____

8. How does the appearance of the clavicle differ in the axial projections compared with the AP/PA projections?

9. What positioning consideration determines how much the x-ray tube should be angled for AP axial and PA axial projections?

10. How many degrees and in which direction should the central ray be directed for the AP axial projection with the patient upright in the lordotic position?

11. What criterion is used to determine if the CR angle was sufficient for the axial projections of the clavicle?

12. True or false. For the AP axial projection, the exposure should occur after the patient has been instructed to suspend respiration following full expiration.

Section 2: Exercise 4: Positioning for the Scapula

This exercise pertains to the essential projections of the scapula. Identify structures, fill in missing words, provide a short answer, choose the correct answer from a list, or choose true or false (explaining any statement you believe to be false) for each question.

1. List the essential projections and positions for the shoulder joint, and describe the positioning steps used for each, as follows:

   Essential projection: _____
   ■ Size of collimated field:

   ■ Key patient/part positioning points:

   ■ Anatomic landmarks and relation to IR:

   ■ CR orientation and entrance point:

Essential projection:_____
■ Size of collimated field:

■ Key patient/part positioning points:

■ Anatomic landmarks and relation to IR:

■ CR orientation and entrance point:

2. What is the purpose of abducting the upper extremity for the AP projection?

3. Which type of respiration should the patient use to obliterate lung detail?
   a. Slow breathing
   b. Suspended full expiration
   c. Suspended full inspiration

4. Which scapular border should be demonstrated free from superimposition with the ribs for the AP projection?
   a. Lateral
   b. Medial
   c. Superior

5. True or false. AP projection images should demonstrate the area of the scapula, including the glenoid cavity and coracoid process, without superimposition with the ribs.

6. True or false. AP projection images should demonstrate the acromion and the inferior angle.

163

7. True or false. For the AP projection, the patient should be rotated toward the affected side for best placement of the scapula parallel with the IR.

8. Identify each lettered structure shown in Fig. 6.16.

A. _____

B. _____

C. _____

D. _____

E. _____

F. _____

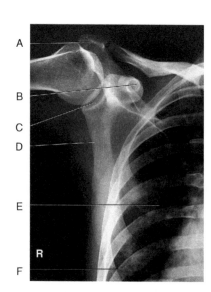

Fig. 6.16 AP scapula.

9. For the lateral projection, what is the significance of arm placement?

10. For the lateral projection, how should the affected arm be placed for best demonstration of the acromion and coracoid processes?

11. True or false. The lateral projection image should demonstrate the lateral and medial borders superimposed.

12. True or false. The lateral projection image should demonstrate the scapular body free from superimposition with the ribs.

13. True or false. The acromion and the inferior angle should be demonstrated in the lateral projection.

14. Identify each lettered structure shown in Fig. 6.17.

A. _____

B. _____

C. _____

D. _____

E. _____

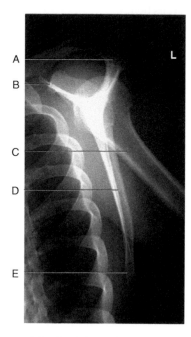

Fig. 6.17 Lateral scapula.

Section 2: Exercise 5: Identifying Projections of the Shoulder Girdle

This exercise provides images from examinations of anatomic structures of the shoulder girdle. Examine each image and identify the projection by name as well as the position and method name, if applicable, and the part of the shoulder girdle that is demonstrated.

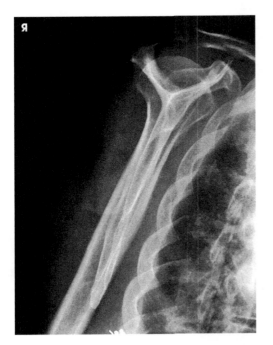

Fig. 6.18

1. Fig. 6.18: _____

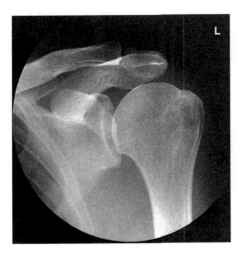

Fig. 6.19

2. Fig. 6.19: _____

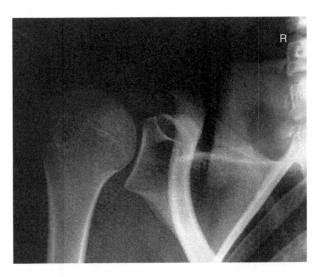

Fig. 6.20

3. Fig. 6.20: _____

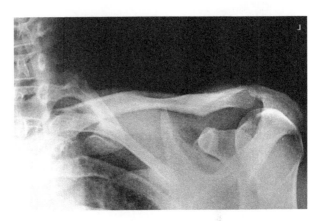

Fig. 6.21

4. Fig. 6.21: (Hint: This projection provides better spatial resolution.) _____

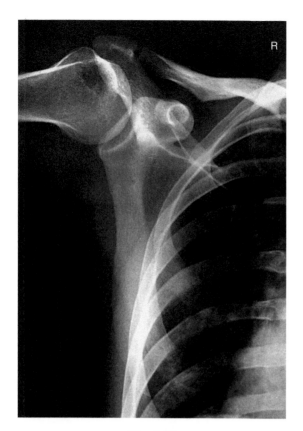

Fig. 6.22

5. Fig. 6.22: _____

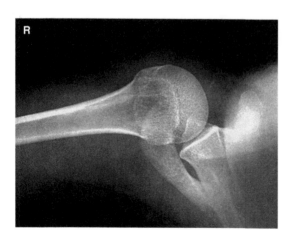

Fig. 6.23

6. Fig. 6.23: _____

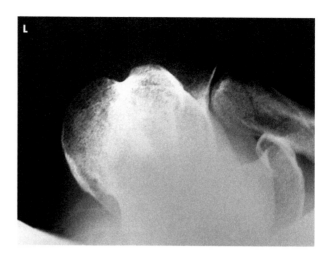

Fig. 6.24

7. Fig. 6.24: _____

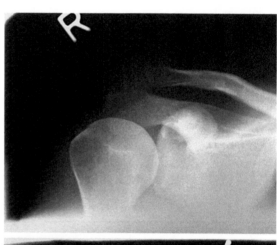

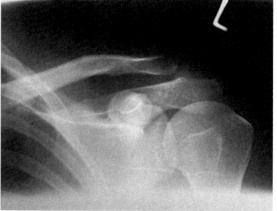

Fig. 6.25

8. Fig. 6.25: _____

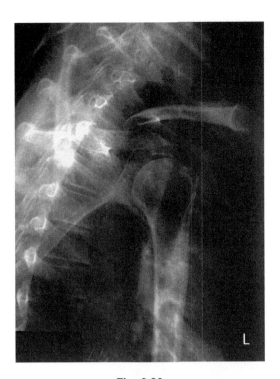

Fig. 6.26

9. Fig. 6.26: _____

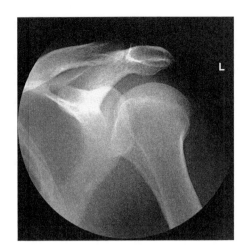

Fig. 6.28

11. Fig. 6.28: _____

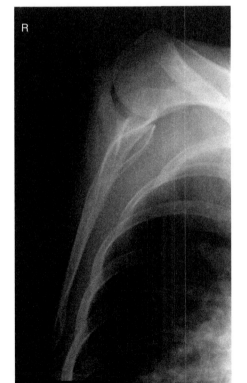

Fig. 6.27

10. Fig. 6.27: _____

167

Section 2: Exercise 6: Shoulder Girdle Image Evaluation

This exercise consists of images of the upper extremity to give you practice evaluating extremity positioning. These images are not from Merrill's Atlas. Each image shows at least one positioning error. Examine each image and answer the questions that follow by providing a short answer or choosing the correct answer from a list.

1. Fig. 6.29 demonstrates an AP projection of the scapula. Explain why this image does not meet the evaluation criteria for this projection.

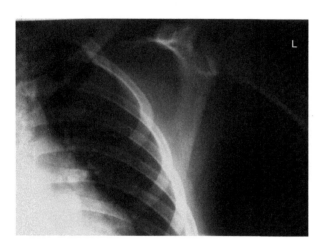

Fig. 6.29

2. Fig. 6.30 is a lateral projection of the scapula to demonstrate the body. Examine the image and state why it does not meet the evaluation criteria for this projection.

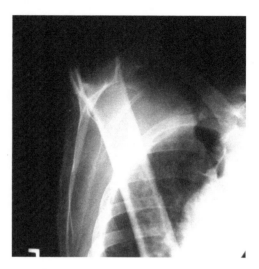

Fig. 6.30 Lateral scapula with error.

3. If a repeat image were attempted for Fig. 6.30, list the corrective measures needed to ensure a quality image.

4. Fig. 6.31 is an AP oblique projection of the shoulder (Grashey method) with a positioning error. What anatomy is not properly demonstrated in this image?

6. Fig. 6.32 is an AP axial projection of the clavicle with an error. What could be done to improve this image?

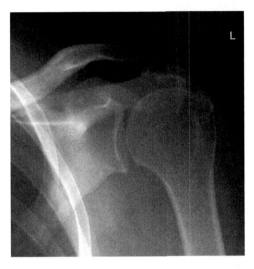

Fig. 6.31 AP oblique projection of the shoulder (Grashey method) with error.

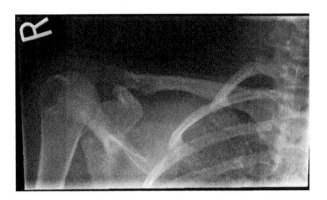

Fig. 6.32 AP axial clavicle with error.

5. What positioning error is the cause of the anatomy not being properly demonstrated in Fig. 6.31?

Answer the following questions by selecting the best choice.

1. Which classification of bone is the scapula?
   a. Flat
   b. Long
   c. Short
   d. Irregular

2. Which classification of bone is the clavicle?
   a. Flat
   b. Long
   c. Short
   d. Irregular

3. What is the name of the fossa on the anterior surface of the scapula?
   a. Subscapular
   b. Infraspinous
   c. Supraspinous
   d. Scapular notch

4. Which border of the scapula extends from the glenoid cavity to the inferior angle?
   a. Medial
   b. Lateral
   c. Superior
   d. Vertebral

5. Which border of the scapula extends from the superior angle to the inferior angle?
   a. Lateral
   b. Medial
   c. Costal
   d. Superior

6. Of which part of the scapula is the acromion an extension?
   a. Body
   b. Spine
   c. Glenoid cavity
   d. Coracoid process

7. Where is the coracoid process located in reference to the body of the scapula?
   a. Medial and superior
   b. Medial and inferior
   c. Lateral and superior
   d. Lateral and inferior

8. Which borders of the scapula unite to form the superior angle?
   1. Medial
   2. Lateral
   3. Superior

   a. 1 and 2 only
   b. 1 and 3 only
   c. 2 and 3 only
   d. 1, 2, and 3

9. Which borders of the scapula unite to form the inferior angle?
   1. Medial
   2. Lateral
   3. Superior

   a. 1 and 2 only
   b. 1 and 3 only
   c. 2 and 3 only
   d. 1, 2, and 3

10. Where is the scapular notch located?
    a. Lateral border
    b. Superior border
    c. Medial border
    d. Dorsal surface

11. Which joint is a ball and socket joint?
    a. Acromioclavicular
    b. Humeroulnar
    c. Scapulohumeral
    d. Sternoclavicular

12. Which portion of the scapula articulates with the humeral head?
    a. Acromion
    b. Coracoid process
    c. Coronoid process
    d. Glenoid fossa

13. Which portion of the scapula articulates with the clavicle?
    a. Acromion
    b. Coracoid process
    c. Coronoid process
    d. Glenoid fossa

14. When performing AP projections of the shoulder, where should the central ray be directed?
    a. 1 inch (2.5 cm) medial to the coracoid process
    b. 1 inch (2.5 cm) inferior to the coracoid process
    c. 2 inches (5 cm) medial to the coracoid process
    d. 2 inches (5 cm) inferior to the coracoid process

15. With reference to the plane of the IR, how should the humeral epicondyles be positioned for the AP projection of the shoulder with the shoulder in external rotation?
    a. Parallel
    b. Perpendicular
    c. 45 degrees lateral oblique
    d. 45 degrees medial oblique

16. With reference to the plane of the IR, how should the humeral epicondyles be positioned for the AP projection of the shoulder with the shoulder in internal rotation?
    a. Parallel
    b. Perpendicular
    c. 45 degrees lateral oblique
    d. 45 degrees medial oblique

17. With reference to the plane of the IR, how should the humeral epicondyles be positioned for the AP projection of the shoulder with the shoulder in neutral rotation?
    a. Parallel
    b. Perpendicular
    c. 45 degrees lateral oblique
    d. 45 degrees medial oblique

18. Which projection of the shoulder best demonstrates the greater tubercle of the humerus in profile?
    a. Transthoracic lateral projection
    b. AP projection with neutral rotation
    c. AP projection with internal rotation
    d. AP projection with external rotation

19. Which projection of the shoulder best demonstrates the humeral head in profile?
    a. Transthoracic lateral projection
    b. AP projection with neutral rotation
    c. AP projection with external rotation
    d. AP projection with internal rotation

20. Which projection of the shoulder best demonstrates the lesser tubercle of the humerus in profile and pointing toward the glenoid cavity?
    a. Transthoracic lateral projection
    b. AP projection with neutral rotation
    c. AP projection with internal rotation
    d. AP projection with external rotation

21. Which projection of the shoulder is being performed when the patient is supine with the right shoulder centered on the IR, a vertical central ray is being directed perpendicular to the center of the IR, and the humeral epicondyles are parallel with the plane of the IR?
    a. Transthoracic lateral projection
    b. PA oblique (scapular Y) projection
    c. AP projection with internal rotation
    d. AP projection with external rotation

22. What should be adjusted from the regular procedure for the transthoracic lateral projection (Lawrence method) of the humerus if the patient is unable to elevate the unaffected arm?
    a. Breathing procedure
    b. Central ray angulation
    c. Placement of the IR
    d. Rotation of the patient

23. Which projection of the upper extremity should be performed to demonstrate a fracture of the proximal humerus when that arm cannot be abducted?
    a. Tangential projection, Fisk modification
    b. AP projection of the shoulder with internal rotation
    c. AP projection of the shoulder with external rotation
    d. Transthoracic lateral projection (Lawrence method) of the humerus

24. When performing the transthoracic lateral projection (Lawrence method) of the humerus, which breathing technique should be used to improve best the image contrast and decrease the exposure necessary to penetrate the body?
    a. Rapid breathing
    b. Shallow breathing
    c. Suspended full expiration
    d. Suspended full inspiration

25. Which projection of the shoulder requires that a horizontal central ray be directed 15 to 30 degrees medially and enter the axilla of the affected arm?
    a. AP projection
    b. PA oblique (scapular Y) projection
    c. Inferosuperior axial projection (Lawrence method)
    d. Transthoracic lateral projection (Lawrence method)

26. What is the proper position of the humerus for the inferosuperior axial projection?
   a. Adducted
   b. Adducted and externally rotated
   c. Abducted to a right angle
   d. Abducted to a right angle and externally rotated

27. How should the central ray be directed for the PA oblique projection (scapular Y) of the shoulder?
   a. Cephalically 10 to 15 degrees
   b. Cephalically 15 to 25 degrees
   c. Cephalically 25 to 30 degrees
   d. Perpendicular to the IR

28. In which body position should the patient be placed to demonstrate the left shoulder with the PA oblique projection (scapular Y)?
   a. Left anterior oblique
   b. Left posterior oblique
   c. Right anterior oblique
   d. Right posterior oblique

29. Which projection of the shoulder joint requires the patient to be rotated until the midcoronal plane forms an angle of 45 to 60 degrees with the plane of the IR?
   a. Transthoracic lateral projection
   b. PA oblique projection (scapular Y)
   c. AP oblique projection (Grashey method)
   d. AP projection with external rotation

30. Where is the humerus generally demonstrated on a PA oblique shoulder (scapular Y) image if the shoulder is normal?
   a. Superimposed on the junction of the acromion and coracoid process
   b. Beneath the acromion
   c. Beneath the coracoid process
   d. Completely separated from the glenoid fossa (open joint space)

31. Where is the humeral head usually seen on a PA oblique (scapular Y) image if the shoulder is anteriorly dislocated?
   a. Superimposed on the junction of the acromion and coracoid process
   b. Beneath the acromion
   c. Beneath the coracoid process
   d. Completely separated from the glenoid fossa (open joint space)

32. Which projection of the shoulder girdle is performed with the patient supine, an IR placed vertically against the superior surface of the shoulder, and the central ray angled 10 to 15 degrees posteriorly (downward from horizontal)?
   a. Tangential for the intertubercular (bicipital) groove
   b. AP axial, lordotic position, for the clavicle
   c. Transthoracic lateral, Lawrence method, for the shoulder
   d. Inferosuperior axial, Lawrence method, for the shoulder joint

33. Which projection demonstrates the scapulohumeral joint space open and the glenoid cavity in profile?
   a. PA oblique projection (scapular Y)
   b. AP projection with external rotation
   c. AP oblique projection (Grashey method)
   d. Inferosuperior axial projection (Lawrence method)

34. What would be the required patient position to demonstrate the left shoulder using the AP oblique projection (Grashey) method?
   a. 10 to 15 degrees RPO
   b. 10 to 15 degrees LPO
   c. 35 to 45 degrees RPO
   d. 35 to 45 degrees LPO

35. When demonstrating the intertubercular (bicipital) groove with the Fisk modification of the tangential projection, how should the affected humerus be positioned?
   a. The humerus should be rotated laterally.
   b. The humerus should be rotated medially.
   c. The vertical humerus should form an angle of 10 to 15 degrees.
   d. The humerus should be abducted to a right angle with the body.

36. If the patient's condition permits, which joint should be demonstrated with the patient in an upright position?
   a. Glenohumeral
   b. Scapulohumeral
   c. Sternoclavicular
   d. Acromioclavicular

37. How many degrees and in which direction should the central ray be directed for the PA axial projection of the clavicle?
   a. 15 to 30 degrees caudad
   b. 15 to 30 degrees cephalad
   c. 25 to 35 degrees caudad
   d. 25 to 35 degrees cephalad

38. How many degrees and in which direction should the central ray be directed for the AP axial projection of the clavicle with the patient supine?
    a. 15 to 30 degrees caudad
    b. 15 to 30 degrees cephalad
    c. 25 to 35 degrees caudad
    d. 25 to 35 degrees cephalad

39. When performing the AP projection of the scapula, the central ray should be directed toward a point

    2 inches (5 cm) _____ to the coracoid process.
    a. Lateral
    b. Medial
    c. Inferior
    d. Superior

40. When performing a lateral projection of the scapula with the patient positioned RAO or LAO, approximately how much body rotation is necessary for the average patient?
    a. 15 to 20 degrees
    b. 25 to 30 degrees
    c. 35 to 40 degrees
    d. 45 to 60 degrees

7 Lower Extremity

OSTEOLOGY AND ARTHROLOGY OF THE LOWER EXTREMITY

Section 1: Exercise 1

Identify each lettered individual bone or group of bones shown in Fig. 7.1.

A. _____

B. _____

C. _____

D. _____

E. _____

F. _____

G. _____

H. _____

I. _____

J. _____

K. _____

L. _____

M. _____

N. _____

O. _____

P. _____

Q. _____

R. _____

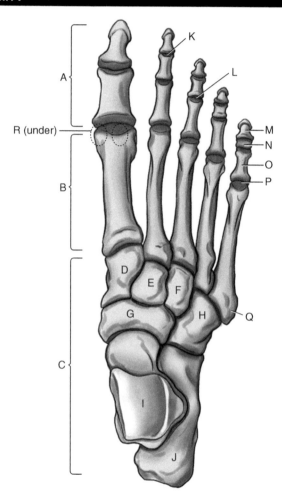

Fig. 7.1 Anterior aspect of the foot.

Section 1: Exercise 2

Identify each lettered individual bone or group of bones shown in Fig. 7.2.

A. _____

B. _____

C. _____

D. _____

E. _____

F. _____

G. _____

H. _____

I. _____

J. _____

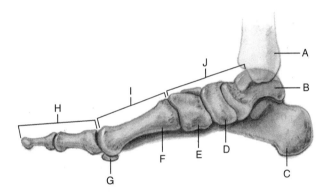

Fig. 7.2 Lateral aspect of a foot.

Section 1: Exercise 3

Identify each lettered structure shown in Fig. 7.3.

A. _____

B. _____

C. _____

D. _____

E. _____

F. _____

G. _____

H. _____

I. _____

J. _____

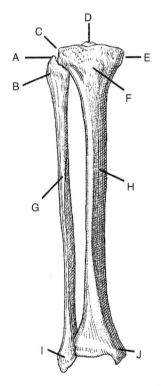

Fig. 7.3 Anterior aspect of a tibia and fibula.

Section 1: Exercise 4

Identify each lettered structure shown in Fig. 7.4.

A. _____

B. _____

C. _____

D. _____

E. _____

F. _____

G. _____

H. _____

I. _____

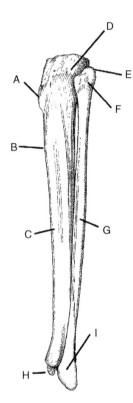

Fig. 7.4 Lateral aspect of a tibia and fibula.

Section 1: Exercise 5

Match the structures found on the tibia or fibula (the bones of the leg) listed in Column A with the descriptions in Column B. Not all descriptions may apply to the listed structures.

Column A

_____ 1. Apex

_____ 2. Crest

_____ 3. Tibia

_____ 4. Fibula

_____ 5. Condyles

_____ 6. Tubercles

_____ 7. Tuberosity

_____ 8. Lateral malleolus

_____ 9. Medial malleolus

_____ 10. Intercondylar eminence

Column B

a. Lateral bone of the leg

b. Enlarged distal end of the fibula

c. The larger of the two bones of the leg

d. Known as the anterior border of the tibia

e. Deep depression between the condyles

f. Conical projection at the head of the fibula

g. Large process at the distal end of the tibia

h. Two prominent processes on the proximal end of the tibia

i. Two peaklike processes arising from the intercondylar eminence

j. Sharp projection between the two superior articular surfaces

k. Prominent process on the anterior surface of the tibia; just below the condyles

Section 1: Exercise 6

Identify each lettered structure shown in Fig. 7.5.

A. _____

B. _____

C. _____

D. _____

E. _____

F. _____

G. _____

H. _____

I. _____

J. _____

Section 1: Exercise 7

Identify each lettered structure shown in Fig. 7.6.

A. _____

B. _____

C. _____

D. _____

E. _____

F. _____

G. _____

H. _____

I. _____

J. _____

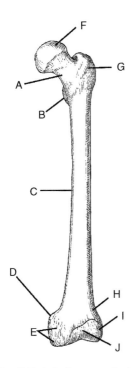

Fig. 7.5 Anterior aspect of a femur.

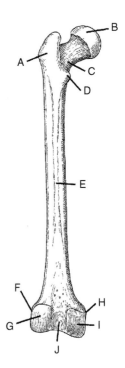

Fig. 7.6 Posterior aspect of a femur.

Section 1: Exercise 8

Identify each lettered structure shown in Fig. 7.7.

A. _____

B. _____

C. _____

D. _____

E. _____

F. _____

G. _____

H. _____

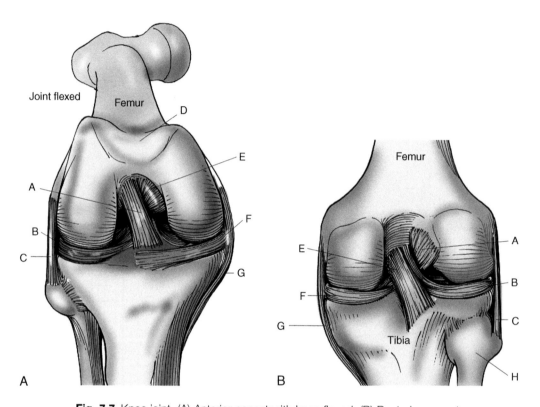

Fig. 7.7 Knee joint. (A) Anterior aspect with knee flexed. (B) Posterior aspect.

Section 1: Exercise 9

Identify each lettered structure shown in Fig. 7.8.

A. _____

B. _____

C. _____

D. _____

E. _____

F. _____

G. _____

H. _____

I. _____

J. _____

Section 1: Exercise 10

Match the structures found on the femur listed in Column A with the descriptions in Column B. Not all descriptions may apply to the listed structures.

Column A	Column B
_____ 1. Head	a. Deep depression between the condyles
_____ 2. Neck	b. Process located on the medial surface, distal femur
_____ 3. Condyles	c. Constricted portion just inferior from the head
_____ 4. Patellar surface	d. Large, rounded eminence on the superior end
_____ 5. Greater trochanter	e. Two large eminences on the distal end
_____ 6. Intercondylar fossa	f. Two large eminences on the proximal end
	g. Large, prominent process superior and lateral on the shaft
	h. Shallow, triangular area on the anterior surface between the condyles

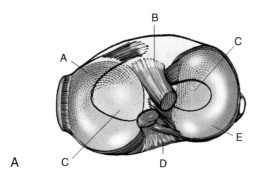

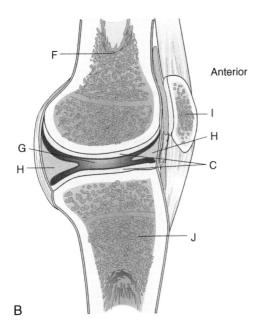

Fig. 7.8 Knee joint. (A) Superior surface of tibia. (B) Sagittal section.

Section 1: Exercise 11

Structures found on the femur, the tibia, or the fibula are listed. In the space provided, write P if that structure is closer to the proximal end or D if that structure is closer to the distal end of the bone on which it is located.

_____ 1. Trochanters

_____ 2. Fibular apex

_____ 3. Fibular head

_____ 4. Tibial plateau

_____ 5. Femoral neck

_____ 6. Femoral head

_____ 7. Tibial condyles

_____ 8. Trochlear groove

_____ 9. Tibial tuberosity

_____ 10. Lateral malleolus

_____ 11. Medial malleolus

_____ 12. Femoral condyles

_____ 13. Intercondylar fossa

_____ 14. Femoral epicondyles

_____ 15. Intercondylar eminence

Section 1: Exercise 12

Match the structures listed in Column A with the bones on which they are found in Column B. Identify each bone if the structure is found on more than one bone.

Column A	Column B
_____ 1. Apex	a. Femur
_____ 2. Head	b. Tibia
_____ 3. Condyles	c. Fibula
_____ 4. Tuberosity	
_____ 5. Trochanters	
_____ 6. Trochlear groove	
_____ 7. Medial malleolus	
_____ 8. Lateral malleolus	
_____ 9. Intercondylar fossa	
_____ 10. Intercondylar eminence	

Section 1: Exercise 13

Match the articulations listed in Column A with the corresponding type of movement listed in Column B. More than one choice from Column B may be used for some articulations, but not all choices from Column B may be used.

Column A	Column B
_____ 1. Knee	a. Gliding
_____ 2. Ankle	b. Flexion
_____ 3. Intertarsal	c. Extension
_____ 4. Interphalangeal	d. Abduction
_____ 5. Tarsometatarsal	e. Adduction
_____ 6. Distal tibiofibular	f. Circumduction
_____ 7. Proximal tibiofibular	g. Rotational (around a single axis)
_____ 8. Metatarsophalangeal	h. Syndesmosis (slight movement)

Section 1: Exercise 14

Match the pathology terms in Column A with the appropriate definition in Column B. Not all choices from Column B should be selected.

Column A

_____ 1. Gout

_____ 2. Bone cyst

_____ 3. Pott fracture

_____ 4. Paget disease

_____ 5. Osteoid osteoma

_____ 6. Congenital

_____ 7. Osteomalacia

_____ 8. Osgood-Schlatter disease

_____ 9. Osteochondroma

_____ 10. Osteoclastoma (giant cell tumor)

Column B

a. Loss of bone density

b. A benign lesion of cortical bone

c. Fluid-filled cyst with a wall of fibrous tissue

d. Thick, soft bone marked by bowing clubfoot and fractures

e. Softening of the bones (rickets) as a result of a vitamin D deficiency

f. Benign bone tumor projection with a cartilaginous cap (exostosis)

g. Incomplete separation or avulsion of the tibial tuberosity

h. Lucent lesion in the metaphysis, usually at the distal femur

i. Abnormal twisting of the foot, usually inward and downward

j. Hereditary form of arthritis in which uric acid is deposited in joints

k. Avulsion fracture of the medial malleolus with the loss of the ankle mortise

Section 1: Exercise 15

This exercise is a comprehensive review of the osteology and arthrology of the lower extremity. Provide a short answer for each question.

1. How many bones are found in one lower extremity?

2. Identify by group name and quantity the bones found in the foot and ankle.

3. How many interphalangeal articulations does one foot have?

4. What types of movement do the interphalangeal joints permit?

5. What type of joint is an interphalangeal joint?

6. With what do the heads of metatarsals articulate?

7. How are metatarsals identified within the foot?

8. Identify by individual name or group the bones found in each section of the foot.

   a. Forefoot: _____

   b. Midfoot: _____

   c. Hindfoot: _____

9. Which metatarsal has a tuberosity that is prominent at its base?

10. List the names of the tarsal bones.

11. Which tarsal bone comprises the heel of the foot?

12. Which is the largest of the tarsal bones?

13. Which tarsal bone articulates superiorly on the calcaneus?

14. Which tarsal bone is located between the calcaneus and the fourth and fifth metatarsals?

15. Which tarsal bone is lateral from the cuneiforms?

16. Which tarsal bone is located between the talus and the cuneiforms?

17. Name the tarsal bones that articulate with metatarsals.

18. Which tarsal bone forms part of the ankle joint?

19. Name the two bones of the leg.

20. Name the lateral bone of the leg.

21. Name the smaller of the bones of the leg.

22. What other term refers to the tibial spine?

23. Which tibial condyle has a facet for articulation with the head of the fibula?

24. Where specifically is the tibial tuberosity located?

25. Name the large bony process that extends both medially and inferiorly from the distal end of the tibia.

26. With what bone does the undersurface of the tibia articulate?

27. List the articulations of the tibia.

28. Name the largest bone of the lower extremity.

29. Where exactly is the intercondylar fossa located?

30. What is (a) the name of the "kneecap" and (b) its bone classification?

a. _____

b. _____

In items 31 to 34, write out the anatomic terms for the abbreviations of the lower extremity.

31. DIP: _____

32. TMT: _____

33. MTP: _____

34. IP: _____

35. Which of the above-listed abbreviations are also used to refer to joints in the hand?

Section 1: Exercise 16

Use the following clues to complete the crossword puzzle.

Across

6. Cushions between tibia and femur
9. Between femoral condyles on posterior aspect (two words)
10. Largest bone of lower extremity
13. Most superior tarsal bone
16. Tarsal located between talus and cuneiforms
17. Bones of the forefoot

Down

1. Lateral tarsal bone
2. Superior, lateral process of femur (two words)
3. Location of fibula in lower leg
4. Articular surfaces on superior tibia
5. Two joints in the lower leg
6. Process on distal end of tibia and fibula
7. Alternative name of the ankle joint
8. Largest tarsal bone
11. Toe bones
12. Processes on proximal tibia
14. Sesamoid that protects knee joint
15. Medial lower leg bone

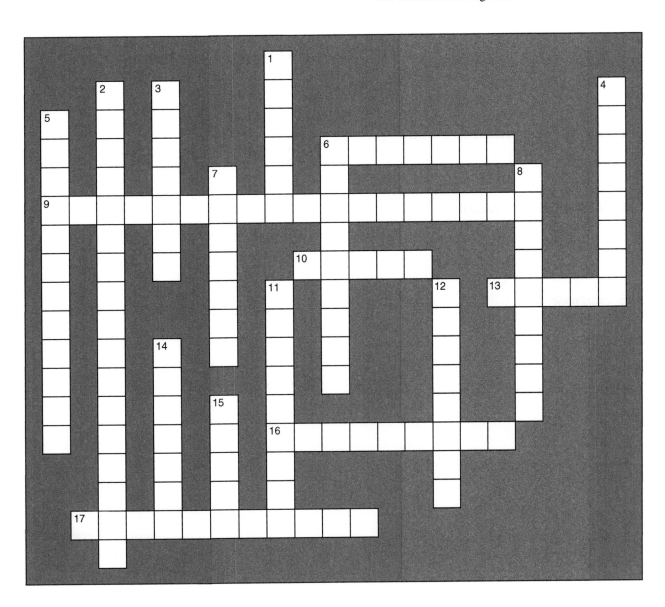

Chapter **7** **Lower Extremity**

POSITIONING OF THE LOWER EXTREMITY

Section 2: Exercise 1: Positioning for the Toes

This exercise pertains to the essential projections of the toes. Identify structures, fill in missing words, provide a short answer, select the correct answer, or choose true or false (explaining any statement you believe to be false) for each item.

1. List the essential projections for the toes, and describe the positioning steps used for each, as follows:

   Essential projection: _____
   - Size of collimated field:

   - Key patient/part positioning points:

   - Anatomic landmarks and relation to IR:

   - CR orientation and entrance point:

   Essential projection: _____
   - Size of collimated field:

   - Key patient/part positioning points:

   - Anatomic landmarks and relation to IR:

   - CR orientation and entrance point:

   Essential projection: _____
   - Size of collimated field:

   - Key patient/part positioning points:

   - Anatomic landmarks and relation to IR:

   - CR orientation and entrance point:

   Essential projection: _____
   - Size of collimated field:

   - Key patient/part positioning points:

   - Anatomic landmarks and relation to IR:

   - CR orientation and entrance point:

186

Chapter **7 Lower Extremity**

Items 2 to 8 pertain to the *AP and AP axial projections.*

2. What is the central ray orientation if the joint spaces of the toes are of primary interest?
   a. Perpendicular
   b. 15 degrees posteriorly (toward the heel)
   c. 15 degrees anteriorly (away from the heel)

3. How should the central ray be directed to demonstrate toes when the plantar surface of the affected foot is in contact with a foam wedge, which should be inclined 15 degrees so that the toes are elevated above a horizontally placed IR?
   a. Perpendicular
   b. 15 degrees posteriorly (toward the heel)
   c. 15 degrees anteriorly (away from the heel)

4. Which of the following projections for toes normally does *not* demonstrate open interphalangeal joints?
   a. AP projection of the toes with the central ray directed perpendicularly
   b. AP axial projection of the toes with a central ray angulation of 15 degrees
   c. AP axial projection of the toes with a 15-degree foam wedge and the central ray directed perpendicularly

Examine the images of the toes shown in Figs. 7.9 and 7.10, and then answer the following questions.

5. Which image best demonstrates interphalangeal joints?

   _____

6. Which image was most likely obtained with the central ray angled 15 degrees posteriorly (toward the heel)?

   _____

7. Which image was most likely obtained with the foot and IR placed parallel with the surface of the table and the central ray directed perpendicular to the foot?

   _____

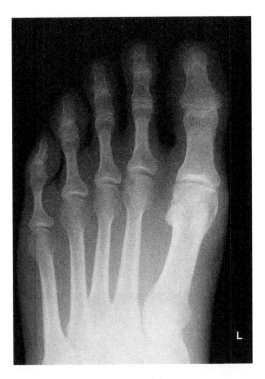

Fig. 7.9 Image of the toes.

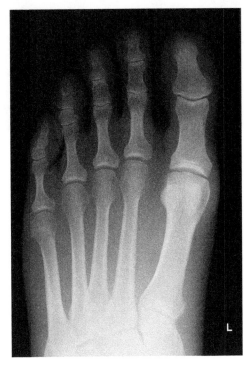

Fig. 7.10 Image of the toes.

8. Identify each lettered bone, group of bones, or joint shown in Fig. 7.11.

A. _____

B. _____

C. _____

D. _____

E. _____

F. _____

G. _____

H. _____

I. _____

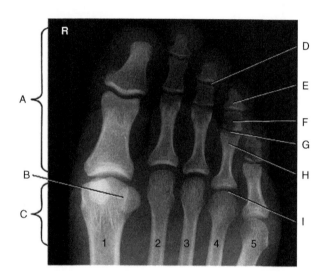

Fig. 7.11 Image of the toes.

Items 9 to 14 pertain to the *AP oblique projection.*

9. For the AP oblique projection demonstrating all of the toes, which way (medially or laterally) should the foot and lower leg be rotated?

_____

10. How many degrees of rotation are needed to rotate the foot properly for the AP oblique projection of toes?

_____

11. Which individual toes are best demonstrated using the AP oblique projection with the foot rotated laterally?

_____

12. For AP oblique projections, the central ray should enter the foot at the _____ joint.

13. True or false. The bases of metatarsals should be included within the image for AP oblique projections.

14. True or false. All phalanges should be seen in the image.

Items 15 to 20 pertain to the *lateral projection.*

15. For lateral projections of the toes, what can be done to prevent the superimposition of toes?

16. For the lateral projection of the great toe, the central ray should enter at the _____ joint of the great toe.

17. For lateral projections of the lesser toes, the central ray should enter at the _____ joint.

18. True or false. For the lateral projection of the great toe, the patient should lie in the lateral recumbent position on the unaffected side.

19. True or false. For the lateral projection of the fifth toe, the patient should lie in the lateral recumbent position on the unaffected side.

20. True or false. Interphalangeal and metatarsophalangeal joint spaces should appear open.

Section 2: Exercise 2: Positioning for the Foot

This exercise reviews the essential projections of the foot. Identify structures, fill in missing words, provide a short answer, select the correct answer, or choose true or false (explaining any statement you believe to be false) for each item.

1. List the essential projections of the foot, and describe the positioning steps used for each, as follows:

    Essential projection: _____
    ■ Size of collimated field:

    ■ Key patient/part positioning points:

    ■ Anatomic landmarks and relation to IR:

    ■ CR orientation and entrance point:

    Essential projection: _____
    ■ Size of collimated field:

    ■ Key patient/part positioning points:

    ■ Anatomic landmarks and relation to IR:

    ■ CR orientation and entrance point:

    Essential projection: _____
    ■ Size of collimated field:

    ■ Key patient/part positioning points:

    ■ Anatomic landmarks and relation to IR:

    ■ CR orientation and entrance point:

Essential projection: _____
■ Size of collimated field:

■ Key patient/part positioning points:

■ Anatomic landmarks and relation to IR:

■ CR orientation and entrance point:

Items 2 to 5 pertain to *AP and AP axial projections*.

2. What other projection term refers to the AP projection?
   a. Axial
   b. Plantodorsal
   c. Dorsoplantar

3. How should the central ray be directed for best demonstration of tarsometatarsal joints with a dorsoplantar projection?

4. Toward what point of the foot should the central ray be directed for AP and AP axial projections?
   a. The base of the third metatarsal
   b. The head of the third metatarsal
   c. The base of the fifth metatarsal
   d. The head of the fifth metatarsal

5. Identify each lettered bone, joint, or group of bones shown in Fig. 7.12.

   A. _____

   B. _____

   C. _____

   D. _____

   E. _____

   F. _____

   G. _____

   H. _____

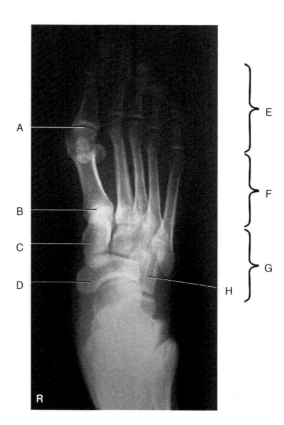

Fig. 7.12 AP axial foot.

Items 6 to 10 pertain to the *AP oblique projection*.

6. In which direction (medially or laterally) should the foot be rotated for the AP oblique projection for best demonstration of the cuboid and its related articulations?

7. What projection of the foot best demonstrates the lateral tarsals with the least superimposition of structures?
   a. AP projection
   b. AP axial projection
   c. AP oblique projection (lateral rotation)
   d. AP oblique projection (medial rotation)

8. For the AP oblique projection, the leg should be rotated medially until the plantar surface of the foot forms an angle of _____ with the IR.
   a. 10 degrees
   b. 20 degrees
   c. 30 degrees
   d. 40 degrees

9. What two metatarsal bases appear overlapped in the image of the AP oblique projection, medial rotation?

10. Identify each lettered bone or joint shown in Fig. 7.13.

    A. _____

    B. _____

    C. _____

    D. _____

    E. _____

    F. _____

    G. _____

    H. _____

    I. _____

    J. _____

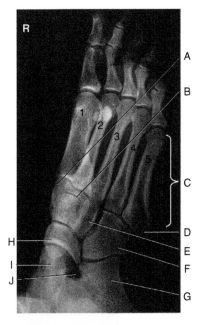

Fig. 7.13 AP oblique foot, medial rotation.

Items 11 to 15 pertain to the *lateral projection*.

11. For patient comfort, which side of the foot (medial or lateral) should be placed in contact with the IR for the lateral projection?

12. With reference to the lower leg, how should the foot be positioned for the lateral projection?

13. Where should the distal fibula be seen in images of the lateral projection of the foot?

14. True or false. The tibiotalar joint must be seen in the lateral projection of the foot.

15. Identify each lettered bone shown in Fig. 7.14.

A. _____

B. _____

C. _____

D. _____

E. _____

F. _____

G. _____

H. _____

I. _____

J. _____

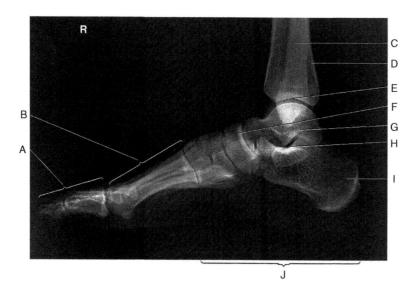

Fig. 7.14 Lateral foot.

Section 2: Exercise 3: Positioning for the Calcaneus

This exercise pertains to the two essential projections of the calcaneus. Identify structures, fill in missing words, provide a short answer, or choose true or false (explaining any statement you believe to be false) for each item.

1. List the essential projections for the calcaneus, and describe the positioning steps used for each, as follows:

   Essential projection: _____
   - Size of collimated field:

   - Key patient/part positioning points:

   - Anatomic landmarks and relation to IR:

   - CR orientation and entrance point:

   Essential projection: _____
   - Size of collimated field:

   - Key patient/part positioning points:

   - Anatomic landmarks and relation to IR:

   - CR orientation and entrance point:

2. With reference to the plane of the IR, the plantar surface of the foot should be _____ for the axial projection.

3. How many degrees and in which direction should the central ray be directed for the axial (plantodorsal) projection?

   _____

4. When performing the axial (plantodorsal) projection, what should the radiographer do to demonstrate a complete calcaneus if the anterior portion of the calcaneus is not seen in the image with the same brightness as the posterior portion?

5. True or false. The plantar surface of the foot should be in contact with the IR for the axial (plantodorsal) projection.

6. True or false. The central ray should enter the dorsal surface of the foot for the axial (plantodorsal) projection.

7. Identify each lettered structure shown in Fig. 7.15.

A. _____

B. _____

C. _____

D. _____

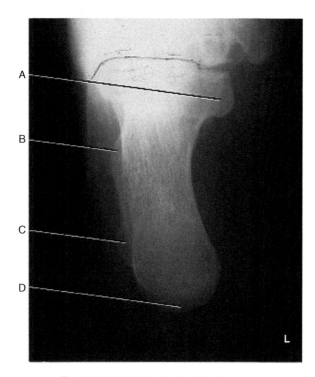

Fig. 7.15 Axial (plantodorsal) calcaneus.

8. Where on the medial surface of the foot should the central ray enter the calcaneus for the lateral projection?

9. Which projection of the calcaneus best demonstrates the sinus tarsi?
   a. Plantodorsal axial
   b. Lateral

10. Identify each lettered structure or joint shown in Fig. 7.16.

A. _____

B. _____

C. _____

D. _____

E. _____

F. _____

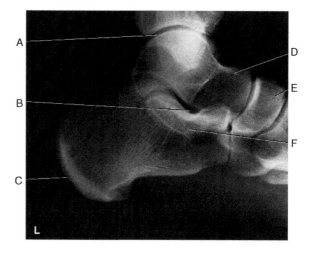

Fig. 7.16 Lateral calcaneus.

Section 2: Exercise 4: Positioning for the Ankle

This exercise pertains to the essential projections of the ankle. Identify structures, fill in missing words, provide a short answer, or choose true or false (explaining any statement you believe to be false) for each item.

1. List the essential projections and positions for the ankle, and describe the positioning steps used for each, as follows:

   Essential projection: _____
   - Size of collimated field:

   - Key patient/part positioning points:

   - Anatomic landmarks and relation to IR:

   - CR orientation and entrance point:

   Essential projection: _____
   - Size of collimated field:

   - Key patient/part positioning points:

   - Anatomic landmarks and relation to IR:

   - CR orientation and entrance point:

   Essential projection: _____
   - Size of collimated field:

   - Key patient/part positioning points:

   - Anatomic landmarks and relation to IR:

   - CR orientation and entrance point:

   Essential projection: _____
   - Size of collimated field:

   - Key patient/part positioning points:

   - Anatomic landmarks and relation to IR:

   - CR orientation and entrance point:

   Essential projection: _____
   - Size of collimated field:

   - Key patient/part positioning points:

   - Anatomic landmarks and relation to IR:

   - CR orientation and entrance point:

Items 2 to 5 pertain to the AP projection.

2. True or false. The AP projection should demonstrate the joint space between the medial malleolus and the talus without any overlapping of structures.

195

3. True or false. The AP projection should demonstrate the distal third of the fibula without superimposition with the talus or tibia.

4. True or false. The AP projection should demonstrate the lateral and medial malleoli.

5. Identify each lettered structure shown in Fig. 7.17.

   A. _____

   B. _____

   C. _____

   D. _____

   E. _____

   F. _____

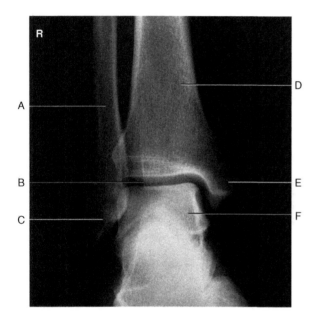

Fig. 7.17 AP ankle.

Items 6 to 10 pertain to the *lateral projection*.

6. Why is dorsiflexion of the foot required for the lateral (mediolateral) projection?

7. True or false. The lateral (mediolateral) projection should demonstrate the fibula over the posterior half of the tibia.

8. True or false. An image of the lateral (mediolateral) projection should demonstrate the lateral malleolus free from superimposition by the talus.

9. True or false. The tuberosity and base of the fifth metatarsal should be demonstrated as a lateral projection image of the ankle.

10. Identify each lettered structure shown in Fig. 7.18.

    A. _____

    B. _____

    C. _____

    D. _____

    E. _____

    F. _____

    G. _____

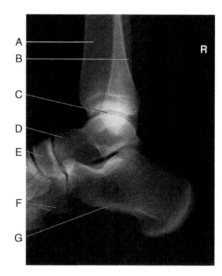

Fig. 7.18 Lateral ankle.

Items 11 and 12 pertain to the *AP oblique projection (medial rotation)* of the ankle.

11. How many degrees and in what direction should the leg and foot be rotated?

12. From the following list, circle the structures and articulations that should be demonstrated in the image of the AP oblique ankle.
    a. Talus
    b. Cuboid
    c. Calcaneus
    d. Distal tibia
    e. Distal fibula
    f. Tibiofibular articulation
    g. Femorotibial articulation
    h. Metatarsophalangeal articulation
    i. Talofibular articulation

Items 13 to 17 pertain to the *AP oblique projection (medial rotation)* of the ankle for demonstrating the mortise joint.

13. From the supine position, how many degrees should the lower extremity and foot be rotated to position the ankle for this projection?

14. With reference to the position of the patient's leg and foot during the procedure, how is it determined that the leg has been rotated the correct number of degrees?

15. True or false. The talofibular joint space should be demonstrated in profile without any bony superimposition.

16. True or false. The foot should be plantar flexed to place the long axis of the foot parallel with the IR.

17. Identify each lettered structure shown in Fig. 7.19.

    A. _____

    B. _____

    C. _____

    D. _____

    E. _____

    F. _____

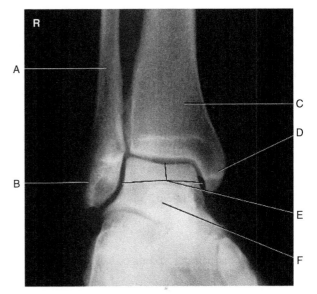

Fig. 7.19 AP oblique ankle, medial rotation.

Items 18 to 20 pertain to AP projections (stress method).

18. State the purpose of performing AP stress studies of the ankle.

19. How can the patient hold the foot in the stress position during AP stress studies?

20. How do images indicate that a patient has a torn ligament affecting the ankle?

Section 2: Exercise 5: Positioning for the Leg

This exercise pertains to the essential projections of the leg. Identify structures, fill in missing words, provide a short answer, select the correct answer, or choose true or false (explaining any statement you believe to be false) for each question.

1. List the essential projections for the leg, and describe the positioning steps used for each, as follows:

   Essential projection: _____
   ■ Size of collimated field:

   ■ Key patient/part positioning points:

   ■ Anatomic landmarks and relation to IR:

   ■ CR orientation and entrance point:

Essential projection: _____
■ Size of collimated field:

■ Key patient/part positioning points:

■ Anatomic landmarks and relation to IR:

■ CR orientation and entrance point:

Items 2 to 5 pertain to the *AP projection.*

2. The placement of the top border of the IR should extend at least _____ inches (_____ cm) above the knee joint to avoid being projected off by beam divergence.
   a. 1 to 1½; 2.5 to 3.8
   b. 2 to 2½; 5 to 6.4
   c. 3 to 3½; 7.6 to 8.9

3. What should the radiographer do if the leg is too long to demonstrate the knee and the ankle joint with the same exposure?
   a. Perform two AP projections to ensure that the entire lower extremity is demonstrated.
   b. Decrease the source-to-image receptor distance (SID) to ensure the beam covers the entire leg.
   c. Angle the central ray along the long axis of the leg to project the joint onto the IR.

4. True or false. The AP projection of the leg should demonstrate the fibula without any overlapping with the tibia.

5. Identify each lettered structure shown in Fig. 7.20.

A. _____

B. _____

C. _____

D. _____

E. _____

F. _____

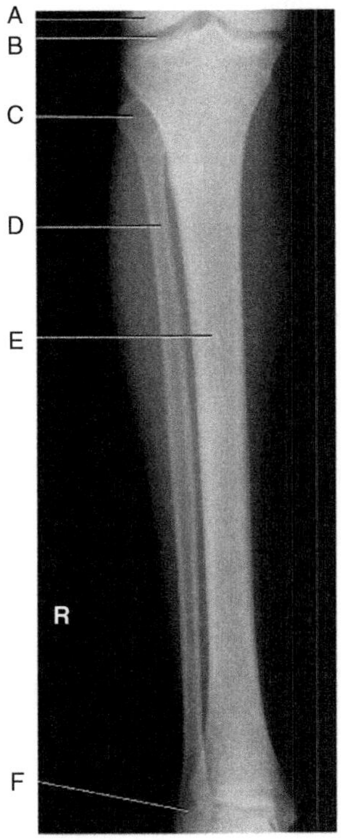

Fig. 7.20 AP tibia and fibula.

Items 6 to 10 pertain to the *lateral projection*.

6. For the lateral projection of the leg, should the patella be positioned perpendicular or parallel with reference to the plane of the IR?

7. What procedure should the radiographer perform if the patient is unable to turn from the supine position toward the affected side to position a fractured leg on the IR for the lateral projection?

8. If a radiographer positions the lower extremity very carefully to ensure that the femoral condyles are physically superimposed, but they do not appear to be well superimposed on the image, what could have caused the image to appear that way?

9. True or false. The lateral projection should demonstrate some interosseous space between the shafts of the fibula and tibia.

10. Identify each lettered structure shown in Fig. 7.21.

A. _____

B. _____

C. _____

D. _____

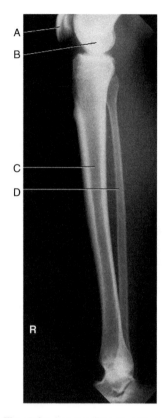

Fig. 7.21 Lateral tibia and fibula.

Section 2: Exercise 6: Positioning for the Knee

This exercise pertains to the essential projections of the knee joint. Identify structures, fill in missing words, provide a short answer, select the correct answer, or choose true or false (explaining any statement you believe is false) for each question.

1. List the essential projections and positions for the knee joint, and describe the positioning steps used for each, as follows:

   Essential projection: _____
   - Size of collimated field:

   - Key patient/part positioning points:

   - Anatomic landmarks and relation to IR:

   - CR orientation and entrance point:

   Essential projection: _____
   - Size of collimated field:

   - Key patient/part positioning points:

   - Anatomic landmarks and relation to IR:

   - CR orientation and entrance point:

Essential projection: _____
- Size of collimated field:

- Key patient/part positioning points:

- Anatomic landmarks and relation to IR:

- CR orientation and entrance point:

Essential projection: _____
- Size of collimated field:

- Key patient/part positioning points:

- Anatomic landmarks and relation to IR:

- CR orientation and entrance point:

Essential projection: _____
- Size of collimated field:

- Key patient/part positioning points:

- Anatomic landmarks and relation to IR:

- CR orientation and entrance point:

Items 2 to 10 pertain to the *AP projection.*

2. List three factors that should be considered when deciding whether or not to use a grid for AP projections.

3. With reference to the knee, where is the centering point used for positioning the IR or centering the collimated field to the knee?
   a. To the apex of the patella
   b. To the most superior point of the patella
   c. ½ inch (1.3 cm) below the apex of the patella
   d. 2 inches (5 cm) below the apex of the patella

4. Where is the patella located on a correctly positioned AP projection of the knee?
   a. Slightly off center to the lateral side of the tibia
   b. Slightly off center to the medial side of the tibia
   c. Slightly off center to the lateral side of the femur
   d. Slightly off center to the medial side of the femur

For the following three situations, choose the central ray angulation that best demonstrates the joint space based on the anterior superior iliac spine (ASIS) to tabletop measurement by writing in the space provided the corresponding letter from the following choices:

Column A	Column B
_____ 5. Less than 7½ inches (19 cm)	a. Perpendicular
_____ 6. Between 7½ and 10 inches (19 and 24 cm)	b. 3 to 5 degrees caudad
	c. 3 to 5 degrees cephalad
_____ 7. More than 10 inches (24 cm)	d. 10 degrees caudad
	e. 10 degrees cephalad

8. On an image of a correctly positioned AP projection of the knee, the patella should be demonstrated:
   a. Projected slightly off of the medial femoral condyle
   b. Projected slightly off of the lateral femoral condyle
   c. In profile just anterior to the distal, anterior femur
   d. Completely superimposed on the femur

201

9. True or false. The AP projection image of a normal knee should demonstrate a femorotibial joint space with equal distances on both sides.

10. Identify each lettered structure shown in Fig. 7.22.

A. _____

B. _____

C. _____

D. _____

E. _____

F. _____

G. _____

H. _____

I. _____

J. _____

K. _____

L. _____

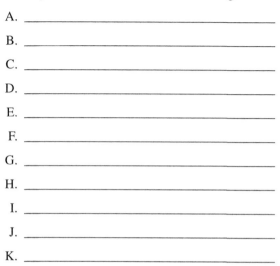

Fig. 7.22 AP knee.

Fig. 7.23 is another AP projection image of the knee. Compare this image with Fig. 7.22 and answer questions 11 to 15.

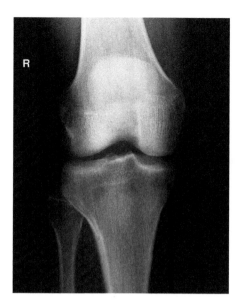

Fig. 7.23 AP knee.

11. How does Fig. 7.23 appear different?
    a. The patella does not superimpose the femur.
    b. The femorotibial joint space is not fully open.
    c. The fibular head does not slightly superimpose the tibia.

12. How did the positioning procedures most likely differ to produce these images?

13. Assuming that the ASIS-to-tabletop measurement for the patient in Fig. 7.22 is greater than 10 inches (24 cm), describe how you believe the central ray was directed to produce the image. Explain why.

14. Assuming that the patient in Fig. 7.23 is the same patient seen in Fig. 7.22, describe how you believe the central ray was directed to produce the image in Fig. 7.23. Explain why.

15. Which image best demonstrates the femorotibial joint space?

Items 16 to 26 pertain to the *lateral projection*.

16. With reference to the plane of the IR, the patella should be _____ (parallel or perpendicular).

17. The knee should be flexed _____ degrees.

18. When a new or healing fracture is present, the knee should be flexed no more than _____ degrees.

19. What could occur if a patient with a healing fracture flexes the knee more than the recommended number of degrees?

20. How many degrees and in what direction should the central ray be directed?

21. Why is the central ray angled cephalad for the lateral projection?

22. The central ray should enter the patient 1 inch (2.5 cm) distal to the _____.

23. Which positioning maneuver relaxes the muscles and shows the maximum volume of the joint cavity?
    a. Fully extending the lower extremity
    b. Flexing the knee 20 to 30 degrees
    c. Placing support pads under the ankle to elevate the lower leg

24. True or false. The femoral condyles should appear superimposed.

25. True or false. The lateral projection demonstrates the patella with slight overlapping with the femoral condyles.

26. Identify each lettered structure shown in Fig. 7.24.

A. _____

B. _____

C. _____

D. _____

E. _____

F. _____

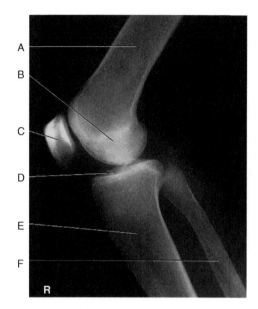

Fig. 7.24 Lateral knee.

Items 27 to 30 pertain to the *weight-bearing AP projection* of the knees.

27. Which physical condition affecting knees is often the reason that weight-bearing AP projections are performed?
    a. Arthritis
    b. Fracture
    c. Torn ligament
    d. Dislocation

28. To what level of the patient should the IR or collimated field be centered?

29. True or false. The patient should slightly flex both knees to maximize the knee joint space.

30. True or false. Both knees should be demonstrated without rotation.

Items 31 to 40 pertain to the *AP oblique projections.*

31. How many degrees should the leg be rotated?
    a. 15 degrees
    b. 30 degrees
    c. 45 degrees
    d. 60 degrees

32. How many degrees and in what direction should the central ray be directed if the patient measures less than 7½ inches (19 cm) from the ASIS to the tabletop?
    a. 0 degrees (perpendicular)
    b. 3 to 5 degrees caudal
    c. 3 to 5 degrees cephalic

33. How many degrees and in what direction should the central ray be directed if the patient measures between 7½ and 10 inches (19 and 24 cm) from the ASIS to the tabletop?
    a. 0 degrees (perpendicular)
    b. 3 to 5 degrees caudal
    c. 3 to 5 degrees cephalic

34. How many degrees and in what direction should the central ray be directed if the patient measures more than 10 inches (24 cm) from the ASIS to the tabletop?
    a. 0 degrees (perpendicular)
    b. 3 to 5 degrees caudal
    c. 3 to 5 degrees cephalic

35. Where on the knee should the central ray enter?
    a. ½ inch (1.3 cm) inferior to the patellar apex
    b. ½ inch (1.3 cm) superior to the patellar apex
    c. 1½ inches (3.8 cm) inferior to the patellar apex
    d. 1½ inches (3.8 cm) superior to the patellar apex

36. Evaluation criteria for AP oblique projections are listed. In the space provided, write M if the statement refers to the medial oblique projection, L if the statement refers to the lateral oblique projection, or B if the statement refers to both oblique projections.

_____ a. Tibial plateaus should be visualized.

_____ b. Knee joint should be seen and open.

_____ c. Soft tissue around the knee should be seen.

_____ d. Medial femoral and tibial condyles should be demonstrated.

_____ e. Lateral femoral and tibial condyles should be demonstrated.

_____ f. Fibula should be superimposed over the lateral half of the tibia.

_____ g. Tibia and fibula should be separated at their proximal articulation.

_____ h. Bony trabecular detail of the distal femur and proximal tibia should be demonstrated.

_____ i. Margin of the patella should project slightly beyond the edge of the femoral lateral condyle.

_____ j. Margin of the patella should project slightly beyond the edge of the femoral medial condyle.

37. Identify the position of the knee demonstrated in Fig. 7.25.

38. Identify the position of the knee demonstrated in Fig. 7.26.

39. Identify each lettered structure shown in Fig. 7.25.

A. _____

B. _____

C. _____

D. _____

E. _____

F. _____

G. _____

H. _____

I. _____

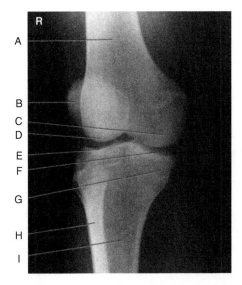

Fig. 7.25 AP oblique knee.

40. Identify each lettered structure shown in Fig. 7.26.

A. _____

B. _____

C. _____

D. _____

E. _____

F. _____

G. _____

H. _____

I. _____

J. _____

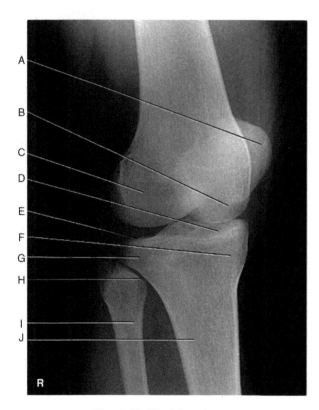

Fig. 7.26 AP oblique knee.

Section 2: Exercise 7: Positioning for the Intercondylar Fossa

This exercise pertains to the two essential projections for the intercondylar fossa. Identify structures, fill in missing words, provide a short answer, choose the correct answer from a list, or choose true or false (explaining any statement you believe to be false) for each item.

1. List the essential projections and positions for the intercondylar fossa, and describe the positioning steps used for each, as follows:

Essential projection:_____ (_____ method)
- Size of collimated field:

- Key patient/part positioning points:

- Anatomic landmarks and relation to IR:

- CR orientation and entrance point:

Essential projection:_____ (_____ method)
- Size of collimated field:

- Key patient/part positioning points:

- Anatomic landmarks and relation to IR:

- CR orientation and entrance point:

Items 2 to 8 pertain to the PA axial projection (Holmblad method).

2. The PA axial projection, first described by Holmblad in 1937, requires the patient to assume a

_____ position.

3. Describe the three ways patients can be positioned.

4. Describe how the IR should be placed.

5. Describe how and where the central ray should be directed.

6. What angle should be formed between the femur and the plane of the IR when the patient is correctly positioned?

7. What structures of the knee are demonstrated with this type of projection?

8. Identify each lettered structure shown in Fig. 7.27.

A. _____

B. _____

C. _____

D. _____

E. _____

F. _____

G. _____

H. _____

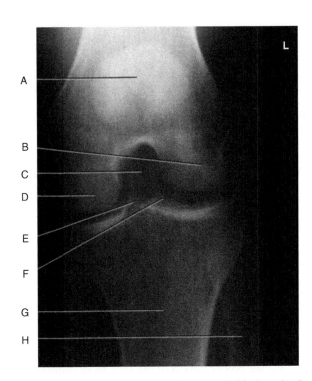

Fig. 7.27 PA axial intercondylar fossa, Holmblad method.

Examine Fig. 7.28 and answer questions 9 to 15, which pertain to the *PA axial projection (Camp-Coventry method).*

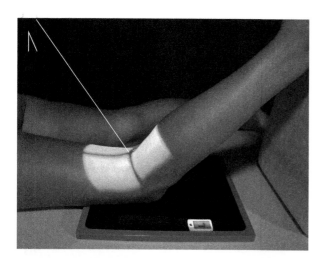

Fig. 7.28 PA axial intercondylar fossa, Camp-Coventry method.

9. Which patient body position should be used when performing this projection?
   a. Prone
   b. Supine
   c. Upright

10. Approximately how many degrees should the knee be flexed?
    a. 20 or 30
    b. 40 or 50
    c. 60 or 70

11. What should the radiographer do to make maintaining the proper flexion of the knee more comfortable for the patient?

12. The central ray should be directed perpendicular to the long axis of the _____.

13. How many degrees and in what direction should the central ray be directed?

14. What factor determines the number of degrees the central ray should be angled?

15. Both PA axial projections (the Holmblad method and the Camp-Coventry method) produce similar results and have identical evaluation criteria. From the following list, circle the seven evaluation criteria that refer to both projections.
    a. Patella should be seen in lateral profile.
    b. Femoral condyles should be superimposed.
    c. Fossa should be open and visualized.
    d. Apex of the patella should not superimpose the fossa.
    e. Soft tissue in the fossa and interspaces should be seen.
    f. Intercondylar eminences and knee joint space should be seen.
    g. No rotation is evident by slight tibiofibular overlap being seen.
    h. Posteroinferior surface of the femoral condyles should be demonstrated.
    i. Bony trabecular detail on the tibial eminences, distal femur, and proximal tibia should be demonstrated.

Section 2: Exercise 8: Positioning for the Patella and Patellofemoral Joint

This exercise reviews the essential projections of the patella and patellofemoral joint. Identify structures, fill in missing words, provide a short answer, or choose true or false (explaining any statement you believe to be false) for each item.

1. List the essential projections and positions for the patella and patellofemoral joint, and describe the positioning steps used for each, as follows:

   Essential projection: _____
   - Size of collimated field:

   - Key patient/part positioning points:

   - Anatomic landmarks and relation to IR:

   - CR orientation and entrance point:

   Essential projection: _____
   - Size of collimated field:

   - Key patient/part positioning points:

   - Anatomic landmarks and relation to IR:

   - CR orientation and entrance point:

   Essential projection: _____ (_____ method)
   - Size of collimated field:

   - Key patient/part positioning points:

   - Anatomic landmarks and relation to IR:

   - CR orientation and entrance point:

   Examine Fig. 7.29 and answer questions 2 to 4, which pertain to the *PA projection.*

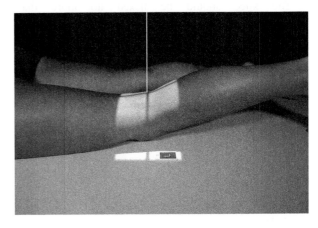

   Fig. 7.29 PA patella.

2. Why is the PA projection preferred over the AP projection?

3. What can be done to alleviate the pressure on the patella caused by the patient's weight?

4. How should the lower extremity be adjusted to place the patella parallel with the IR?

Items 5 to 7 pertain to the *lateral projection*.

5. True or false. The lateral side of the affected knee should be in contact with the table or IR.

6. The knee should be flexed no more than _____ degrees.

7. What might occur if the patient flexes the knee more than the recommended number of degrees?

Items 8 to 17 pertain to the tangential projection (Settegast method).

8. Describe three ways the patient can be positioned on a radiographic table for the tangential projection (Settegast method).

9. Why is it preferable to place the patient in the prone position for the tangential projection?

10. What projection of the patella should be performed before a tangential projection is attempted? Explain why.

11. When the patient is placed in the prone position and is unable to maintain a steady lower leg after flexing the knee, what can be done to help the patient hold the position?

12. Describe how and where the central ray should be directed.

13. What determines the number of degrees the central ray is angled?

14. True or false. The patellofemoral articulation is seen in slight overlap with the anterior surfaces of the femoral condyles.

15. True or false. The patella should be seen in profile.

16. True or false. The bony trabecular detail of the femoral condyles should be demonstrated.

17. Identify each lettered structure shown in Fig. 7.30.

    A. _____

    B. _____

    C. _____

    D. _____

    E. _____

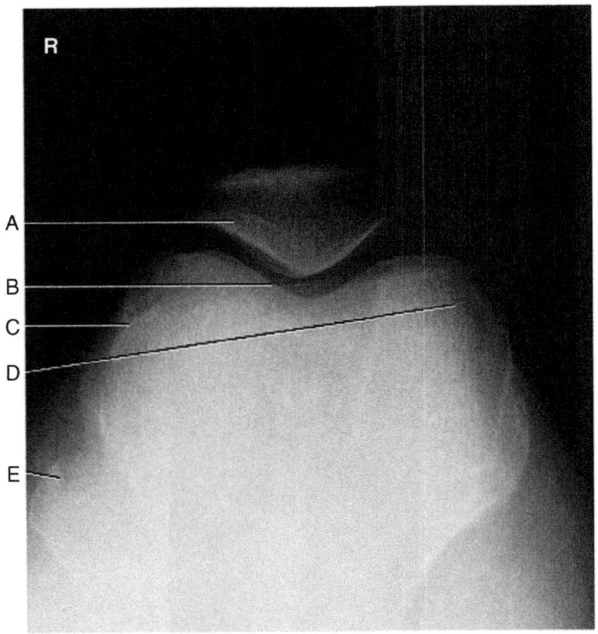

Fig. 7.30 Tangential patella, Settegast method.

Section 2: Exercise 9: Positioning for the Femur

This exercise pertains to the essential projection of the femur. Identify structures, fill in missing words, provide a short answer, choose the correct answer from a list, or choose true or false (explaining any statement you believe to be false) for each item.

1. List the essential projections for the femur, and describe the positioning steps used for each. Be sure to include how to position for the proximal and distal portions of the femur. Use the following format.

Essential projection: _____
- Size of collimated field:

- Key patient/part positioning points:

- Anatomic landmarks and relation to IR:

- CR orientation and entrance point:

Essential projection: _____
- Size of collimated field:

- Key patient/part positioning points:

- Anatomic landmarks and relation to IR:

- CR orientation and entrance point:

Items 2 to 8 pertain to the *AP projection.*

2. How many degrees and in which direction should the lower extremity be rotated to demonstrate the proximal femur?
   a. 3 to 5 degrees medially
   b. 10 to 15 degrees medially
   c. 3 to 5 degrees laterally
   d. 10 to 15 degrees laterally

3. Why should the lower extremity be rotated?

4. How should the femoral neck appear in the AP projection of the proximal femur?

5. Describe how the lesser trochanter should appear in the AP projection of the proximal femur.

6. What portion of an orthopedic appliance should be demonstrated on the image?

7. True or false. Gonadal shielding should not be used because it may superimpose the femoral head.

8. Identify each lettered structure shown in Fig. 7.31.

A. _____

B. _____

C. _____

D. _____

E. _____

F. _____

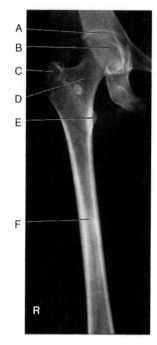

Fig. 7.31 AP proximal femur.

Items 9 to 15 pertain to the *lateral projection*.

9. How should the pelvis be positioned to demonstrate the proximal femur?
   a. True lateral
   b. From true lateral, the pelvis should be rolled anteriorly about 10 to 15 degrees
   c. From true lateral, the pelvis should be rolled posteriorly about 10 to 15 degrees

10. How should the pelvis be positioned to demonstrate the distal femur?
    a. True lateral
    b. From true lateral, the pelvis should be rolled anteriorly about 10 to 15 degrees
    c. From true lateral, the pelvis should be rolled posteriorly about 10 to 15 degrees

11. Concerning IR placement/collimated field location, (a) to what level on the patient should the upper border of an IR or collimated field be placed when demonstrating the proximal femur, and (b) to what level of the patient should the lower border of the IR or collimated field be placed when demonstrating the distal femur?

12. Concerning the placement of the unaffected (uppermost) extremity, (a) where should it be placed when demonstrating the proximal femur, and (b) where should it be placed when demonstrating the distal femur?

13. When demonstrating the distal femur and including the knee, how many degrees should the knee be flexed?

14. From the following list, circle the four evaluation criteria that indicate the femur was correctly positioned when including the knee in a lateral projection of the distal femur.
    a. The patella should be seen in profile.
    b. The patella should superimpose the femur.
    c. The patellofemoral joint space should be open.
    d. The greater trochanter should be seen in profile.
    e. The anterior surface of the femoral condyles should be superimposed.
    f. The inferior surface of the femoral condyles should not be superimposed.

15. Identify each lettered structure shown in Fig. 7.32.

    A. _____

    B. _____

    C. _____

    D. _____

    E. _____

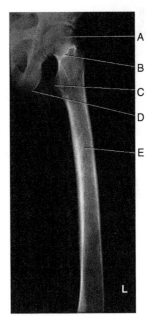

Fig. 7.32 Lateral proximal femur.

Section 2: Exercise 10: Lower Extremity Image Evaluation

This exercise consists of images of the lower extremity to give you practice in evaluating extremity positioning. These images are not from Merrill's Atlas. Each image shows at least one positioning error. Examine each image and answer the questions that follow by providing a short answer or choosing the correct answer from a list.

1. Fig. 7.33 shows an AP oblique projection image of the toes. Examine the image and state why it does not meet the evaluation criteria for this projection.

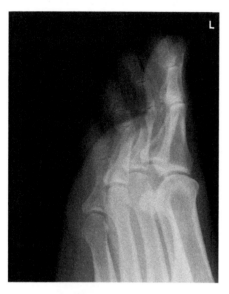

Fig. 7.33 AP oblique toes with improper positioning.

Fig. 7.34 is an inferior-quality AP projection of the ankle. Examine the image and answer the questions that follow.

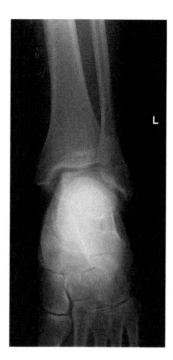

Fig. 7.34 AP ankle with improper positioning.

2. Explain why the image does not meet the evaluation criteria for this projection.

3. What positioning error most likely produced this image?

4. Fig. 7.35 is an AP oblique projection image of inferior quality demonstrating the mortise joint. Examine the image and state why it does not meet the evaluation criteria for this projection.

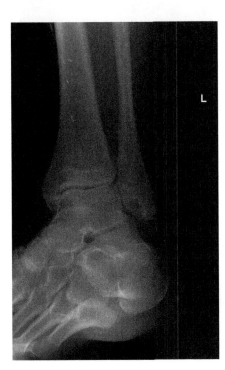

Fig. 7.35 AP oblique ankle, medial rotation, with improper positioning.

Fig. 7.36 is a lateral projection image of the knee that does not meet all of the evaluation criteria. Examine the image and answer the questions that follow.

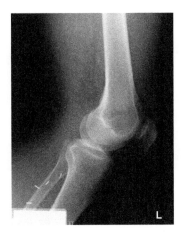

Fig. 7.36 Lateral knee with improper positioning.

5. From the following list, circle the three evaluation criteria for lateral projections that this image does not meet.
   a. The femoropatellar space should be open.
   b. The femoral condyles should be superimposed.
   c. The knee should be flexed approximately 20 to 30 degrees.
   d. The fibular head and tibia should be slightly super-imposed.
   e. The joint space between femoral condyles and tibia should be open.

6. What central ray angulation was most likely used to make this image? Explain your answer.

7. Fig. 7.37 is a lateral projection of the foot with an error. Examine this image and explain why it does not meet the evaluation criteria for this projection.

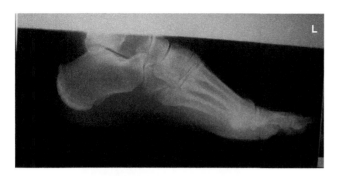

Fig. 7.37 Lateral foot with error.

8. Before making the exposure for Fig. 7.37, what should the radiographer have done to prevent this error?

Fig. 7.38 is a lateral projection of the ankle with improper positioning. Examine this image and answer the questions that follow.

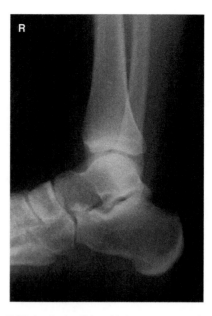

Fig. 7.38 Lateral ankle with improper positioning.

9. State why this image does not meet the evaluation criteria for this projection.

10. Explain what positioning maneuver would correct the error.

POSITIONING OF THE LONG BONE MEASUREMENT

Section 3: Exercise 1: Positioning for Long Bone Measurement

Answer the following questions by selecting the best choice.

1. List imaging methods used to evaluate extremity length discrepancy.

2. What area of the body is more frequently imaged for long bone measurement?

3. How many exposures should be made of each extremity?

4. Why might movement by the patient cause the examination need to be repeated?

5. What type of projection should be performed?

6. With reference to the affected lower extremity, where should the metal ruler be placed when only one extremity is imaged?

7. If the right side is shorter than the left side, which side should be imaged?

8. Identify the centering point for each of the following joints:

   a. Hip: _____

   b. Knee: _____

   c. Ankle: _____

9. Why does orthoroentgenography produce more accurate long bone measurements than single-exposure examinations?

10. How is bone length determined with orthoroentgenography?

11. For simultaneous bilateral projections of lower extremities, where should the central ray be directed for each exposure?

12. What body plane of the patient should be centered on the table for simultaneous bilateral projections of the lower extremities?

217

13. With reference to the lower extremities, where should the metal ruler be placed when both lower extremities are simultaneously imaged?

14. How many times should the patient be positioned when simultaneous bilateral projections of the lower extremities are made?

15. For simultaneous bilateral projections of the lower extremities, what procedure should be performed to correct an examination when bones of different lengths cause bilateral distortion?

16. List two advantages that obtaining long bone measurements with computed tomography has over the conventional radiographic approach.

17. How many exposures are taken when performing a teleoroentgenogram?

18. What is the primary difference when performing an orthoroentgenogram versus a scanogram?

19. Describe the recommended order in which the exposures are performed during an orthoroentgenogram technique.

20. During digital imaging, what is the term that describes the post-processing of three images into a single image of the entire extremity?

Answer the following questions by selecting the best choice.

1. How many and what kind of bones comprise the foot and ankle?
   a. 14 phalanges, 5 metatarsals, and 7 tarsals
   b. 14 phalanges, 7 metatarsals, and 5 tarsals
   c. 7 phalanges, 5 metatarsals, and 14 tarsals
   d. 7 phalanges, 14 metatarsals, and 5 tarsals

2. Which bone classification are tarsals?
   a. Flat
   b. Long
   c. Short
   d. Irregular

3. What is the most distal part of a metatarsal?
   a. Base
   b. Head
   c. Tuberosity
   d. Styloid process

4. Where in the foot is the tuberosity that is easily palpable?
   a. Distal portion of the first metatarsal
   b. Distal portion of the fifth metatarsal
   c. Proximal portion of the first metatarsal
   d. Proximal portion of the fifth metatarsal

5. Which tarsal bone is the most superior tarsal bone?
   a. Talus
   b. Cuboid
   c. Navicular
   d. Calcaneus

6. Which tarsal bone is the largest of the tarsal bones?
   a. Talus
   b. Cuboid
   c. Navicular
   d. Calcaneus

7. Which tarsal bone is located on the lateral side of the foot between the calcaneus and the fourth and fifth metatarsals?
   a. Talus
   b. Cuboid
   c. Navicular
   d. Lateral cuneiform

8. Which tarsal bone is located on the medial side of the foot between the talus and the three cuneiforms?
   a. Talus
   b. Cuboid
   c. Navicular
   d. Calcaneus

9. Which bone articulates medially with the cuboid?
   a. First metatarsal
   b. Medial cuneiform
   c. Intermediate cuneiform
   d. Lateral cuneiform

10. Which bones comprise the midfoot?
    a. Talus and cuboid
    b. Talus and calcaneus
    c. Metatarsals and toes
    d. Navicular, cuboid, and cuneiforms

11. Which bone articulates with the superior surface of the calcaneus?
    a. Tibia
    b. Talus
    c. Fibula
    d. Navicular

12. Which bones articulate distally with the tarsal navicular?
    a. Phalanges
    b. Cuneiforms
    c. Metatarsals
    d. Talus and calcaneus

13. Which bones articulate distally with the three cuneiforms?
    a. Navicular
    b. Phalanges
    c. Metatarsals
    d. Talus and calcaneus

14. Which bones articulate with the metatarsals?
    a. Calcaneus and cuboid
    b. Calcaneus and navicular
    c. Cuneiforms and cuboid
    d. Cuneiforms and navicular

15. Which cuneiform is the largest cuneiform?
    a. Medial
    b. Intermediate
    c. Third
    d. Later

16. Where in the foot are the cuneiforms located?
    a. Between the cuboid and the calcaneus
    b. Between the cuboid and the metatarsals
    c. Between the navicular and the calcaneus
    d. Between the navicular and the metatarsals

17. Which articulation is an ellipsoid-type joint?
    a. Intertarsal
    b. Interphalangeal
    c. Tarsometatarsal
    d. Metatarsophalangeal

219

18. Which articulation of the foot is a gliding-type joint?
    a. Mortise
    b. Intertarsal
    c. Interphalangeal
    d. Tarsometatarsal

19. Which two tarsal bones articulate with each other by way of three facets?
    a. Talus and cuboid
    b. Talus and calcaneus
    c. Navicular and cuboid
    d. Navicular and calcaneus

20. Which part of the talus articulates with the distal tibia?
    a. Styloid
    b. Tubercle
    c. Trochlea
    d. Epicondyle

21. Which type of joint is the ankle joint?
    a. Hinge
    b. Gliding
    c. Ellipsoid
    d. Ball-and-socket

22. Where is the medial malleolus located in the leg?
    a. Distal tibia
    b. Distal fibula
    c. Proximal tibia
    d. Proximal fibula

23. Where is the lateral malleolus located in the leg?
    a. Distal tibia
    b. Distal fibula
    c. Proximal tibia
    d. Proximal fibula

24. What structure is located on the proximal end of the fibula?
    a. Base
    b. Apex
    c. Tuberosity
    d. Trochanter

25. Where is the intercondylar eminence located?
    a. Distal tibia
    b. Distal femur
    c. Proximal tibia
    d. Proximal femur

26. Where are the tibial plateaus located?
    a. Distal tibia
    b. Distal femur
    c. Proximal tibia
    d. Proximal femur

27. On which border of the tibia is the crest located?
    a. Lateral
    b. Medial
    c. Anterior
    d. Posterior

28. Which term refers to the sharp ridge on the anterior border of the tibia?
    a. Apex
    b. Crest
    c. Tubercle
    d. Eminence

29. Which term refers to the prominent process on the anterior surface of the proximal tibia that is just inferior to the condyles?
    a. Apex
    b. Styloid
    c. Eminence
    d. Tuberosity

30. Which joint is formed by the articulation of the head of the fibula with the lateral condyle of the tibia?
    a. Knee
    b. Ankle
    c. Distal tibiofibular
    d. Proximal tibiofibular

31. Which type of joint is the proximal tibiofibular joint?
    a. Hinge
    b. Gliding
    c. Ellipsoid
    d. Ball-and-socket

32. Which structure is located on the head of the fibula?
    a. Apex
    b. Condyle
    c. Lateral malleolus
    d. Medial malleolus

33. With which structure does the head of the fibula articulate?
    a. Lateral malleolus
    b. Medial malleolus
    c. Lateral tibial condyle
    d. Medial tibial condyle

34. Which term refers to the inferior tip of the patella?
    a. Base
    b. Apex
    c. Styloid
    d. Tubercle

35. Which part of the patella is the base?
    a. Apex
    b. Lateral border
    c. Medial border
    d. Superior border

36. Where on the femur is the greater trochanter located?
    a. Lateral and inferior
    b. Lateral and superior
    c. Medial and inferior
    d. Medial and superior

37. Where on the femur is the lesser trochanter located?
    a. Lateral and anterior
    b. Lateral and posterior
    c. Medial and anterior
    d. Medial and posterior

38. Where is the fovea capitis located?
    a. Distal tibia
    b. Distal femur
    c. Proximal tibia
    d. Proximal femur

39. Where is the intercondylar fossa located?
    a. Distal tibia
    b. Distal femur
    c. Proximal tibia
    d. Proximal femur

40. Which femoral structures articulate with the tibia?
    a. Condyles
    b. Tubercles
    c. Trochanters
    d. Epicondyles

41. With which structure does the head of the femur articulate?
    a. Condyle
    b. Trochanter
    c. Epicondyle
    d. Acetabulum

42. How many degrees and in what direction should the central ray be directed for the AP axial projection of the toes?
    a. 10 degrees caudad (toward the toes)
    b. 10 degrees cephalad (toward the heel)
    c. 15 degrees caudad (toward the toes)
    d. 15 degrees cephalad (toward the heel)

43. How many degrees and in what direction should the foot be rotated for the AP oblique projection to demonstrate the second toe?
    a. 15 to 25 degrees medially
    b. 15 to 25 degrees laterally
    c. 30 to 45 degrees medially
    d. 30 to 45 degrees laterally

44. How and toward what centering point should the central ray be directed for the AP oblique projection to demonstrate all five toes?
    a. Perpendicular to the proximal interphalangeal (PIP) joint of the third digit
    b. Perpendicular to the third metatarsophalangeal joint
    c. 15 degrees posterior (toward the heel) to the PIP of the third digit
    d. 15 degrees posterior (toward the heel) to the third metatarsophalangeal joint

45. How many degrees and in what direction should the foot be rotated for the AP oblique projection for the best demonstration of the great toe?
    a. 10 to 15 degrees medially
    b. 10 to 15 degrees laterally
    c. 30 to 45 degrees medially
    d. 30 to 45 degrees laterally

46. What other projection term refers to the AP projection of the foot?
    a. Plantodorsal
    b. Dorsoplantar
    c. Inferosuperior
    d. Superoinferior

47. How many degrees and in what direction should the central ray be directed for the AP axial projection of the foot?
    a. 10 degrees caudad (toward the toes)
    b. 10 degrees cephalad (toward the heel)
    c. 15 degrees caudad (toward the toes)
    d. 15 degrees cephalad (toward the heel)

48. Which projection of the foot best demonstrates the cuboid and its articulations?
    a. Lateral
    b. Dorsoplantar
    c. AP oblique (lateral rotation)
    d. AP oblique (medial rotation)

49. How many degrees and in what direction should the foot be rotated for the AP oblique projection of the foot?
    a. 15 degrees laterally
    b. 30 degrees medially
    c. 45 degrees laterally
    d. 45 degrees medially

221

50. What is the appropriate collimated field size for the AP projection of the foot?
   a. 1 inch (2.5 cm) on all sides of the foot shadow, including 1 inch (2.5 cm) superior to the medial malleolus
   b. 1 inch (2.5 cm) of all sides, including 1 inch (2.5 cm) beyond the calcaneus and distal tips of the toes
   c. 1 inch (2.5 cm) past the posterior and inferior heel shadow, including the medial malleolus and fifth metatarsal
   d. 10 inches wide by 12 inches long (25 cm wide by 30 cm long)

51. Where should the central ray be directed for the AP oblique projection of the foot?
   a. To the base of the third metatarsal
   b. To the head of the third metatarsal
   c. To the metatarsophalangeal joint of the third digit
   d. To the proximal interphalangeal joint of the third digit

52. Regardless of the condition of the patient, which positioning maneuver should be performed to position the foot for the lateral projection?
   a. Plantar flex the foot.
   b. Rotate the leg laterally until the knee is against the table.
   c. Ensure that the plantar surface is in contact with the IR.
   d. Ensure that the plantar surface is perpendicular to the IR.

53. How should the central ray be directed for the best demonstration of the tarsometatarsal joint spaces of the midfoot for the AP projection of the foot?
   a. Perpendicularly
   b. 10 degrees posteriorly (toward the heel)
   c. 15 degrees posteriorly (toward the heel)
   d. 20 degrees posteriorly (toward the heel)

54. Which projection of the foot best demonstrates the sinus tarsi?
   a. AP projection
   b. Lateral projection
   c. AP oblique projection (lateral rotation)
   d. AP oblique projection (medial rotation)

55. Which projection of the foot best demonstrates most of the tarsals with the least amount of superimposition?
   a. AP projection
   b. Lateral projection
   c. AP oblique projection (lateral rotation)
   d. AP oblique projection (medial rotation)

56. Which projection of the foot best demonstrates the bases of the fourth and fifth metatarsals free from superimposition?
   a. AP projection
   b. Lateral projection
   c. AP oblique projection (lateral rotation)
   d. AP oblique projection (medial rotation)

57. Which projection of the foot should demonstrate the metatarsals nearly superimposed on each other?
   a. AP projection
   b. Lateral projection
   c. AP oblique projection (lateral rotation)
   d. AP oblique projection (medial rotation)

58. Which two projections comprise the typical series that best demonstrates the calcaneus?
   a. AP (dorsoplantar) and lateral projections
   b. AP (dorsoplantar) and medial oblique projections
   c. Axial (plantodorsal) and lateral projections
   d. Axial (plantodorsal) and medial oblique projections

59. How many degrees and in what direction should the central ray be directed for the axial (plantodorsal) projection of the calcaneus?
   a. 10 degrees caudad
   b. 10 degrees cephalad
   c. 40 degrees caudad
   d. 40 degrees cephalad

60. What procedural compensation is required for the plantodorsal axial projection of the calcaneus when the patient cannot dorsiflex the foot sufficiently to place the plantar surface vertical?
   a. Elevate the leg on sandbags to achieve the correct position.
   b. Refer the patient to CT.
   c. Decrease the angle of the central ray.
   d. Reverse the angle of the central ray.

61. At which level on the plantar surface should the central ray enter the foot for the axial (plantodorsal) projection of the calcaneus?
   a. Midpoint of the calcaneus
   b. Tuberosity of the calcaneus
   c. Base of the third metatarsal
   d. Head of the third metatarsal

62. Where should the central ray be directed for the lateral projection of the calcaneus?
   a. Toward the midpoint of the foot
   b. Toward the midpoint of the calcaneus
   c. Toward the base of the third metatarsal
   d. Toward the head of the third metatarsal

63. Where should the central ray enter for the lateral projection of the ankle?
    a. At the lateral malleolus
    b. At the medial malleolus
    c. At the midpoint of the calcaneus
    d. At the base of the third metatarsal

64. How many degrees and in which direction should the foot and leg be rotated for the best demonstration of the mortise joint for the AP oblique projection of the ankle?
    a. 15 to 20 degrees laterally
    b. 15 to 20 degrees medially
    c. 40 to 45 degrees laterally
    d. 40 to 45 degrees medially

65. Which projection of the ankle best demonstrates the talofibular joint space free from bony superimposition?
    a. AP projection
    b. Lateral projection
    c. AP oblique projection (lateral rotation)
    d. AP oblique projection (medial rotation)

66. Which articulation should be seen in profile with the AP oblique projection (medial rotation) of the ankle?
    a. Subtalar
    b. Tibiofibular
    c. Talocalcaneal
    d. Distal tibiofibular

67. With reference to the plane of the IR, how should the malleoli be positioned for the AP oblique projection of the ankle for the best demonstration of the mortise joint spaces open?
    a. Parallel
    b. Perpendicular
    c. 45 degrees lateral rotation
    d. 45 degrees medial rotation

68. Which projection of the ankle should be performed for the best demonstration of a ligamentous tear?
    a. AP projection with inversion
    b. AP projection with dorsiflexion
    c. AP oblique projection (lateral rotation)
    d. AP oblique projection (medial rotation)

69. How long should the collimated field be for the AP and AP oblique projections of the ankle?
    a. 1 inch (2.5 cm) above and below the malleoli
    b. 3 inches (7.6 cm) above and below the malleoli
    c. 8 inches (20 cm)
    d. 10 inches (25 cm)

70. Which projection of the knee best demonstrates the femorotibial joint space open if the patient measures more than 10 inches (24 cm) between the ASIS and the tabletop?
    a. AP oblique projection (medial rotation)
    b. AP projection with perpendicular central ray
    c. AP projection with the central ray angled 3 to 5 degrees caudad
    d. AP projection with the central ray angled 3 to 5 degrees cephalad

71. For the lateral projection of the knee, how many degrees should the knee be flexed?
    a. 10 to 20 degrees
    b. 20 to 30 degrees
    c. 30 to 40 degrees
    d. 40 to 50 degrees

72. How many degrees of angulation should be formed between the femur and the radiographic table for the PA axial projection (Holmblad method) of the knee?
    a. 20 degrees
    b. 45 degrees
    c. 70 degrees
    d. 90 degrees

73. Which of the following projections of the knee best demonstrates the intercondylar fossa?
    a. AP projection
    b. Lateral projection
    c. AP oblique projection (medial rotation)
    d. PA axial projection (Holmblad method)

74. How many degrees and in what direction should the central ray be directed for the lateral projection of the knee?
    a. Perpendicular
    b. 5 to 7 degrees caudad
    c. 5 to 7 degrees cephalad
    d. 10 degrees cephalad

75. Which structure of the knee is best demonstrated with the tangential projection?
    a. Patella
    b. Intercondylar fossa
    c. Joint space of the knee
    d. Intercondylar eminence

76. Which structure of the knee is best demonstrated with the PA axial projection (the Holmblad method)?
    a. Patella
    b. Tibial crest
    c. Tibiofibular articulation
    d. Femoral intercondylar fossa

77. Which projection of the knee best demonstrates the proximal tibiofibular articulation without bony superimposition?
   a. AP projection
   b. Lateral projection
   c. AP oblique projection (lateral rotation)
   d. AP oblique projection (medial rotation)

78. Which projection of the knee best demonstrates the femoropatellar space open?
   a. Lateral projection
   b. AP oblique projection (lateral rotation)
   c. AP oblique projection (medial rotation)
   d. PA axial projection (Holmblad method)

79. Which of the following evaluation criteria indicates that the knee is properly positioned for a lateral projection?
   a. The femoral condyles are superimposed.
   b. The proximal tibiofibular articulation is open.
   c. The patella is parallel with the IR.
   d. The femoral condyles are parallel with the IR.

80. What should be done to prevent the knee joint space from being obscured by the magnified shadow of the medial femoral condyle when the lateral projection of the knee is performed?
   a. Use foam wedges to support the leg.
   b. Direct the central ray perpendicularly.
   c. Direct the central ray 5 to 7 degrees cephalad.
   d. Decrease the SID.

81. Which of the following evaluation criteria indicates that the knee is properly positioned for the AP projection?
   a. The femorotibial joint space is open.
   b. The femoral condyles are perpendicular.
   c. The proximal tibiofibular articulation is open.
   d. The patella is perpendicular to the IR.

82. Where should the patella be demonstrated on the image of the AP oblique projection of the knee with medial rotation?
   a. Over the lateral condyle of the femur
   b. Over the medial condyle of the femur
   c. Centered between the femoral condyles
   d. Superimposed with the tibiofibular articulation

83. Where should the patella be demonstrated on the image of the AP oblique projection of the knee with lateral rotation?
   a. Over the lateral femoral condyle
   b. Over the medial femoral condyle
   c. Centered between the femoral condyles
   d. Superimposed with the femorotibial joint

84. For the lateral projection of the patella, which positioning maneuver reduces the femoropatellar joint space?
   a. Straightening the leg
   b. Superimposing the tibial condyles
   c. Superimposing the femoral condyles
   d. Flexing the knee more than 10 degrees

85. Which area of the knee should the central ray enter for the PA axial projection (Holmblad method)?
   a. Anterior
   b. Posterior
   c. Lateral condyle
   d. Medial condyle

86. Which of the following projections of the knee best demonstrates the femoral intercondylar fossa?
   a. AP projection
   b. Lateral projection
   c. AP oblique projection (medial rotation)
   d. PA axial projection (Camp-Coventry method)

87. Which projection of the knee should be used to demonstrate the patella completely superimposed on the femur?
   a. AP projection
   b. Lateral projection
   c. AP oblique projection (lateral rotation)
   d. AP oblique projection (medial rotation)

88. Which projection of the knee should be used to demonstrate the patella in profile?
   a. AP projection
   b. Lateral projection
   c. AP oblique projection (lateral rotation)
   d. AP oblique projection (medial rotation)

89. For a patient prone on the radiographic table with the knee centered to the midline and the knee flexed until the lower leg forms a 40-degree angle with the table, how should the central ray be directed to demonstrate the femoral intercondylar fossa?
   a. Caudally 3 to 5 degrees
   b. Cephalically 3 to 5 degrees
   c. Caudally 40 degrees
   d. Cephalically 40 degrees

90. For which projection of the knee should the patient be prone on the table, with the knee flexed until the leg forms an angle of 40 degrees with the table, and the central ray directed perpendicular to the long axis of the leg, entering the back side of the knee?
   a. Tangential projection (Settegast method)
   b. Tangential projection (Hughston method)
   c. PA axial projection (Holmblad method)
   d. PA axial projection (Camp-Coventry method)

91. How should the central ray be directed for the bilateral weight-bearing AP projection of the knees?
    a. Perpendicularly
    b. Caudally 3 to 5 degrees
    c. Cephalically 3 to 5 degrees
    d. Cephalically 10 degrees

92. Which projection of the knee can be accomplished with the patient upright, the affected knee flexed and its anterior surface in contact with a vertically placed IR, and the horizontally directed central ray entering the posterior aspect of the knee?
    a. Tangential projection (Settegast method)
    b. AP projection, weight-bearing
    c. PA axial projection (Holmblad method)
    d. PA axial projection (Camp-Coventry method)

93. Which positioning factor determines the number of degrees the central ray should be angled for the tangential projection (Settegast method) to demonstrate the patella?
    a. Part thickness
    b. Degree of knee flexion
    c. Object-to-image distance
    d. SID

94. How should the central ray be directed for the AP projection of the femur?
    a. Perpendicularly
    b. Caudally 3 to 5 degrees
    c. Cephalically 3 to 5 degrees
    d. Cephalically 15 degrees

95. Which positioning maneuver should be performed to place the femoral neck in profile for the AP projection of the proximal femur?
    a. Flex the lower extremity.
    b. Rotate the lower extremity laterally 10 to 15 degrees.
    c. Rotate the lower extremity medially 10 to 15 degrees.
    d. Elevate the unaffected side of the pelvis 10 to 15 degrees.

96. Which positioning maneuver should be performed to prevent the femoral neck from appearing foreshortened in the AP projection of the proximal femur?
    a. Angle the central ray 10 to 15 degrees caudad.
    b. Angle the central ray 10 to 15 degrees cephalad.
    c. Rotate the lower extremity laterally 10 to 15 degrees.
    d. Rotate the lower extremity medially 10 to 15 degrees.

97. For the AP projection of the femur on typical adults, what should be done to ensure that both joints of the femur are demonstrated?
    a. Rotate the lower extremity laterally 15 degrees.
    b. Increase the SID.
    c. Use lead masking to divide the IR in half.
    d. Perform a second exposure with another IR.

98. For which lower extremity projection should the lower extremity be rotated medially 10 to 15 degrees?
    a. AP projection of the proximal femur
    b. AP projection of the distal femur
    c. AP oblique projection of the foot (medial rotation)
    d. AP oblique projection of the knee (medial rotation)

99. For which lower extremity projection should the pelvis be rotated 10 to 15 degrees from true lateral?
    a. AP projection of the distal femur
    b. AP projection of the proximal femur
    c. Lateral projection of the distal femur
    d. Lateral projection of the proximal femur

100. For the lateral projection of the femur, how should the pelvis be positioned to demonstrate only the knee joint with the distal femoral shaft?
    a. True lateral
    b. From supine, unaffected side elevated 15 degrees
    c. From true lateral, rotated anteriorly 10 to 15 degrees
    d. From true lateral, rotated posteriorly 10 to 15 degrees

101. What is the purpose of orthoroentgenography?
    a. To measure the length of long bones
    b. To identify the location of a foreign body
    c. To measure the calcium content of long bones
    d. To measure the length of the vertebral column

102. Which parameters should be moved when exposures for long bone measurement are made?
    a. X-ray tube and patient
    b. X-ray tube and IR
    c. Metal ruler and patient
    d. Metal ruler and IR

103. Which special device must be used for long bone measurement examinations?
    a. Leg brace
    b. Metal ruler
    c. Wedge filter
    d. Upright IR holder

104. For exposures made at the knee joint, the central ray should be directed to which of the following levels?
   a. Tibial tuberosity
   b. Base of the patella
   c. Widest point of the femoral epicondyles
   d. Depression between the femoral and tibial condyles

105. For orthoroentgenography, how many exposures should be made of each extremity?
   a. One
   b. Two
   c. Three
   d. Four

106. For simultaneous bilateral projections of the lower extremities, how many exposures should be made?
   a. Two
   b. Three
   c. Four
   d. Six

107. Which procedure must be performed to ensure accuracy in long bone measurement examinations?
   a. Use the smaller focal spot size.
   b. Do not move the extremities between exposures.
   c. Make all exposures with the patient upright.
   d. Use a SID of 72 inches (183 cm).

108. Long bone measurement may be accomplished by which of the following?
   1. MRI
   2. Microdose DR
   3. Nuclear Medicine
   4. US
   5. CT

   a. 1, 2, 3, 5
   b. 1, 2, 3, 4
   c. 2, 3, 4, 5
   d. 1, 2, 4, 5

8 Pelvis and Hip

CHAPTER 8: SECTION 1

OSTEOLOGY AND ARTHROLOGY OF THE PELVIS, HIP, AND PROXIMAL FEMORA

Section 1: Exercise 1

Identify each lettered structure shown in Fig. 8.1.

A. ______________________________

B. ______________________________

C. ______________________________

D. ______________________________

E. ______________________________

F. ______________________________

G. ______________________________

H. ______________________________

I. ______________________________

J. ______________________________

K. ______________________________

L. ______________________________

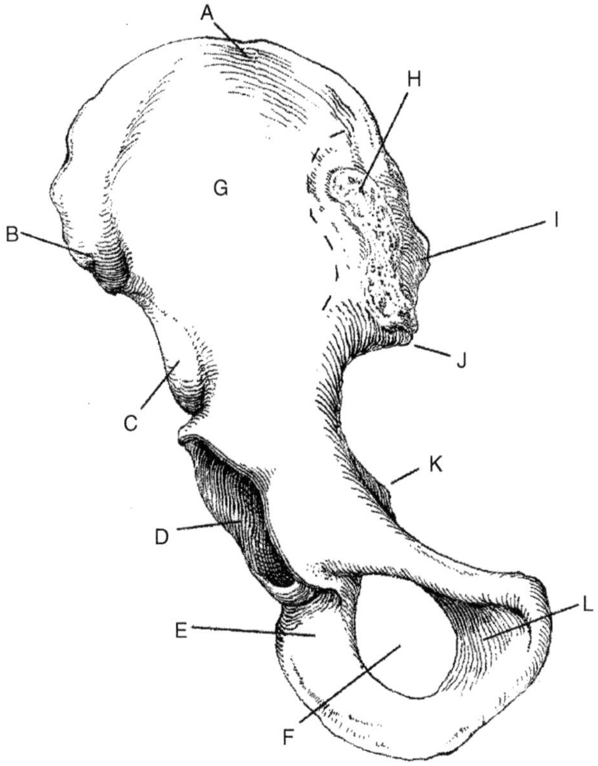

Fig. 8.1 Anterior aspect of the right os coxae (hip bone).

Section 1: Exercise 2

Identify each lettered structure shown in Fig. 8.2.

A. _____

B. _____

C. _____

D. _____

E. _____

F. _____

G. _____

H. _____

I. _____

J. _____

K. _____

L. _____

M. _____

N. _____

O. _____

P. _____

Q. _____

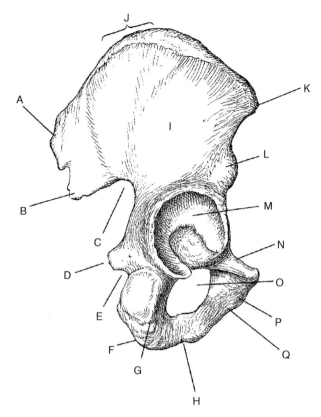

Fig. 8.2 Lateral aspect of the right os coxae (hip bone).

Section 1: Exercise 3

Identify each lettered structure shown in Fig. 8.3.

A. _____

B. _____

C. _____

D. _____

E. _____

F. _____

G. _____

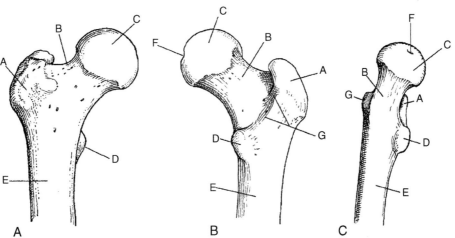

Fig. 8.3 Three views of the proximal femur. (A) Anterior view. (B) Posterior view. (C) View of the medial aspect.

Section 1: Exercise 4

Identify each lettered structure shown in Fig. 8.4.

A. _____

B. _____

C. _____

D. _____

E. _____

F. _____

G. _____

H. _____

I. _____

J. _____

K. _____

L. _____

M. _____

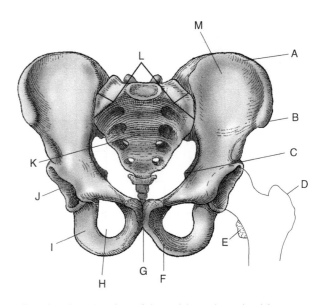

Fig. 8.4 Anterior view of the pelvis and proximal femora.

Use the following clues to complete the crossword puzzle. All answers refer to the bones and joints of the pelvis.

Across

2. Femoral process
4. Serves as a base for the trunk
8. Inferior process
9. Posterior pelvic articulations
13. Large opening
14. Ridgelike process
16. Hip bone
18. Projects from the pubic bone

Down

1. Superior process
3. Hip socket
5. Articulation
6. Forms posterior aspect of pelvis
7. Found above the acetabulum
10. Opening in bone
11. Articulates with the sacrum
12. Has a body and two rami
15. Sharp bony process
17. Winglike portion of ilium

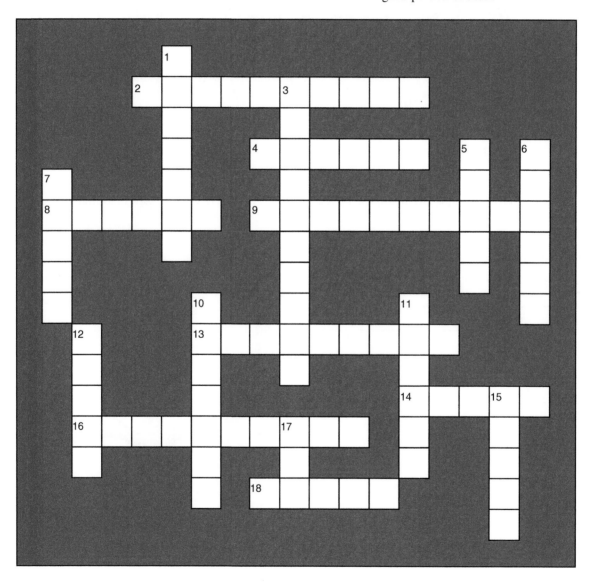

Section 1: Exercise 6

Match the pathology terms in Column A with the appropriate definition in Column B. Not all choices from Column B should be selected.

Column A

_____ 1. Osteoporosis

_____ 2. Osteopetrosis

_____ 3. Osteoarthritis

_____ 4. Paget disease

_____ 5. Chondrosarcoma

_____ 6. Slipped epiphysis

_____ 7. Multiple myeloma

_____ 8. Ankylosing spondylitis

_____ 9. Congenital hip dysplasia

_____ 10. Legg-Calvé-Perthes disease

Column B

a. Loss of bone density

b. Benign tumor consisting of cartilage

c. Increased density of atypically soft bone

d. Malignant tumor arising from cartilage cells

e. Thick, soft bone marked by bowing and fractures

f. Flattening of the femoral head as a result of vascular interruption

g. Rheumatoid arthritis variant involving the sacroiliac (SI) joints and spine

h. Malformation of the acetabulum causing displacement of the femoral head

i. Proximal portion of femur dislocated from distal portion at the proximal epiphysis

j. Form of arthritis marked by progressive cartilage deterioration in synovial joints and vertebrae

k. Malignant neoplasm of plasma cells involving the bone marrow and causing destruction of bone

Section 1: Exercise 7

This exercise is a comprehensive review of the osteology and arthrology of the pelvis and the proximal femur. Fill in missing words, provide a short answer, select the answer from a list, or choose true or false (explaining any statement you believe to be false) for each item.

1. The structure of the body that serves as a base for the trunk and as a girdle for the attachment of the lower

   extremities is known as the _____.

2. Which bones form the pelvis?
   a. Two hip bones only
   b. Two hip bones and sacrum only
   c. Two hip bones, sacrum, and coccyx only
   d. Two hip bones, sacrum, coccyx, and femora

3. Which three names refer to the major bone that makes up the right or left half of the pelvis?
   a. Ilium, hip bone, and ischium
   b. Ilium, pubis, and innominate
   c. Os coxae, pubis, and ischium
   d. Ilium, pubis, and ischium

4. Which two prominent structures found on the ilium are frequently used as radiographic positioning reference points?
   a. Iliac crest and inferior superior iliac spine
   b. Iliac crest and anterior superior iliac spine (ASIS)
   c. Pubic symphysis and inferior superior iliac spine
   d. Pubic symphysis and ASIS

5. Which bone/portion of the hip bone consists of a body and two rami?
   a. Ala
   b. Ilium
   c. Pubis
   d. Ischium

6. Which bone/portion of the hip bone extends inferiorly from the acetabulum and joins with the inferior ramus of the pubic bone?
   a. Ilium
   b. Pubis
   c. Ischium
   d. Acetabulum

7. What part of the hip bone forms the broad, curved portion called the ala?

8. What bones of the hip bone form the obturator foramen?

9. What structure of the hip bone is formed by the fusion of three bones?

10. What structures form the posterior part of the pelvis?

11. Name the two parts a pelvis is divided into by the brim of the pelvis.

12. With reference to the brim of the pelvis, identify the location of the greater (false) pelvis and the lesser (true) pelvis as either "above" or "below."

    a. Greater pelvis: _____

    b. Lesser pelvis: _____

13. The region between the inlet and the outlet of the true pelvis is called the _____.

14. Which gender (male or female) has a pelvis with a larger and more rounded outlet?

15. Which gender (male or female) has a broader and shallower pelvis?

16. Which two large processes are located at the proximal end of the femur?
    a. Greater tubercle and lesser tubercle
    b. Greater tubercle and lesser trochanter
    c. Greater trochanter and lesser tubercle
    d. Greater trochanter and lesser trochanter

17. Which process is located at the superolateral aspect of the proximal femoral shaft?
    a. Lesser tubercle
    b. Lesser trochanter
    c. Greater tubercle
    d. Greater trochanter

18. Name the two areas of the proximal femur that are common sites for fractures in elderly patients.

19. In a typical adult, in which direction (anterior or posterior) does the femoral neck project away from the long axis of the femur?

20. Identify the major articulations of the pelvis by name or abbreviation, and give the quantity for each.

21. What are the two palpable bony points of localization for the hip joint?

22. Describe how to use the two points identified in question 21 to locate the femoral neck.

23. True or false. The greater sciatic notch is located on the anterior border of the ilium.

24. True or false. In the seated position, the weight of the body rests on two ischial tuberosities.

25. True or false. The highest point of the greater trochanter is in the same transverse plane as the midpoint of the hip joint.

POSITIONING OF THE PELVIS AND PROXIMAL FEMORA

Section 2: Exercise 1: Projections for the Pelvis and Femoral Necks

This exercise pertains to the essential projections of the pelvis and femoral necks. Provide a short answer, select the answer from a list, or identify structures for each item.

1. List the essential projections for the pelvis and femoral necks, and describe the positioning steps used for each, as follows:

   Essential projection: _____

   _____

   ■ Size of collimated field:

   ■ Key patient/part positioning points:

   ■ Anatomic landmarks and relation to IR:

   ■ CR orientation and entrance point:

   Essential projection: _____

   _____ (_____

   _____ method)

   ■ Size of collimated field:

   ■ Key patient/part positioning points:

   ■ Anatomic landmarks and relation to IR:

   ■ CR orientation and entrance point:

Questions 2 to 13 refer to the AP *projection* of the pelvis and proximal femora.

2. Describe how the patient's lower extremities should be positioned.

3. What is the rationale for positioning of the lower extremities?

4. How is rotation of the pelvis detected in an AP projection image?
   a. The lesser trochanters are well demonstrated if the pelvis is rotated.
   b. The femoral necks are seen in their entirety if the pelvis is rotated.
   c. The alae of the ilia are asymmetric if the pelvis is rotated.

5. Which plane of the body should be positioned on the midline of the table and grid?
   a. Horizontal
   b. Midsagittal
   c. Midcoronal

6. With reference to the patient, where should the IR be centered?

Chapter **8 Pelvis and Hip**

Examine the AP images in Figs. 8.5 and 8.6 and answer the questions that follow.

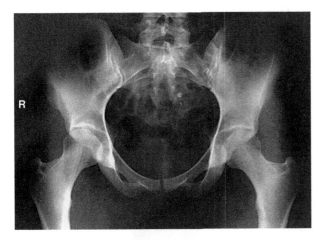

Fig. 8.5 AP pelvis.

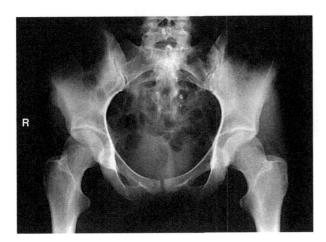

Fig. 8.6 AP pelvis.

7. Which structures in these two images appear different?

8. Which image demonstrates correct positioning of the proximal femora?

9. State the image characteristics that lead you to believe the patient was properly positioned for that image.

10. Describe how the lower extremities were positioned in Fig. 8.5.

11. Describe how the lower extremities were positioned in Fig. 8.6.

12. From the following list, circle the 11 evaluation criteria that indicate the pelvis was properly positioned for an AP projection.
    a. The iliac alae should be symmetric.
    b. The obturator foramina should be symmetric.
    c. The ischial spines should be equally demonstrated.
    d. The greater trochanters should be fully demonstrated.
    e. Both ilia should be equidistant to the edge of the image.
    f. The entire pelvis should be included along with the proximal femora.
    g. The sacrum and coccyx should be aligned with the pubic symphysis.
    h. The lower vertebral column should be centered to the middle of the image.
    i. Both greater trochanters should be equidistant to the edge of the image.
    j. Each greater trochanter should be seen superimposed with the femoral neck.
    k. The femoral necks should be demonstrated in their full extent without superimposition.
    l. The femoral necks should not be well demonstrated to their full extent because of superimposition.
    m. If seen, the lesser trochanters should be demonstrated on the lateral borders of the femora.
    n. If seen, the lesser trochanters should be demonstrated on the medial borders of the femora.

Chapter **8 Pelvis and Hip**

13. Identify each lettered structure shown in Fig. 8.7.

A. _____   F. _____

B. _____   G. _____

C. _____   H. _____

D. _____   I. _____

E. _____   J. _____

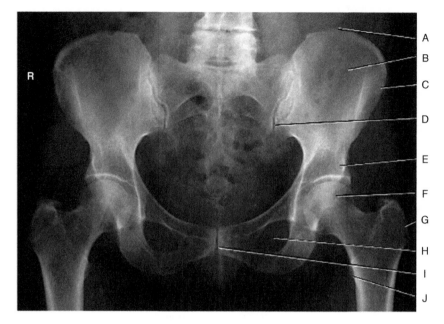

Fig. 8.7 AP pelvis.

Questions 14 to 25 pertain to the *AP oblique projection (modified Cleaves method)* of the femoral necks.

Examine Fig. 8.8 as you answer the following questions.

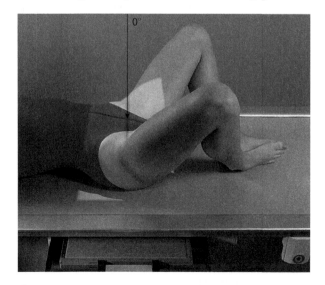

Fig. 8.8 AP oblique femoral necks, modified Cleaves method.

14. What other name commonly refers to the AP oblique projection, modified Cleaves method?

15. How much should the hips and knees be flexed?

16. After the patient's knees and hips are flexed, how many degrees from vertical should the thighs be abducted?

17. What is the purpose of abducting the thighs as required?

18. What breathing instructions should be given to the patient?

19. Describe how and where the central ray should be directed.

20. Where should each lesser trochanter appear in the image?
    a. Superimposed on the femur
    b. On the lateral side of the femur
    c. On the medial side of the femur

21. True or false. The patient may be positioned either supine or upright.

22. True or false. The gonads should not be shielded for the AP oblique projection.

23. True or false. The AP oblique projection should not be performed on a patient who is suspected to have a fractured femoral neck.

24. True or false. The greater trochanter should be seen in profile on the lateral side of the proximal femur.

25. True or false. This projection can be modified to demonstrate only one hip area.

Section 2: Exercise 2: Projections for Demonstrating the Hip

This exercise reviews the essential projections of the hip. Identify structures, provide a short answer, select from a list, or choose true or false (explaining any statement you believe to be false) for each item.

1. List the essential projections for the hip, and describe the positioning steps used for each, as follows:

   Essential projection: _____

   _____

   ■ Size of collimated field:

   ■ Key patient/part positioning points:

   ■ Anatomic landmarks and relation to IR:

   ■ CR orientation and entrance point:

   Essential projection: _____

   _____ (_____

   _____ method)
   ■ Size of collimated field:

   ■ Key patient/part positioning points:

- Anatomic landmarks and relation to IR:

- CR orientation and entrance point:

Essential projection: _____

_____ (_____

_____ method)
- Size of collimated field:

- Key patient/part positioning points:

- Anatomic landmarks and relation to IR:

- CR orientation and entrance point:

Examine Fig. 8.9 as you answer the following questions. Items 2 to 10 pertain to the *AP projection.*

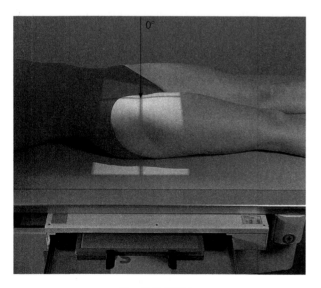

Fig. 8.9 AP hip.

2. Why should a radiographer ensure that the distance from the ASIS to the tabletop on each side of the pelvis is the same?
   a. To ensure that the pelvis is not rotated
   b. To align the midsagittal plane to the midline of the table
   c. To demonstrate the lesser trochanter beyond the medial border of the femur

3. Which positioning maneuver should be performed to place the femoral neck parallel with the plane of the IR?
   a. Abduct the femur laterally 15 to 20 degrees.
   b. Abduct the femur medially 15 to 20 degrees.
   c. Rotate the foot and lower extremity laterally 15 to 20 degrees.
   d. Rotate the foot and lower extremity medially 15 to 20 degrees.

4. What procedure should help the patient keep the affected lower leg in the required position?
   a. Place a compression band across the pelvis.
   b. Place a foam cushion or folded blanket under the pelvis.
   c. Place a support under the knee and a sandbag across the ankle.

5. Describe how to find the centering point where the central ray should enter the patient.

6. Which trochanter (greater or lesser) is not usually demonstrated beyond the border of the femur?

7. True or false. The entire pubis of the affected side should be demonstrated.

8. True or false. The exposure should be performed with the patient breathing shallowly.

9. True or false. An initial radiographic study of a fractured hip may include an AP projection of the pelvic girdle and proximal femora to demonstrate bilateral hip joints.

10. Identify each lettered structure shown in Fig. 8.10.

A. _____

B. _____

C. _____

D. _____

E. _____

F. _____

G. _____

H. _____

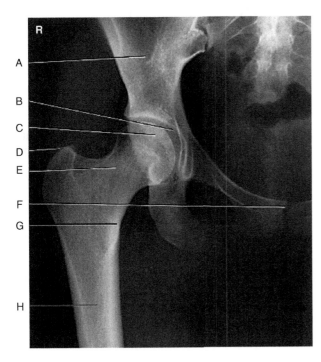

Fig. 8.10 AP hip.

Examine Fig. 8.11 as you answer the following questions. Items 11 to 16 pertain to the *Lauenstein method and Hickey method for lateral projections.*

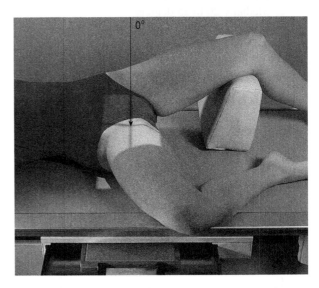

Fig. 8.11 Mediolateral hip, Lauenstein method.

11. A lateral projection image obtained by the Lauenstein method or the Hickey method is used to demonstrate the hip joint and the relationship of the head of the femur with the:
    a. Acetabulum
    b. Femoral shaft
    c. Greater trochanter

12. Describe how the affected thigh and leg should be positioned for lateral projections of the hip.

13. Describe how the unaffected lower extremity should be positioned.

14. How should the central ray be directed for the Lauenstein method of a lateral hip projection?
   a. Perpendicularly
   b. Caudally 20 to 25 degrees
   c. Medially 20 to 25 degrees
   d. Cephalically 20 to 25 degrees

15. How should the central ray be directed for the Hickey method of a lateral hip projection?
   a. Perpendicularly
   b. Caudally 20 to 25 degrees
   c. Medially 20 to 25 degrees
   d. Cephalically 20 to 25 degrees

16. Identify each lettered structure shown in Fig. 8.12.

   A. _____

   B. _____

   C. _____

   D. _____

   E. _____

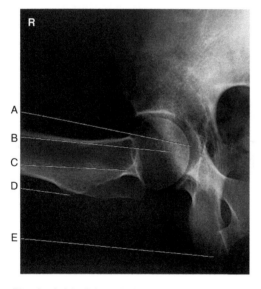

Fig. 8.12 Mediolateral hip, Lauenstein method.

Examine Fig. 8.13 as you answer the following questions. Items 17 to 30 pertain to the *axiolateral projection, Danelius-Miller method.*

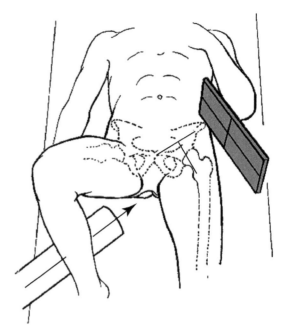

Fig. 8.13 Axiolateral hip, Danelius-Miller method.

17. List two common names used to denote the axiolateral projection (Danelius-Miller method) of the hip.

18. Describe an acceptable method for locating the femoral neck.

19. Why should a firm pillow or folded blanket be placed under the pelvis?

20. Describe how the unaffected lower extremity should be positioned.

21. Describe the placement of the IR.

22. Describe how and where the central ray should be directed.

23. With reference to the femoral neck, how should the lead strips of the grid be placed?
    a. Horizontally, parallel with the long axis of the femoral neck
    b. Vertically, perpendicular with the long axis of the femoral neck

24. What breathing instructions should be given to the patient?
    a. Breathe slowly and deeply.
    b. Stop breathing for the exposure.

25. What is the general rule concerning demonstration of any orthopedic appliance with this projection?
    a. Any orthopedic appliance should be completely demonstrated.
    b. Ensure that the orthopedic appliance does not superimpose the acetabulum.

26. True or false. The pelvis should be rotated approximately 15 to 20 degrees.

27. True or false. The foot and lower extremity should be rotated laterally 15 to 20 degrees.

28. True or false. The entire lesser trochanter should be demonstrated on the lateral surface of the femur.

29. True or false. A small area of soft tissue overlap from the thigh of the unaffected lower extremity is permitted.

30. Identify each lettered structure shown in Fig. 8.14.

    A. _____

    B. _____

    C. _____

    D. _____

    E. _____

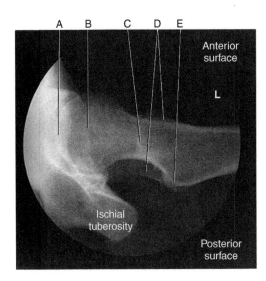

Fig. 8.14 Axiolateral hip, Danelius-Miller method.

Section 2: Exercise 3: Projection for Demonstrating the Acetabulum

This exercise reviews the essential projection for demonstration of the acetabulum. Provide a short answer, select the correct answer, or identify labeled structures on images for the following questions.

1. List the essential projection for the acetabulum, and describe the positioning steps used as follows:

   Essential projection: _____

   _____ (_____

   _____ method)
   - Size of collimated field:

   - Key patient/part positioning points:

   - Anatomic landmarks and relation to IR:

   - CR orientation and entrance point:

2. The internal oblique position places the affected side

   _____.

3. The external oblique position places the affected side

   _____.

4. What specific portion of the acetabulum and pelvis is demonstrated by the internal oblique position of the Judet method?

5. What specific portion of the acetabulum and pelvis is demonstrated by the external oblique position of the Judet method?

242

Questions 6 to 9 pertain to Fig. 8.15.

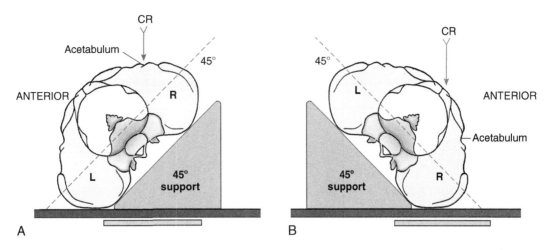

Fig. 8.15 (A) and (B), AP oblique acetabulum, Judet method.

6. Which figure (A or B) depicts the proper patient position to demonstrate a suspected fracture of the right iliopubic column and posterior rim of the acetabulum?

7. Which figure (A or B) depicts the proper patient position to demonstrate a suspected fracture of the ilioischial column and anterior rim of the acetabulum?

8. Where should the central ray enter the patient as positioned in Fig. 8.15A?

9. Where should the central ray enter the patient as positioned in Fig. 8.15B?

10. Identify each lettered structure shown in Fig. 8.16.

A. _____

B. _____

C. _____

D. _____

E. _____

F. _____

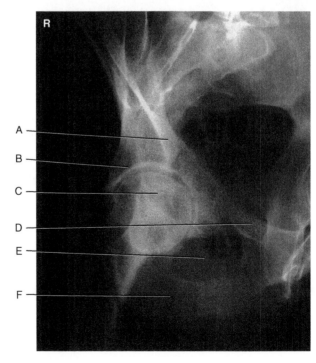

Fig. 8.16 AP oblique (Judet method), internal oblique.

243

11. Identify each lettered structure shown in Fig. 8.17.

A. _____

B. _____

C. _____

D. _____

E. _____

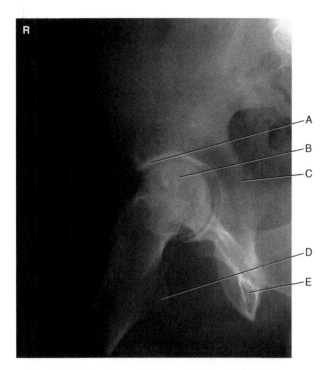

Fig. 8.17 AP oblique (Judet method), external oblique.

Section 2: Exercise 4: Projections for Demonstrating the Anterior Pelvic Bones

The AP axial "outlet" projection (Taylor method) and the AP axial "inlet" projection (Bridgeman method) are used to image the anterior pelvic bones. The following questions pertain to these projections.

1. Which projection demonstrates the superior and inferior rami of the pubic bones superimposed medially?

2. To demonstrate the pubic and ischial rami without foreshortening, the _____ method should be used.

3. Explain how the central ray orientation for the AP axial "outlet" projection (Taylor method) differs between male and female patients.

4. The superoinferior axial "inlet" projection (Bridgeman method) requires the central ray be directed

   _____.

5. Where does the central ray enter the patient for the superoinferior axial "inlet" projection (Bridgeman method)?
   a. 2 inches (5 cm) inferior to the pubic symphysis
   b. At the pubic symphysis
   c. At the ASIS
   d. At the iliac crests

6. Where does the central ray enter the patient for the AP axial "outlet" projection (Taylor method)?
   a. 2 inches (5 cm) distal to the superior border of the pubic symphysis
   b. 2 inches (5 cm) proximal to the superior border of the pubic symphysis
   c. At the ASIS
   d. At the pubic symphysis

7. Identify each lettered structure shown in Fig. 8.18.

A. _____

B. _____

8. Identify each lettered structure shown in Fig. 8.19.

A. _____

B. _____

C. _____

D. _____

E. _____

F. _____

G. _____

H. _____

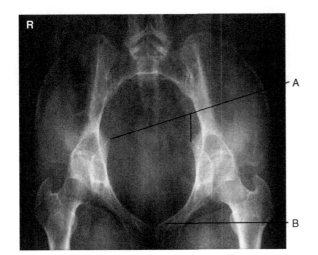

Fig. 8.18 AP axial pelvic bones, Bridgeman method.

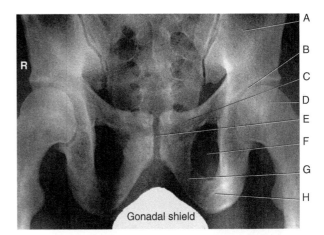

Fig. 8.19 AP axial pelvic bones, Taylor method.

Section 2: Exercise 5: Pelvic Girdle Image Evaluation

This exercise provides images of the pelvic girdle to provide an opportunity to apply your critique and evaluation skills. These images are not from Merrill's Atlas. Each image has at least one error. Examine each image and answer the associated questions.

1. Explain why the image in Fig. 8.20 must be repeated.

Fig. 8.21 is an image of an AP pelvis. Examine this image and answer the questions that follow.

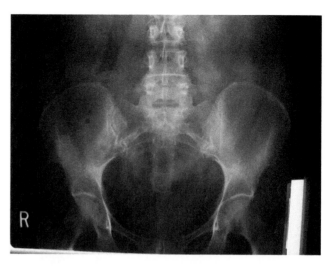

Fig. 8.21 AP pelvis with improper positioning.

2. Explain why Fig. 8.21 does not meet the evaluation criteria for this projection.

3. What positioning error likely produced this image?

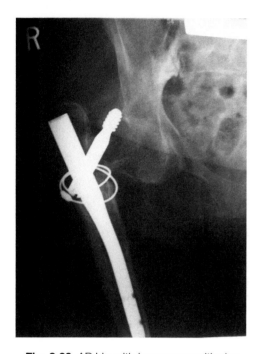

Fig. 8.20 AP hip with improper positioning.

4. Explain why Fig. 8.22 does not meet the evaluation criteria for the AP projection of the pelvis.

Fig. 8.23 is a lateral projection of the hip (Lauenstein method) with a positioning error. Examine the image and answer the following questions.

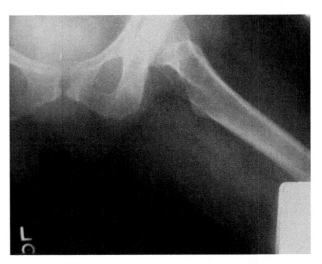

Fig. 8.23 Lateral hip with improper positioning.

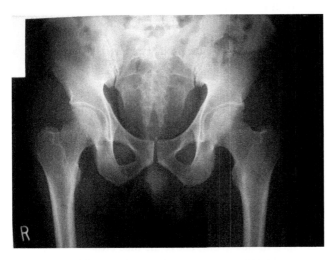

Fig. 8.22 AP pelvis with improper positioning.

5. What positioning error likely produced the image in Fig. 8.22?

6. Which of the following evaluation criteria are not met in this image?
   a. Hip joint centered to the image
   b. Hip joint, acetabulum, and femoral head demonstrated
   c. Femoral neck overlapped by the greater trochanter
   d. Evidence of proper collimation

7. Which of the following likely caused the error demonstrated in Fig. 8.23?
   a. Central ray and IR centered too low
   b. Central ray and IR centered too high
   c. Incorrect AEC detector used
   d. Leg was not abducted enough

Answer the following questions by selecting the best choice.

1. Which structure of the pelvis articulates with the femur?
   a. Acetabulum
   b. Inferior aperture
   c. Auricular surface
   d. Obturator foramen

2. Which bones of the pelvis comprise the acetabulum?
   a. Ilium and pubis only
   b. Ilium and ischium only
   c. Pubis and ischium only
   d. Pubis, ischium, and ilium

3. On which bone is the ala located?
   a. Ilium
   b. Pubis
   c. Femur
   d. Ischium

4. Which of the following pelvic structures is not used as a positioning palpation point?
   a. Iliac crest
   b. Ischial spine
   c. Pubic symphysis
   d. ASIS

5. Which portions of the hip bone join to form the obturator foramen?
   a. Ilium and pubis only
   b. Ilium and ischium only
   c. Pubis and ischium only
   d. Pubis, ischium, and ilium

6. What is the name of the border that extends on the hip bone from the posterior superior iliac spine to the ASIS?
   a. Iliac crest
   b. Greater sciatic notch
   c. Iliac auricular surface
   d. Brim of the lesser pelvis

7. What is the name of the process that separates the greater sciatic notch from the lesser sciatic notch on the hip bone?
   a. Ischial spine
   b. Ischial ramus
   c. Inferior ramus of the pubis
   d. Superior ramus of the pubis

8. Which parts of the hip bones support the weight of the body when a person is in the sitting position?
   a. Ischial spines
   b. Ischial tuberosities
   c. Inferior rami of the pubes
   d. Posterior inferior iliac spines

9. Where in the pelvis is the body of the pubis located?
   a. It forms part of the acetabulum.
   b. It forms part of the pubic symphysis.
   c. It is between the inferior and superior rami of the pubis.
   d. It is between the ischial ramus and the inferior ramus of the pubis.

10. In average-sized patients, where should the IR be centered for the AP projection of the pelvis?
    a. To the level of the iliac crest
    b. To the level of the pubic symphysis
    c. 2 inches (5 cm) below the greater trochanter
    d. Approximately 2 inches (5 cm) inferior to ASIS and 2 inches (5 cm) superior to pubic symphysis

11. Where on the midline of the patient should the central ray enter for the AP projection of the pelvis?
    a. 2 inches (5 cm) above the iliac crest
    b. 2 inches (5 cm) above the pubic symphysis
    c. At the level of the ASIS
    d. 2 inches (5 cm) above the level of the ASIS

12. Which positioning maneuver should be performed to place the femoral necks parallel with the IR for an AP projection of the pelvis?
    a. Rotate the lower extremities laterally 15 to 20 degrees.
    b. Rotate the lower extremities medially 15 to 20 degrees.
    c. Flex the hips 15 to 20 degrees and extend the lower extremities.
    d. Flex the hips and abduct the femora laterally 15 to 20 degrees.

13. How should the central ray be directed for the AP oblique projection (modified Cleaves method) to demonstrate bilateral hips?
    a. Perpendicularly
    b. Cephalically 20 degrees
    c. Cephalically 40 degrees
    d. Parallel with the long axis of the femora

14. For which projection of the lower extremities or pelvis should the hips be flexed and the femora be abducted from the midline of the patient?
    a. AP projection of the hip
    b. AP projection of the pelvis
    c. AP oblique projection (modified Cleaves method) for femoral necks
    d. Axiolateral projection (Danelius-Miller method) of the hip

15. Where on the midline of the patient should the central ray be directed for the AP oblique projection (modified Cleaves method)?
    a. To the level of the iliac crests
    b. 1 inch (2.5 cm) above the pubic symphysis
    c. To the level of the ASIS
    d. 2 inches (5 cm) above the ASIS

16. All of the following projections can be used to image a patient with a suspected intertrochanteric fracture, *except for the:*
    a. AP projection of the hip
    b. AP projection of the pelvis
    c. Lateral projection (Lauenstein method) of the hip
    d. Axiolateral projection (Danelius-Miller method) of the hip

17. For the AP oblique projection (modified Cleaves method), what is the purpose of abducting the femora the required number of degrees?
    a. To position the pelvis in the true lateral position
    b. To prevent superimposing the acetabulum with the pelvis
    c. To position the femoral necks parallel with the IR
    d. To prevent superimposing the femoral head with the acetabulum

18. Which structure should be centered to the midline of the table when the AP oblique projection (modified Cleaves method) is adapted to demonstrate only one hip?
    a. Femoral body
    b. Pubic symphysis
    c. Greater trochanter
    d. ASIS

19. For which projection of an individual hip should the unaffected hip be flexed and the thigh be raised out of the way of the central ray?
    a. AP projection
    b. Lateral projection (Lauenstein method)
    c. AP oblique projection (modified Cleaves method)
    d. Axiolateral projection (Danelius-Miller method)

20. For which projection of the hip should the central ray be directed horizontally into the medial aspect of the affected thigh?
    a. AP projection
    b. Lateral projection (Lauenstein method)
    c. AP oblique projection (modified Cleaves method)
    d. Axiolateral projection (Danelius-Miller method)

21. Which of the following best demonstrates suspected fractures of the acetabulum?
    a. AP axial "inlet" projection (Bridgeman method)
    b. AP axial "outlet" projection (Taylor method)
    c. AP oblique projection (Judet method)
    d. Axiolateral projection (Danelius-Miller method)

22. Which of the following positions would be used to demonstrate the posterior rim of the left acetabulum?
    a. 45-degree RPO
    b. 45-degree LPO
    c. 45-degree RAO
    d. 45-degree LAO

23. What specific portion of the acetabulum is demonstrated by the AP oblique projection, external oblique position (Judet method)?
    a. Posterior rim
    b. Anterior rim
    c. Medial border
    d. Lateral border

24. Which of the following would best demonstrate the pubic and ischial rami without foreshortening?
    a. AP axial "inlet" projection (Bridgeman method)
    b. AP axial "outlet" projection (Taylor method)
    c. AP oblique projection (Judet method)
    d. Axiolateral projection (Danelius-Miller method)

25. What is the proper central ray orientation for the AP axial projection (Taylor method) for female patients?
    a. 20 to 35 degrees caudad
    b. 20 to 35 degrees cephalad
    c. 30 to 45 degrees caudad
    d. 30 to 45 degrees cephalad

26. When performing an AP projection of the pelvis and proximal femora, all of the following should be clearly seen EXCEPT:
    a. the entire pelvis and proximal femora.
    b. both ilia and greater trochanters equidistant from the edge of the image.
    c. the lesser trochanters, which, if seen, are visible on the lateral border of the femora.
    d. no rotation of pelvis.

27. When performing an AP oblique projection modified Cleaves method, all of the following should be clearly seen EXCEPT:
    a. no rotation of the pelvis, as demonstrated by a symmetric appearance.
    b. the acetabulum, femoral head, and femoral neck.
    c. the lesser trochanter on the medial side of the femur.
    d. the femoral neck without superimposition by the lesser trochanter; excess abduction causes the lesser trochanter to obstruct the neck.

28. Where does the central ray enter the patient for the AP projection of the hip?
    a. Approximately 1 inch (2.5 cm) distal on a line drawn perpendicular from the midpoint of a line between the ASIS and the pubic symphysis
    b. Approximately 1.5 inches (3.8 cm) distal on a line drawn perpendicular from the midpoint of a line between the ASIS and the pubic symphysis
    c. Approximately 2 inches (5 cm) distal on a line drawn perpendicular from the midpoint of a line between the ASIS and the pubic symphysis
    d. Approximately 2.5 inches (6.4 cm) distal on a line drawn perpendicular from the midpoint of a line between the ASIS and the pubic symphysis

29. When performing the AP oblique projection modified Cleaves method, how many degrees should the patient abduct the thighs from vertical plane?
    a. 30
    b. 35
    c. 40
    d. 45

30. Which examination is contraindicated for patients with suspected fracture or pathologic condition?
    a. Modified Cleaves method
    b. Danelius-Miller method
    c. Clements and Nakayama
    d. AP Pelvis

9 Vertebral Column

OSTEOLOGY AND ARTHROLOGY OF THE VERTEBRAL COLUMN

Section 1: Exercise 1

Refer to Fig. 9.1 and match the vertebral curvatures listed in Column A with the characteristic or classification terms in Column B. Each curvature has three terms associated with it. Terms are used more than once.

Column A		Column B
____ ____ ____	1. Cervical	a. Primary curve
____ ____ ____	2. Thoracic	b. Secondary curve
____ ____ ____	3. Lumbar	c. Lordotic curve
____ ____ ____	4. Pelvic	d. Kyphotic curve
		e. Convex anteriorly
		f. Concave anteriorly

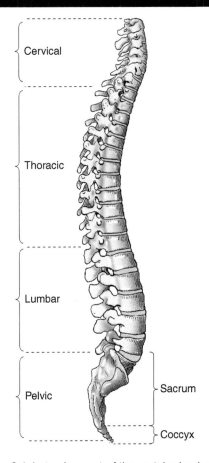

Fig. 9.1 Lateral aspect of the vertebral column.

251

Section 1: Exercise 2

Examine Fig. 9.2 and identify the abnormal curvatures of the vertebral column.

1. Identify each abnormal curvature shown in Fig. 9.2.

   A. _____

   B. _____

   C. _____

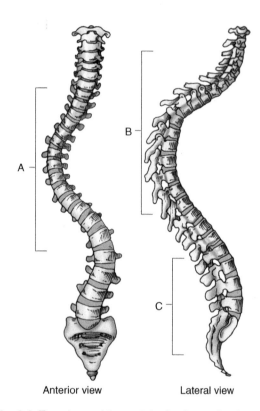

Anterior view   Lateral view

Fig. 9.2 Two views of the vertebral column showing abnormal curvatures.

Section 1: Exercise 3

This exercise pertains to the cervical vertebrae. Identify structures for each question.

1. Identify each lettered structure shown in Fig. 9.3.

   A. _____

   B. _____

   C. _____

   D. _____

   E. _____

   F. _____

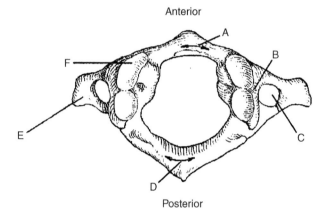

Anterior

Posterior

Fig. 9.3 Superior aspect of atlas (C1).

2. Identify each lettered structure shown in Fig. 9.4.

A. _____

B. _____

C. _____

D. _____

E. _____

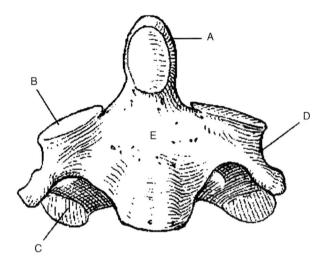

Fig. 9.4 Anterior aspect of axis (C2).

3. Identify each lettered structure shown in Fig. 9.5.

A. _____

B. _____

C. _____

D. _____

E. _____

F. _____

G. _____

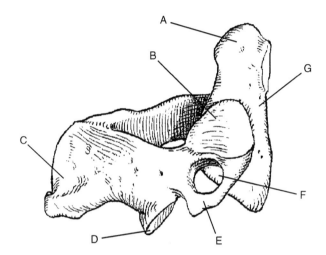

Fig. 9.5 Lateral aspect of axis (C2).

4. Identify each lettered structure shown in Fig. 9.6.

A. _____   E. _____

B. _____   F. _____

C. _____   G. _____

D. _____   H. _____

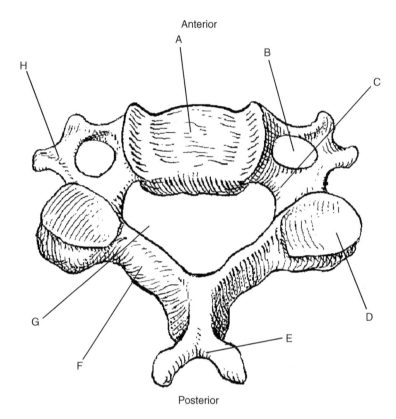

Fig. 9.6 Superior aspect of a typical cervical vertebra.

5. Identify each lettered structure shown in Fig. 9.7.

A. _____

B. _____

C. _____

D. _____

E. _____

F. _____

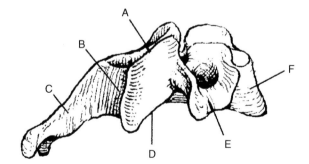

Fig. 9.7 Lateral aspect of a typical cervical vertebra.

This exercise pertains to the thoracic vertebrae. Identify structures for each question.

1. Identify each lettered structure shown in Fig. 9.8.

A. _____

B. _____

C. _____

D. _____

E. _____

F. _____

G. _____

H. _____

I. _____

2. Identify each lettered structure shown in Fig. 9.9.

A. _____

B. _____

C. _____

D. _____

E. _____

F. _____

G. _____

H. _____

I. _____

J. _____

K. _____

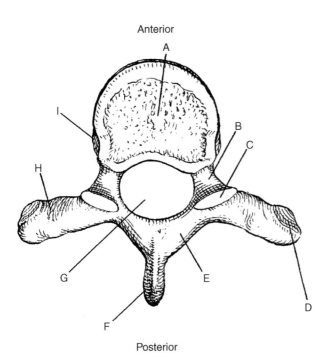

Fig. 9.8 Superior aspect of a thoracic vertebra.

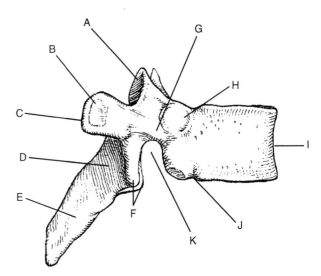

Fig. 9.9 Lateral aspect of a thoracic vertebra.

Section 1: Exercise 5

This exercise pertains to the lumbar vertebrae. Identify structures for each question.

1. Identify each lettered structure shown in Fig. 9.10.

   A. _____

   B. _____

   C. _____

   D. _____

   E. _____

   F. _____

   G. _____

   H. _____

   I. _____

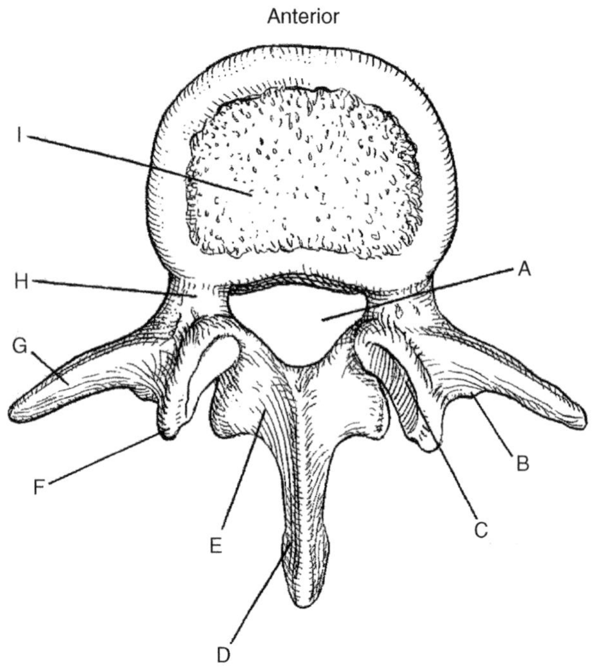

2. Identify each lettered structure shown in Fig. 9.11.

   A. _____

   B. _____

   C. _____

   D. _____

   E. _____

   F. _____

   G. _____

   H. _____

   I. _____

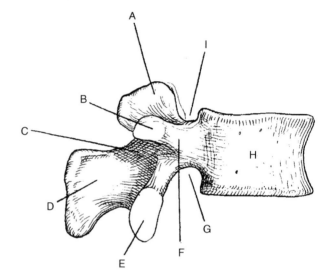

Fig. 9.11 Lateral aspect of a lumbar vertebra.

Fig. 9.10 Superior aspect of a lumbar vertebra.

Section 1: Exercise 6

This exercise pertains to the sacrum and coccyx. Identify structures for each question.

1. Identify each lettered structure shown in Fig. 9.12.

   A. _____

   B. _____

   C. _____

   D. _____

   E. _____

   F. _____

2. Identify each lettered structure shown in Fig. 9.13.

   A. _____

   B. _____

   C. _____

   D. _____

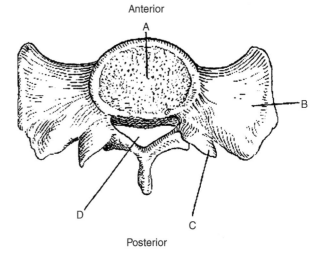

Fig. 9.13 Superior aspect of the sacrum.

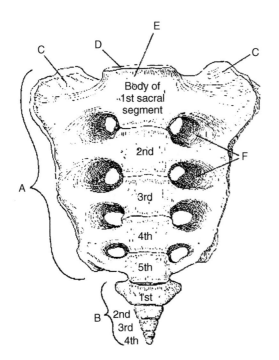

Fig. 9.12 Anterior aspect of the sacrum and coccyx.

Section 1: Exercise 7

Use the following clues to complete the crossword puzzle. All answers refer to the vertebral column.

Across
3. Thoracic depressions
6. C2 name
8. Number of cervical vertebrae
10. Articular processes
12. Holds up the skull
13. Articulates with thoracic vertebrae
15. Lumbar curvature
17. Forms posterior vertebral arch
20. Two tips
21. Inferior to the sacrum
22. Between thoracic and sacrum

Down
1. Number of lumbar vertebrae
2. Extends posteriorly from a vertebral body
4. Lateral vertebral curvature
5. Cylindric vertebral portion
6. Occipitocervical joint
7. Most superior vertebrae
9. Thoracic curvature
11. Just below cervical
14. Odontoid process
16. Number of thoracic vertebrae
18. Vertebral cartilage pad
19. Articulates with both ilia

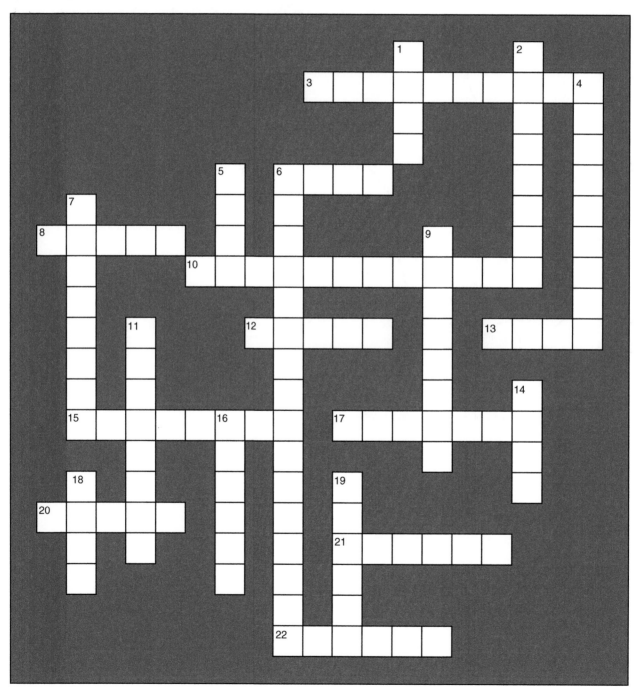

Section 1: Exercise 8

Match the pathology terms in Column A with the appropriate definition in Column B. Not all choices from Column B should be selected.

Column A

_____ 1. Tumor

_____ 2. Fracture

_____ 3. Lordosis

_____ 4. Scoliosis

_____ 5. Kyphosis

_____ 6. Metastases

_____ 7. Subluxation

_____ 8. Spina bifida

_____ 9. Osteoporosis

_____ 10. Spondylolysis

_____ 11. Paget disease

_____ 12. Jefferson fracture

_____ 13. Spondylolisthesis

_____ 14. Multiple myeloma

_____ 15. Hangman fracture

_____ 16. Compression fracture

_____ 17. Ankylosing spondylitis

_____ 18. Scheuermann disease

_____ 19. Clay shoveler's fracture

_____ 20. Herniated nucleus pulposus

Column B

a. Loss of bone density

b. Breaking down of a vertebra

c. Incomplete or partial dislocation

d. Kyphosis with onset in adolescence

e. Disruption in the continuity of bone

f. Comminuted fracture of the ring of C1

g. Increased density of atypically soft bone

h. Abnormally increased concavity of the spine

i. Malignant tumor arising from cartilage cells

j. Thick, soft bone marked by bowing and fractures

k. Transfer of a cancerous lesion from one area to another

l. Fracture of the anterior arch of C2 as a result of hyperextension

m. Abnormally increased convexity in the thoracic curvature

n. New tissue growth where cell proliferation is uncontrolled

o. Rheumatoid arthritis variant involving the sacroiliac (SI) joints and spine

p. Lateral deviation of the spine with possible vertebral rotation

q. Failure of the posterior encasement of the spinal cord to close

r. Rupture or prolapse of the nucleus pulposus into the spinal canal

s. Forward displacement of a vertebra over a lower vertebra, usually L5-S1

t. Fracture that causes compaction of bone and a decrease in the length or width

u. Avulsion fracture of the spinous process in the lower cervical and upper thoracic region

v. Malignant neoplasm of plasma cells involving the bone marrow and causing destruction of bone

Section 1: Exercise 9

Match the parts of the vertebra listed in Column A with the descriptions in Column B.

Column A

_____ 1. Body

_____ 2. Laminae

_____ 3. Pedicles

_____ 4. Zygapophyses

_____ 5. Spinous process

_____ 6. Transverse process

Column B

a. Process extending laterally and posteriorly from the body

b. Process extending posteriorly from the junction of both laminae

c. Process extending laterally from the pedicle-lamina junction

d. Articular processes

e. Solid anterior part of a vertebra

f. Connects the transverse process with the spinous process

Section 1: Exercise 10

This exercise is a comprehensive review of the osteology and arthrology of the vertebral column. Provide a short answer for each question.

1. List four functions of the vertebral column.

2. As viewed from the lateral aspect, name (from superior to inferior) the four vertebral curvatures.

3. State how vertebral curvatures are classified as either primary or secondary curvatures.

4. Name the two vertebral curvatures that are classified as primary curvatures.

5. Name the two vertebral curvatures that are classified as secondary curvatures.

6. What is the name of the opening formed by the vertebral arch and the body of a vertebra?

7. What other name refers to C1?

8. What other name refers to C2?

9. What other name refers to C7?

10. What two typical vertebral parts are missing from the first cervical vertebra?

11. How are the transverse processes of cervical vertebrae significantly different from those of other typical vertebrae?

12. Which cervical vertebra has the dens?

13. What other term refers to the dens?

14. How many cervical vertebrae are in the vertebral column?

15. With reference to the midsagittal plane, how do zygapophyseal articulations of the cervical vertebrae open?

16. With reference to the midsagittal plane, how do cervical intervertebral foramina open?

17. Which section of the vertebral column has costovertebral joints?

18. Which section of the vertebral column has facets and demifacets?

19. Which bones articulate with thoracic facets and demifacets?

20. With reference to the midsagittal plane, how do zygapophyseal articulations of the thoracic vertebrae open?

21. With reference to the midsagittal plane, how do thoracic intervertebral foramina open?

22. With reference to the midsagittal plane, how do zygapophyseal articulations of the lumbar vertebrae open?

23. With reference to the midsagittal plane, how do lumbar intervertebral foramina open?

24. What structure of the vertebral column articulates with both ilia?

25. With reference to the midsagittal plane, how many degrees and in which direction do SI joints open?

For questions 26 to 28, write out the terms beside their abbreviations.

26. EAM: _____

27. HNP: _____

28. OML: _____

29. IOML: _____

POSITIONING OF THE VERTEBRAL COLUMN

Section 2: Exercise 1: Positioning for the Cervical Spine

Seven essential projections are used to demonstrate the anatomy of the cervical spine. This exercise pertains to those projections. Identify structures, fill in missing words, provide a short answer, select the correct answer from a list, or choose true or false (explaining any statement you believe to be false) for each item.

1. List the essential projections for the cervical spine, and describe the positioning steps used for each, as follows:

   Essential projection: _____
   (_____ method)
   - Size of collimated field:

   - Key patient/part positioning points:

   - Anatomic landmarks and relation to IR:

   - CR orientation and entrance point:

   Essential projection: _____
   - Size of collimated field:

   - Key patient/part positioning points:

   - Anatomic landmarks and relation to IR:

   - CR orientation and entrance point:

   Essential projection: _____
   _____
   - Size of collimated field:

   - Key patient/part positioning points:

   - Anatomic landmarks and relation to IR:

   - CR orientation and entrance point:

   Essential projection: _____
   (_____ method)
   - Size of collimated field:

   - Key patient/part positioning points:

   - Anatomic landmarks and relation to IR:

   - CR orientation and entrance point:

   Essential projection: _____
   (_____ positions)
   - Size of collimated field:

   - Key patient/part positioning points:

   - Anatomic landmarks and relation to IR:

   - CR orientation and entrance point:

263

Essential projection: _____
- Size of collimated field:

- Key patient/part positioning points:

- Anatomic landmarks and relation to IR:

- CR orientation and entrance point:

Essential projection: _____
- Size of collimated field:

- Key patient/part positioning points:

- Anatomic landmarks and relation to IR:

- CR orientation and entrance point:

Items 2 to 5 pertain to the *AP projection (Fuchs method)*. Examine Figs. 9.14 and 9.15 as you answer the following questions.

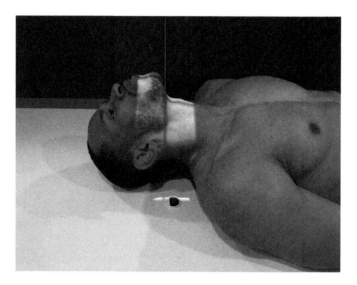

Fig. 9.14 AP dens: Fuchs method.

2. True or false. The AP projection (Fuchs method) should be used to demonstrate an upper cervical fracture in trauma patients.

3. True or false. In the image of the AP projection (Fuchs method), the entire dens should be seen within the foramen magnum.

4. What two structures are aligned for the AP projection (Fuchs method) of the dens?

5. Identify each lettered structure shown in Fig. 9.15.

A. _____

B. _____

C. _____

D. _____

E. _____

F. _____

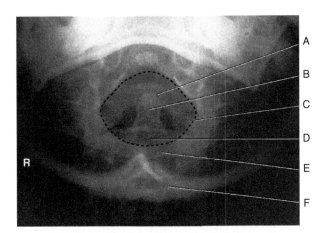

Fig. 9.15 AP dens: Fuchs method.

Items 6 to 9 pertain to the *AP projection (open mouth)*. Examine Fig. 9.16 as you answer the following questions.

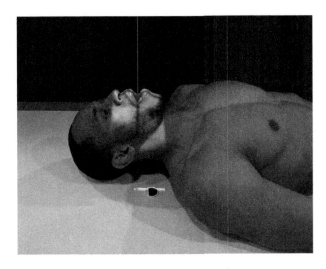

Fig. 9.16 AP atlas and axis.

6. Why should the patient be asked to phonate "ah" softly during the exposure?

7. In the image produced by the AP projection (open mouth), which cranial structure should be superimposed with the occlusal surface of the upper central incisors?
   a. Mastoid process
   b. Base of the skull
   c. External occipital protuberance

8. Which areas of cervical vertebrae should be clearly demonstrated with the AP projection (open mouth)?
   a. Intervertebral foramina
   b. Cervical zygapophyseal articulations
   c. Articulations between C1 and C2

9. Identify each lettered structure shown in Fig. 9.17.

A. _____

B. _____

C. _____

D. _____

E. _____

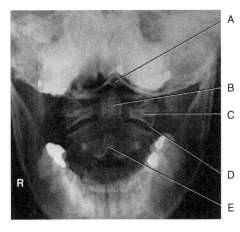

Fig. 9.17 Open-mouth atlas and axis.

Items 10 to 15 pertain to the *AP axial projection*.

10. What should the patient be instructed to do to prevent superimposition of the mandible and the mid-cervical vertebrae?

11. How is it determined that the chin has been correctly extended?

12. How many degrees and in what direction should the central ray be directed?

13. The AP axial projection for cervical vertebrae should demonstrate the vertebrae from _____ to _____.
    a. C1; C7
    b. C1; T2
    c. C3; C7
    d. C3; T2

14. From the following list, circle the two evaluation criteria indicating that the patient was properly positioned without rotation for the AP axial projection.
    a. The spinous processes should be equidistant to the pedicles and aligned with the midline of the cervical bodies.
    b. The mandibular angles and mastoid processes should be equidistant to the vertebrae.
    c. The intervertebral foramina farthest from the IR should be "open."
    d. The superimposed rami of the mandible should be anterior to vertebral bodies.

15. Identify the labeled structures shown in Fig. 9.18.

    A. _____

    B. _____

    C. _____

    D. _____

    E. _____

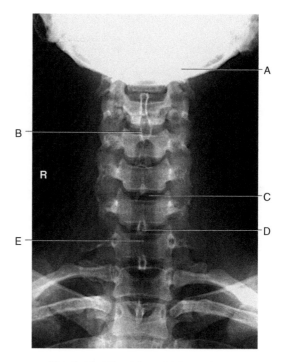

Fig. 9.18 AP axial cervical vertebrae.

Items 16 to 21 pertain to the *lateral projection, Grandy method.* Examine Fig. 9.19 as you answer the following questions.

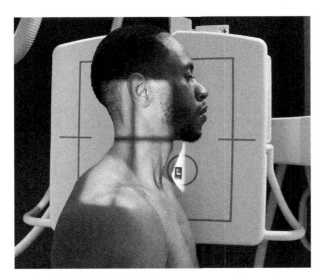

Fig. 9.19 Lateral cervical vertebrae, Grandy method.

16. Which of the cervical vertebrae should be demonstrated with lateral projections?

17. What positioning maneuver is used to prevent the mandible from superimposing the vertebrae?

18. What breathing instructions should be given to the patient?

19. What should the radiographer do to help overcome the effects of a large object-to-image receptor distance (OID) created with the lateral projection?

20. What should the radiographer do if the C7 vertebra is not well visualized on a lateral projection image?

21. Identify each lettered structure shown in Fig. 9.20.

A. _____

B. _____

C. _____

D. _____

E. _____

F. _____

G. _____

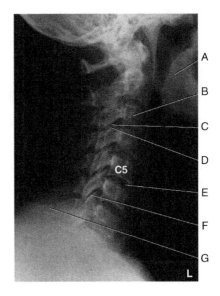

Fig. 9.20 Lateral cervical vertebrae.

Items 22 to 27 pertain *to hyperextension and hyperflexion lateral projections.* Examine Figs. 9.21 and 9.22 as you answer the following questions.

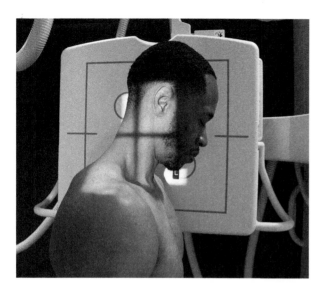

Fig. 9.21 Lateral cervical vertebrae, hyperflexion.

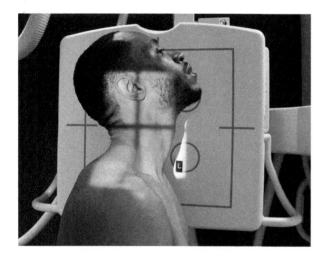

Fig. 9.22 Lateral cervical vertebrae, hyperextension.

22. Describe how the patient's head and neck should be adjusted from the neutral lateral position for the hyperflexion position.

23. Describe how the patient's head and neck should be adjusted from the neutral lateral position for the hyperextension position.

24. In an image with the patient in the hyperflexion position, how is it determined that the patient's neck has been flexed far enough?

25. In an image with the patient in the hyperextension position, how is it determined that the patient's neck has been extended far enough?

26. What cervical vertebrae should be clearly demonstrated in images produced with the patient in the hyperflexion and hyperextension positions?

27. Indicate how the cervical spinous processes should appear in images with the patient in the (a) hyperflexion lateral position and (b) hyperextension lateral position.

    a. _____

    _____

    b. _____

    _____

Items 28 to 40 pertain to the AP *axial oblique projection.* Examine Fig. 9.23 as you answer the following questions.

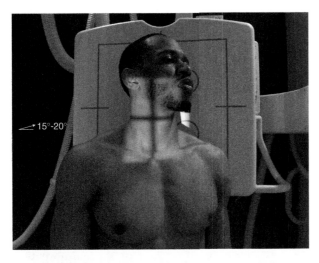

15°-20°

Fig. 9.23 AP axial oblique intervertebral foramina.

28. AP axial oblique projections are used for the best demonstration of the pedicles and:
    a. zygapophyseal joints.
    b. intervertebral foramina.
    c. superior articular facets.
    d. spinous processes.

29. Why should the patient be instructed to lift and extend the chin?

30. Explain how the positioning of the cervical vertebrae is affected if the patient turns the head until the mid-sagittal plane of the skull is parallel with the plane of the IR.

31. How many degrees and in what direction should the central ray be directed?

32. Why is the central ray directed in the manner indicated in the answer to question 31?

33. If an AP axial oblique projection is performed with the patient in a recumbent posterior oblique position, should the direction and angulation of the central ray be different from that recommended for an upright patient?

34. Why should a support be placed under the patient's head for the AP axial oblique projection with the patient in a recumbent posterior oblique body position?

35. What breathing instructions should be given to the patient?

36. Which of the following procedures should be avoided when positioning a patient for an AP axial oblique projection?
    a. Slightly protruding the chin
    b. Turning the chin to the side
    c. Rotating the body 45 degrees

37. From the following list, circle the five evaluation criteria indicating that the patient was properly positioned for an AP axial oblique projection.
   a. The occipital bone should not overlap C1.
   b. The cervical zygapophyseal joints should be well demonstrated.
   c. The chin should be elevated and not overlap C1 and C2.
   d. All seven cervical vertebrae and T1 should be included.
   e. The intervertebral disk spaces should be open and well demonstrated.
   f. The intervertebral foramina should be open, with foramina nearest the IR well demonstrated.
   g. The intervertebral foramina should be open, with foramina farthest from the IR well demonstrated.

Fig. 9.24 shows an AP axial oblique projection image. Examine the image and answer the questions that follow.

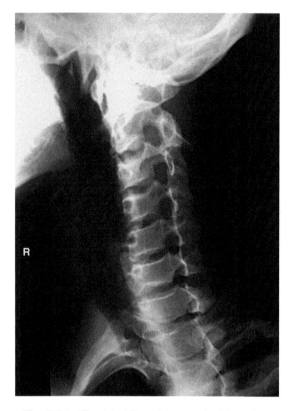

Fig. 9.24 AP axial oblique intervertebral foramina.

38. In what body position is the patient?

39. The intervertebral foramina of which side (left or right) are best demonstrated?

40. Is the anatomy demonstrated closer to or farther from the IR?

Items 41 to 48 pertain to PA *axial oblique projections.* Examine Fig. 9.25 as you answer the following questions.

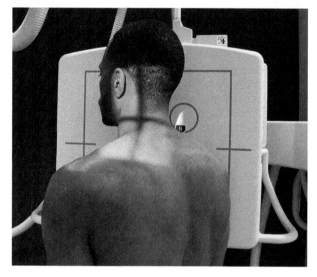

Fig. 9.25 PA axial oblique intervertebral foramina.

41. With the patient positioned in the right anterior oblique (RAO) position, the intervertebral foramina best demonstrated are those on the patient's

_____ (right or left) side.

42. When the patient is in the standing position, to what level of the patient should the IR be centered?
   a. C3
   b. C5
   c. C7

43. How many degrees should the entire body of the patient be rotated?
   a. 25
   b. 35
   c. 45

44. How many degrees and in what direction should the central ray be angled?
    a. 15 to 20 degrees cephalic
    b. 15 to 20 degrees caudal
    c. 25 to 30 degrees cephalic
    d. 25 to 30 degrees caudal

45. Through which cervical vertebra should the central ray be directed?
    a. C3
    b. C4
    c. C5

Fig. 9.26 shows a PA axial oblique projection image. Examine the image and answer the questions that follow.

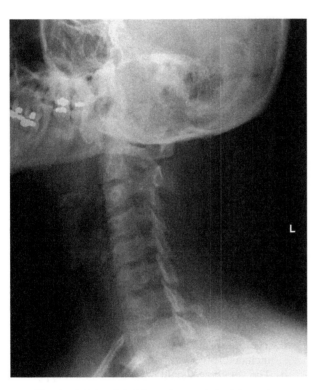

Fig. 9.26 PA axial oblique intervertebral foramina.

46. What position is shown in the image?

47. The intervertebral foramina of which side (left or right) are best demonstrated?

48. Are the open intervertebral foramina demonstrated in this image closer to or farther from the IR?

Section 2: Exercise 2: Positioning for the Cervicothoracic Region

A lateral projection using the swimmer's technique can be performed to demonstrate the cervicothoracic region. This exercise pertains to this projection. Identify structures, fill in missing words, provide a short answer, select an answer from a list, or choose true or false (explain any statement you believe to be false) for each item.

Items 1 to 13 pertain to the *swimmer's technique* for demonstrating the cervicothoracic region. Examine Figs. 9.27 and 9.28 as you answer the following questions.

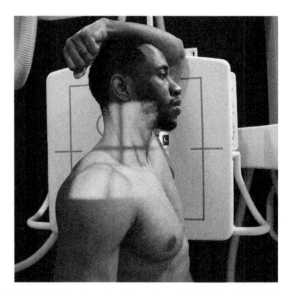

Fig. 9.27 Lateral cervicothoracic projection (swimmer's), upright position.

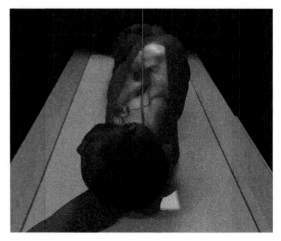

Fig. 9.28 Lateral cervicothoracic region (swimmer's), recumbent position.

271

1. The swimmer's technique is performed when _____.

2. Which body plane should be centered to the midline of the grid?

3. With reference to the patient, where should the IR be centered?

4. Describe how the patient's arms should be positioned.

5. Describe how the patient's shoulders should be positioned.

6. List the two ways that the patient's respiration can be controlled.

7. Which two ways can the central ray be directed for the swimmer's technique?
   a. Perpendicular or 3 to 5 degrees caudad
   b. Perpendicular or 3 to 5 degrees cephalad
   c. 5 degrees caudad or 5 degrees cephalad

8. For the swimmer's technique, the patient may be positioned either _____.

9. When the patient is positioned recumbent, where should the body be supported to maintain the long axis of the cervicothoracic vertebrae in a horizontal position?

10. With reference to the patient, to what specific location should the central ray be directed?
    a. Disk space of C1 and C2
    b. Disk space of C4 and C5
    c. Disk space of C7 and T1
    d. Disk space of T1 and T2

11. According to Monda's recommendation, how many degrees and in which direction should the central ray be directed?
    a. 3 to 5 degrees caudad
    b. 3 to 5 degrees cephalad
    c. 5 to 15 degrees caudad
    d. 5 to 15 degrees cephalad

12. From the following list, circle the four evaluation criteria indicating that the patient was properly positioned for a lateral projection of the cervicothoracic region.
    a. The exposure must have penetrated the shoulder area.
    b. The shoulders should be seen separated from each other.
    c. The area from approximately C5-T4 should be included.
    d. The vertebrae should be lateral and not appreciably rotated.
    e. The spinous processes should be seen centered on vertebral bodies.
    f. The intervertebral foramina should be open, with foramina nearest the IR well demonstrated.
    g. The intervertebral foramina should be open, with foramina farthest from the IR well demonstrated.

272

13. Identify each lettered structure shown in Fig. 9.29.

A. _____

B. _____

C. _____

D. _____

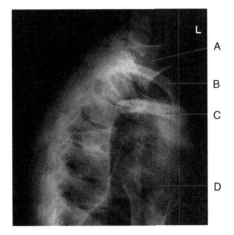

Fig. 9.29 Lateral cervicothoracic region.

Section 2: Exercise 3: Positioning for the Thoracic Vertebrae

This exercise pertains to the two essential projections for the thoracic vertebrae. Identify structures, fill in missing words, provide a short answer, select an answer from a list, or choose true or false (explaining any statement you believe to be false) for each question.

1. List the essential projections for the thoracic spine, and describe the positioning steps used for each, as follows:

   Essential projection: _____
   ■ Size of collimated field:

   ■ Key patient/part positioning points:

   ■ Anatomic landmarks and relation to IR:

   ■ CR orientation and entrance point:

   Essential projection: _____
   ■ Size of collimated field:

   ■ Key patient/part positioning points:

   ■ Anatomic landmarks and relation to IR:

   ■ CR orientation and entrance point:

273

Items 2 to 15 pertain to the *AP projection.* Examine Fig. 9.30 as you answer the following questions.

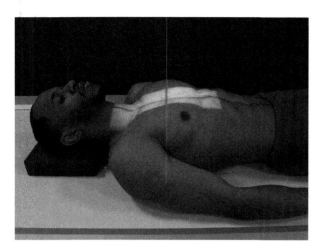

Fig. 9.30 AP thoracic vertebrae.

2. If the supine position is used, what should be done to reduce the normal thoracic kyphosis of the patient?
   a. Flex the patient's hips and knees.
   b. Extend the patient's lower extremities.
   c. Place cushions under the patient's lower back.

3. Which vertebra should be in the center of the collimated field/IR?
   a. T3
   b. T5
   c. T7
   d. T12

4. Where exactly on the anterior side of the patient's chest should the central ray enter?

5. With reference to the patient, where should the upper edge of the IR/collimated field be placed?

6. List the two options for patient respiration instructions and explain the rationale for each.

7. Which part of the x-ray tube (the anode or cathode) should be positioned over the patient's head? Explain why.

8. For the supine patient, why should the patient's head rest directly on the table or on a thin pillow instead of a thick foam cushion or thick pillow?

9. What should the radiographer do to ensure the appearance of a more even exposure when performing a single-image AP projection of the thoracic spine?

274

Chapter **9 Vertebral Column**

Figs. 9.31 and 9.32 both show AP projection images; however, they are not identical in appearance. Compare the images and answer the questions that follow.

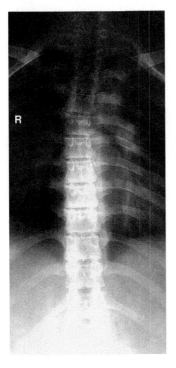

Fig. 9.31 AP thoracic vertebrae.

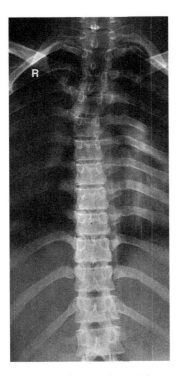

Fig. 9.32 AP thoracic vertebrae.

10. Which image best demonstrates all 12 thoracic vertebrae?

11. Which image used the anode heel effect of the x-ray tube to its maximum advantage?

12. In which image was the anode of the x-ray tube positioned above the patient's head?

13. In which image was the cathode of the x-ray tube positioned above the patient's head?

14. From the following list, circle the five evaluation criteria indicating that the patient was correctly positioned and the exposure was properly performed for the AP projection.
    a. The ribs should appear posteriorly superimposed.
    b. All 12 thoracic vertebrae should be included.
    c. The thoracic zygapophyseal joints should be best demonstrated.
    d. The x-ray beam should be collimated to the thoracic spine.
    e. The spinous processes should appear at the midline of the vertebral bodies.
    f. The vertebral column should be aligned to the middle of the image.
    g. The spinous processes should appear without superimposition of vertebral bodies.

275

15. Identify each lettered structure shown in Fig. 9.33.

A. _____

B. _____

C. _____

D. _____

E. _____

F. _____

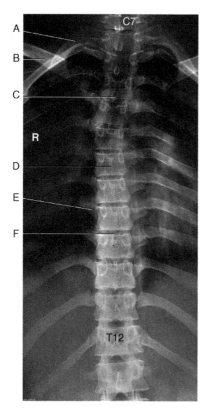

Fig. 9.33 AP thoracic vertebrae.

Items 16 to 36 pertain to the *lateral projection*. Examine Fig. 9.34 as you answer the following questions.

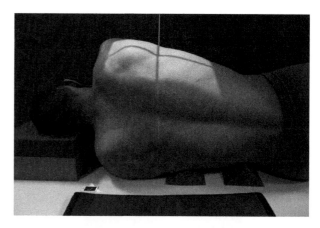

Fig. 9.34 Lateral thoracic vertebrae.

16. Why is it preferable to place the patient in the left lateral position instead of the right lateral position?

17. For the lateral recumbent position, what is the purpose of placing a firm pillow under the patient's head?

18. To what level of the patient should the superior border of the IR/collimated field be placed?

19. Which posterior body landmark coincides with T7 for centering the IR?

20. Describe how the patient's arms should be positioned and explain why.

21. What is the purpose of placing a radiolucent support under the lower thoracic region when the patient is in the lateral recumbent position?

22. How many degrees and in which direction should the central ray be directed if the thoracic vertebrae are not parallel with the table when a female patient is in the lateral recumbent position? A male patient?

23. If an angled central ray is used, why should it be angled more for men than for women?

24. With reference to the patient's breathing, when should the exposure be made?

25. Why should a sheet of leaded rubber be placed on the table posterior to the patient when the IR is exposed and the patient is in a lateral recumbent position?

26. How can it be determined by looking at ribs in the image that the patient was rotated?

27. What additional projection may be performed if the upper thoracic vertebrae are not well demonstrated with a routine lateral projection?

28. When the thoracic vertebrae are parallel with the plane of the IR, the central ray should be directed

_____ (perpendicularly, cephalad, caudad).

29. True or false. A lead apron should be placed over the patient's pelvis.

30. True or false. The central ray should be directed to enter the posterior half of the thorax at the level of T7.

31. True or false. Normal breathing by the patient reduces the amount of scattered radiation that reaches the IR.

32. True or false. Scattered radiation may cause the automatic exposure control system to terminate the exposure prematurely.

33. True or false. If the exposure is terminated prematurely, the vertebral bodies will appear too light in the image.

34. True or false. The upper thoracic vertebrae, specifically T1 and T2, are not usually demonstrated in the full lateral view.

35. From the following list, circle the six evaluation criteria indicating that the patient was correctly positioned and the exposure was properly performed for the lateral projection.
    a. The thoracic zygapophyseal joints should be open.
    b. Soft tissue and bony trabecular detail should be evident.
    c. The intervertebral disk spaces should be open.
    d. The ribs should appear posteriorly superimposed.
    e. The spinous processes should appear at the midline of the patient.
    f. The vertebrae should be clearly seen through rib and lung shadows.
    g. Twelve thoracic vertebrae should be centered on the IR.
    h. The x-ray beam should be tightly collimated to reduce scatter radiation.

36. Identify each structure labeled in Fig. 9.35.

A. _____

B. _____

C. _____

D. _____

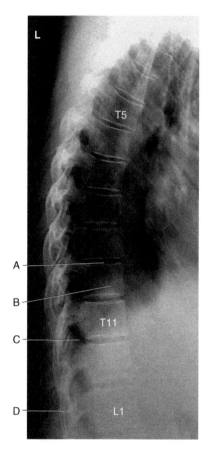

Fig. 9.35 Lateral thoracic vertebrae.

Section 2: Exercise 4: Positioning for the Lumbar Vertebrae

This exercise pertains to the essential projections of the lumbar vertebrae. Identify structures, fill in missing words, provide a short answer, select an answer from a list, or choose true or false (explaining any statement you believe to be false) for each question.

1. List the essential projections for the lumbar vertebrae and lumbosacral junction, and describe the positioning steps used for each, as follows:

   Essential projection: _____
   - Size of collimated field:

   - Key patient/part positioning points:

   - Anatomic landmarks and relation to IR:

   - CR orientation and entrance point:

   Essential projection: _____
   - Size of collimated field:

   - Key patient/part positioning points:

   - Anatomic landmarks and relation to IR:

   - CR orientation and entrance point:

   Essential projection: _____
   - Size of collimated field:

   - Key patient/part positioning points:

   - Anatomic landmarks and relation to IR:

   - CR orientation and entrance point:

   Essential projection: _____
   - Size of collimated field:

   - Key patient/part positioning points:

   - Anatomic landmarks and relation to IR:

   - CR orientation and entrance point:

   Essential projection: _____
   (_____ method)
   - Size of collimated field:

   - Key patient/part positioning points:

   - Anatomic landmarks and relation to IR:

   - CR orientation and entrance point:

Items 2 to 11 pertain to the *AP projection* with the patient in the supine position. Examine Fig. 9.36 as you answer the following questions.

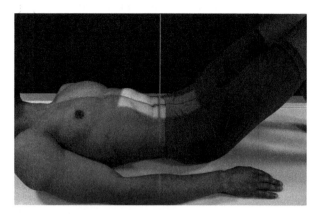

Fig. 9.36 AP lumbar vertebrae

2. Why should the patient empty the urinary bladder before the AP projection is performed?

3. What source-to-image receptor distance (SID) is recommended? Why?

4. How should the patient's arms be positioned to prevent the forearms from inadvertently superimposing the lower abdomen?

5. Why should the patient be instructed to flex the hips and knees in the supine position?

6. When using a 14- × 17-inch (35- × 43-cm) IR or a longer collimated field, the central ray should be

   centered to _____.

7. From the following list, select the parts of the lumbar vertebrae that should be demonstrated in an AP projection image.
   a. Lumbar bodies
   b. Intervertebral disk spaces
   c. Open intervertebral foramina
   d. Laminae
   e. Interpediculate spaces
   f. Open zygapophyseal joints
   g. Spinous processes
   h. Transverse processes

8. How much of the vertebral column should be clearly demonstrated in the image?

9. The width of the collimation should extend to the

   _____.

10. Explain why a patient wearing a pair of undershorts with an elastic waistband should be asked to remove or lower the garment.

11. Identify each lettered structure of the lumbar vertebrae in Fig. 9.37.
    A. _____
    B. _____
    C. _____
    D. _____
    E. _____
    F. _____
    G. _____
    H. _____
    I. _____

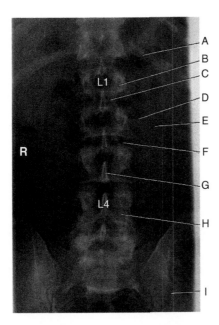

Fig. 9.37 AP lumbar vertebrae.

Items 12 to 22 pertain to the *lateral projection* with the patient in the left lateral recumbent body position. Examine Fig. 9.38 as you answer the following questions.

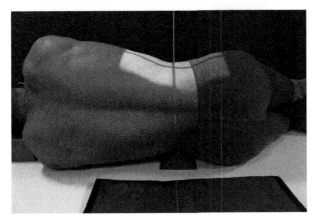

Fig. 9.38 Lateral lumbar vertebrae.

12. What body plane should be centered to the midline of the table?

13. For a patient with a thin body build and a narrow waist, what can a radiographer do to make the lumbar vertebral column closer to parallel with the table?

14. Which breathing instruction should be given to the patient?
    a. Breathe slowly.
    b. Stop breathing after expiration.
    c. Stop breathing after inspiration.

15. How should the central ray be directed when the long axis of the lumbar vertebral column is parallel with the table?
    a. Caudad
    b. Cephalad
    c. Perpendicular

16. For males, how many degrees and in what direction should the central ray be directed when the long axis of the lumbar vertebral column is not parallel with the table? For females?

17. How much of the vertebral column should be included in the image?

18. What lumbar anatomy should be demonstrated with the lateral projection?
    a. Lumbar zygapophyseal joints
    b. Intervertebral foramina
    c. Pars interarticularis
    d. All of the above

19. How should lumbar intervertebral disk spaces appear in the image of the lateral projection?

281

20. True or false. The patient's knees should be exactly superimposed to prevent rotation.

21. True or false. A sheet of leaded rubber should be placed on the table just posterior to the patient's lumbar column.

22. Identify each lettered structure of the vertebral column shown in Fig. 9.39.

    A. _____

    B. _____

    C. _____

    D. _____

    E. _____

    F. _____

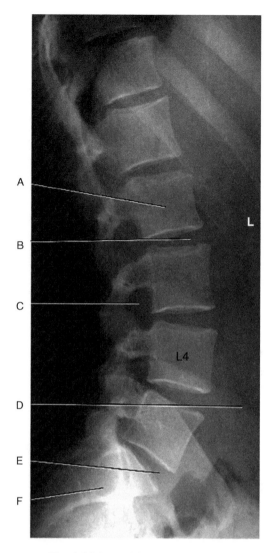

Fig. 9.39 Lateral lumbar vertebrae.

Chapter **9 Vertebral Column**

Items 23 to 28 pertain to the *localized lateral projection* that demonstrates the lumbosacral junction. Refer to Fig. 9.40, which shows a patient in the lateral recumbent position for a lateral projection of L5-S1, as you answer the following questions.

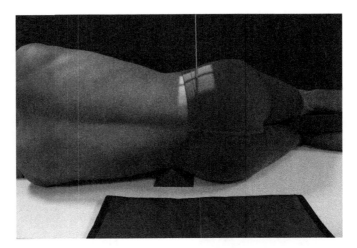

Fig. 9.40 Lateral L5-S1.

23. When positioning the typical patient, where is the lumbosacral junction located?

24. To what level of the patient should the IR/collimated field be centered?

25. What positioning factor determines whether the central ray needs to be angled or directed perpendicularly?
    a. Whether the legs are extended or hips flexed
    b. Whether or not the vertebral column is horizontal with the table
    c. Whether or not the arms are perpendicular to the long axis of the torso

26. Where should the perpendicular central ray enter the patient?
    a. At the level of the iliac crests
    b. 2 inches (5 cm) superior to the iliac crest
    c. 2 inches (5 cm) posterior to the anterior superior iliac spine (ASIS) and 1.5 inches (3.8 cm) inferior to the iliac crest

27. When the central ray needs to be angled, how many degrees and in what direction should it be directed for males? For females?

28. Identify each lettered structure of the vertebral column shown in Fig. 9.41.

A. _____

B. _____

C. _____

D. _____

E. _____

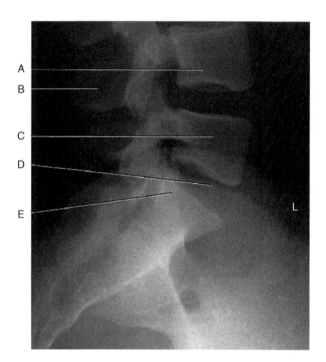

Fig. 9.41 Lateral L5-S1.

Items 29 to 46 pertain to AP *oblique projections* with the patient recumbent. Examine Figs. 9.42 and 9.43 as you answer the following questions.

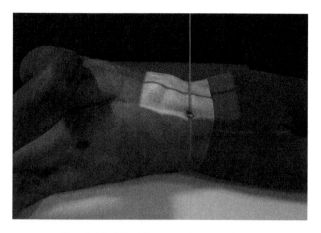

Fig. 9.42 AP oblique lumbar vertebrae.

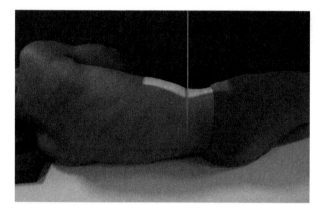

Fig. 9.43 AP oblique lumbar vertebrae.

29. Lumbar articular facets for vertebrae L1-L4 form an angle of _____ to _____ degrees.

30. The facets of the last lumbar vertebra form an average angle of _____ degrees.

31. The lumbar zygapophyseal articulations of the _____ side are demonstrated when the patient is rotated with the left side elevated off of the table.

32. On what vertebra should the IR/collimated field be centered for demonstrating the lumbar region?

33. Where exactly should the central ray enter the patient?

34. What is the significance of seeing the "Scottie dog" in the image?

35. Identify each lettered structure of the "Scottie dog" in Fig. 9.44.

   A. _____

   B. _____

   C. _____

   D. _____

   E. _____

   F. _____

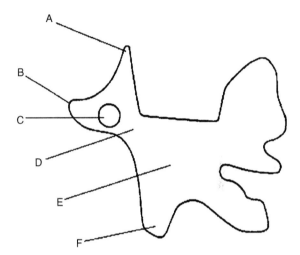

Fig. 9.44 Parts of the "Scottie dog."

36. On which side (right or left) are the lumbar zygapophyseal joints best demonstrated when the patient is positioned left posterior oblique (LPO)?

37. How much of the vertebral column should be included in the image?

38. What positioning error most likely occurred if the lumbar zygapophyseal joint is not well demonstrated and the pedicle is quite anterior on the vertebral body?
    a. The patient was rotated too much.
    b. The patient was not rotated enough.
    c. The vertebral column was not parallel with the table.

39. What positioning error most likely occurred if the lumbar zygapophyseal joint is not well demonstrated and the pedicle is quite posterior on the vertebral body?
    a. The patient was rotated too much.
    b. The patient was not rotated enough.
    c. The vertebral column was not parallel with the table.

40. True or false. The vertebral column should remain parallel with the tabletop to keep T12-L1 and L1-L2 joint spaces open.

41. True or false. The patient should be instructed to breathe slowly and deeply to blur overlying soft tissue shadows.

42. True or false. Demonstrating the "Scottie dog" means that the lumbar intervertebral foramina are open and well demonstrated.

43. True or false. The "eye" in the "Scottie dog" is the pedicle on the side closer to the IR.

44. True or false. The central ray should be directed caudally when the vertebral column is not parallel with the plane of the IR.

45. True or false. An oblique body position of up to 60 degrees from the plane of the IR may be needed to demonstrate the L5-S1 zygapophyseal joint and articular processes.

46. Identify each lettered structure of the vertebral column shown in Fig. 9.45.

    A. _____

    B. _____

    C. _____

    D. _____

    E. _____

    F. _____

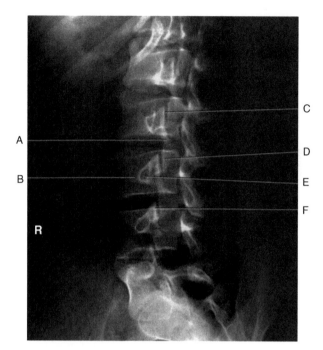

Fig. 9.45 AP oblique lumbar vertebrae.

Questions 47 to 53 pertain to the *AP axial projection (Ferguson method)* of the lumbosacral junction. Examine Fig. 9.46 as you answer the following questions.

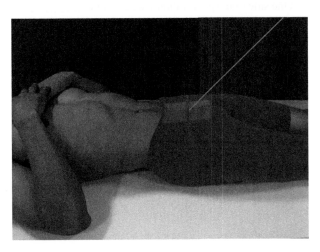

Fig. 9.46 AP axial projection of the lumbosacral junction and sacroiliac joints.

47. How should the patient's lower limbs be positioned?

48. What vertebral joints are demonstrated with the AP axial projection?

49. Through what joint should the central ray be directed?

50. Where on the midsagittal plane of the patient's anterior surface should the central ray enter?

51. How many degrees and in what direction should the central ray be directed for a man? For a woman?

52. What breathing instructions should be given to the patient?

53. Identify each labeled structure in Fig. 9.47.

A. _____

B. _____

C. _____

D. _____

E. _____

F. _____

G. _____

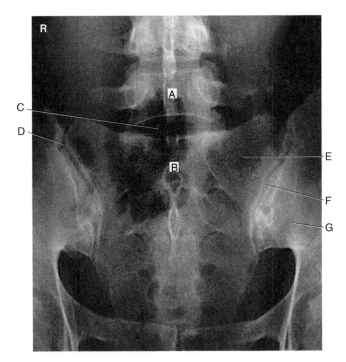

Fig. 9.47 AP axial projection of the lumbosacral junction and sacroiliac joints (Ferguson method).

Section 2: Exercise 5: Positioning for the Sacroiliac Joints, the Sacrum, and the Coccyx

This exercise pertains to the one essential projection for the SI joints and the two each for the sacrum and coccyx. Identify structures, fill in missing words, provide a short answer, select an answer from a list, or choose true or false (explaining any statement you believe to be false) for each item.

1. List the essential projection for the SI joints, and describe the positioning steps used, as follows:

   Essential projection: _____
   - Size of collimated field:

   - Key patient/part positioning points:

   - Anatomic landmarks and relation to IR:

   - CR orientation and entrance point:

Items 2 to 6 pertain to the *AP oblique projection* for the SI joints. Examine Fig. 9.48 as you answer the following questions.

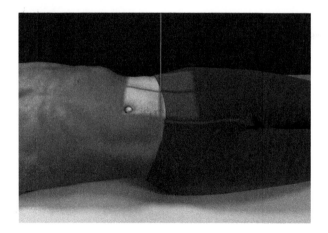

Fig. 9.48 AP oblique sacroiliac joint.

2. True or false. The affected side of the patient should be elevated.

3. One side of the pelvis should be elevated _____ to _____ degrees.

4. Where is the sagittal plane located that should be used to position the patient to the midline of the table?

5. What breathing instructions should be given to the patient?

6. Where on the patient's body should the central ray enter?

Items 7 to 12 pertain to the essential *projections for the sacrum.* Examine Figs. 9.49 and 9.50 as you answer the following questions.

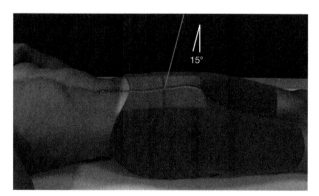

Fig. 9.49 AP axial sacrum.

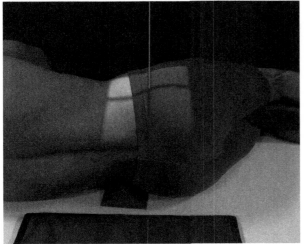

Fig. 9.50 Lateral sacrum.

7. List the essential projections for the sacrum, and describe the positioning steps used for each, as follows:

Essential projection: _____
- Size of collimated field:

- Key patient/part positioning points:

- Anatomic landmarks and relation to IR:

- CR orientation and entrance point:

Essential projection: _____
- Size of collimated field:

- Key patient/part positioning points:

- Anatomic landmarks and relation to IR:

- CR orientation and entrance point:

Essential projection: _____
- Size of collimated field:

- Key patient/part positioning points:

- Anatomic landmarks and relation to IR:

- CR orientation and entrance point:

8. Why is the AP axial projection preferred to the PA axial projection?

9. Why should the central ray be directed at a certain angle for the AP axial projection instead of being perpendicular to the IR?

10. What breathing instructions should be given to the patient?

11. How many degrees and in which direction should the central ray be directed when performing the AP axial sacrum?

12. Identify each lettered structure of the sacrum shown in Fig. 9.51.

A. _____

B. _____

C. _____

D. _____

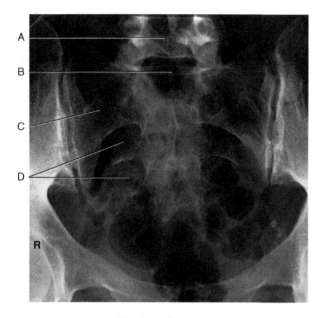

Fig. 9.51 Sacrum.

Items 13 to 20 pertain to the *essential projections for the coccyx.* Examine Figs. 9.52 and 9.53 as you answer the following questions.

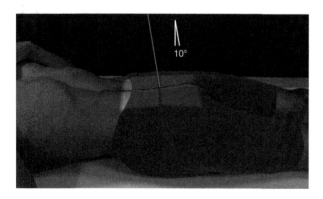

Fig. 9.52 AP coccyx.

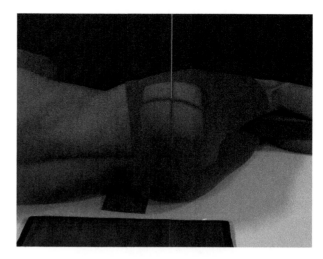

Fig. 9.53 Lateral coccyx.

13. List the essential projections for the coccyx, and describe the positioning steps used for each, as follows:

Essential projection: _____
■ Size of collimated field:

■ Key patient/part positioning points:

■ Anatomic landmarks and relation to IR:

■ CR orientation and entrance point:

Essential projection: _____
■ Size of collimated field:

■ Key patient/part positioning points:

■ Anatomic landmarks and relation to IR:

■ CR orientation and entrance point:

Essential projection: _____
- Size of collimated field:

- Key patient/part positioning points:

- Anatomic landmarks and relation to IR:

- CR orientation and entrance point:

14. Why is the AP axial projection preferred to the PA axial projection?

15. Should gonadal shielding be used for female patients? Explain your answer.

16. How should coccygeal segments appear in the AP and PA axial images?
    a. They should overlie the sacral segments.
    b. They should be superimposed with the symphysis pubis.
    c. They should be centered on the IR without rotation or superimposition.

17. For the lateral projection, which object should be placed behind the patient on the tabletop to improve image quality?
    a. Foam cushion
    b. Folded blanket
    c. Sheet of leaded rubber

18. When the patient is in the lateral recumbent position for the lateral projection, approximately how far posterior from the ASIS should the patient be centered on the IR?

19. To what level of the patient should the IR be centered for the lateral projection?

20. What breathing instructions should be given to the patient?

Section 2: Exercise 6: Thoracolumbar Spine: Scoliosis

This exercise pertains to the methods used to image patients with scoliosis. Provide a short answer, select an answer from a list, or choose true or false (explaining any statement you believe to be false) for each item. Examine Fig. 9.54 as you answer the following questions.

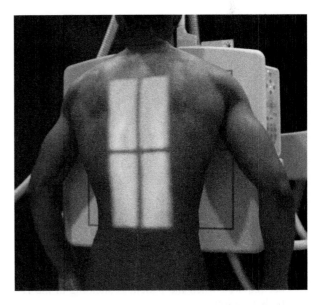

Fig. 9.54 PA thoracolumbar vertebrae for scoliosis.

1. List the two methods used to image patients with scoliosis.

2. How many images are necessary to complete the Ferguson series?
   a. 2
   b. 3
   c. 4

3. List the projections that might be used to evaluate scoliosis using the Frank et al. method.

4. What type of positioning maneuver is used to differentiate between primary and secondary curves in scoliosis imaging procedures?

5. True or false. Primary curves will not change on lateral bending studies.

6. True or false. The patient should be in the supine position for the Ferguson series.

7. True or false. The AP projection is preferred to reduce radiation dose to the breasts.

8. True or false. Images from previous examinations should be checked to determine the appropriate amount of collimation of the width of the field size.

9. True or false. In the first image, the patient should be standing with a support block under the convex side of the vertebral curve.

10. True or false. Lead-impregnated gonadal shielding is not required when the patient is standing in the PA body position.

11. True or false. A compression band may be used to hold the patient firmly against the grid.

12. How much of the vertebral column should be demonstrated on the images?

13. Why is a PA projection preferred to an AP projection?

14. To expose the length of the 36-inch (90-cm) IR, what recommended SID should be used?

15. Fig. 9.55 shows a frontal view of a patient who has scoliosis. If this is the first image obtained with the Ferguson method for performing a scoliosis series, under which side of the patient should a support block be placed for the patient to stand on for the second image?

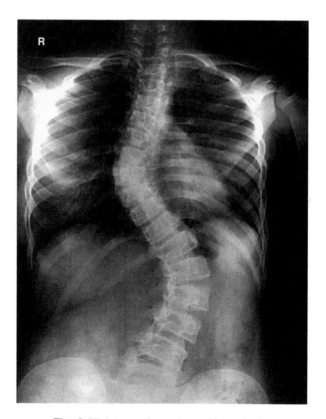

Fig. 9.55 Image of a patient with scoliosis.

292

Section 2: Exercise 7: Identifying Projections of the Vertebral Column

This exercise has photographs that show patients being positioned for various projections of the vertebral column. Examine each photograph and identify the projection by name and the part of the vertebral column that is being demonstrated.

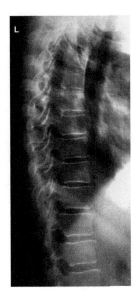

Fig. 9.56

1. Fig. 9.56: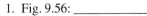

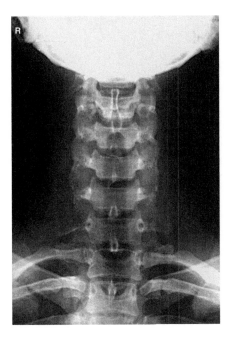

Fig. 9.57

2. Fig. 9.57: _____

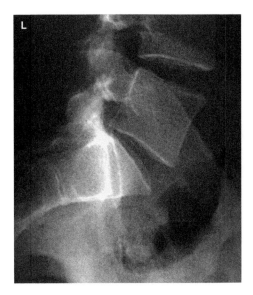

Fig. 9.58

3. Fig. 9.58: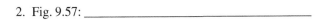

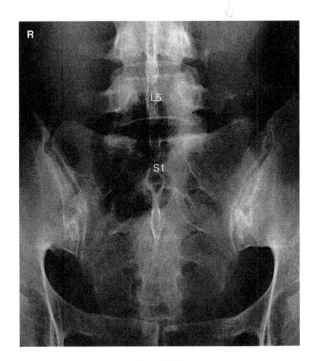

Fig. 9.59

4. Fig. 9.59: _____

293

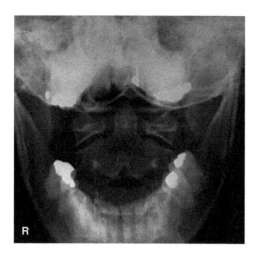

Fig. 9.60

5. Fig. 9.60: _____

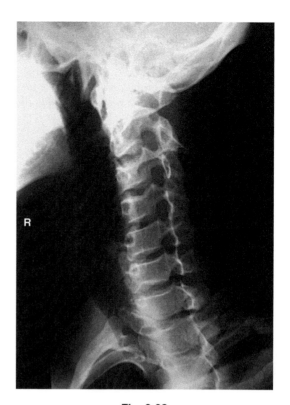

Fig. 9.62

7. Fig. 9.62, RPO position: _____

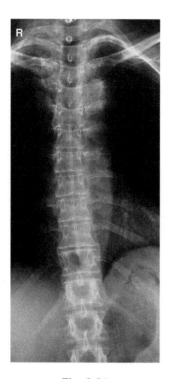

Fig. 9.61

6. Fig. 9.61: _____

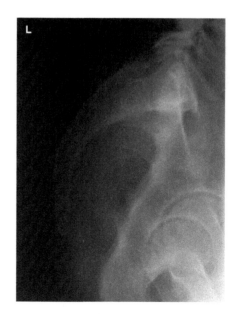

Fig. 9.63

8. Fig. 9.63: _____

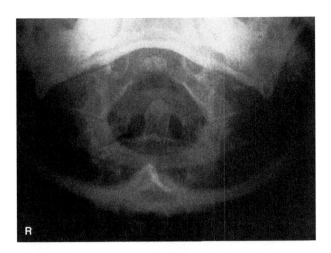

Fig. 9.64

9. Fig. 9.64: _____

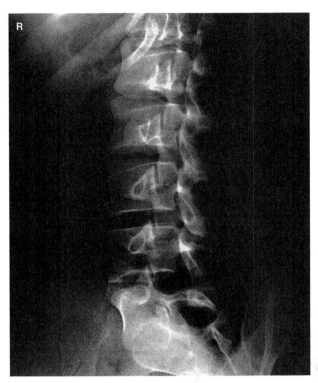

Fig. 9.66

11. Fig. 9.66, RPO position: _____

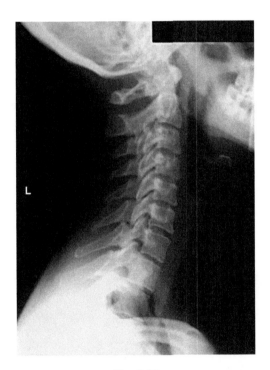

Fig. 9.65

10. Fig. 9.65: _____

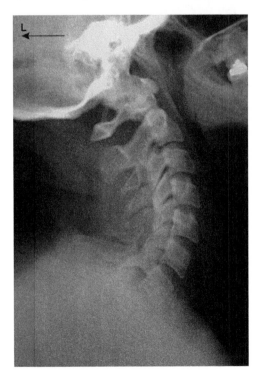

Fig. 9.67

12. Fig. 9.67: _____

Chapter **9** **Vertebral Column**

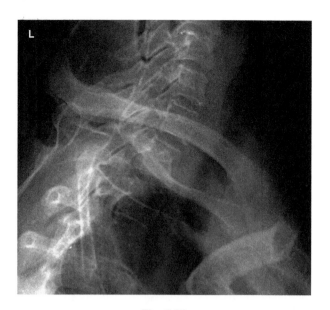

Fig. 9.68

13. Fig. 9.68: _____

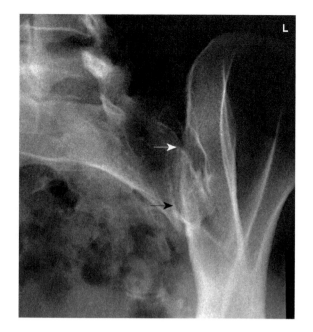

Fig. 9.70

15. Fig. 9.70, RPO position: _____

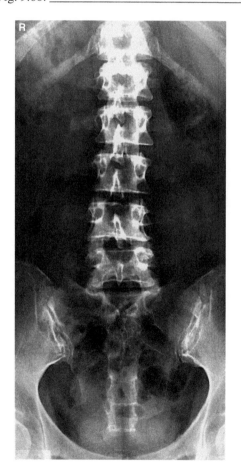

Fig. 9.69

14. Fig. 9.69: _____

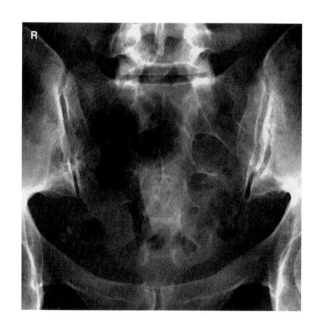

Fig. 9.71

16. Fig. 9.71: _____

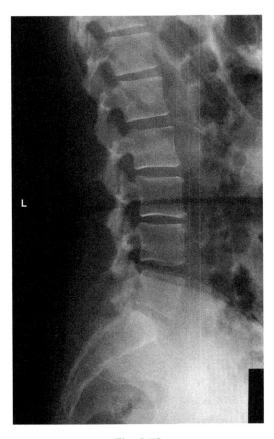

Fig. 9.72

17. Fig. 9.72: _____

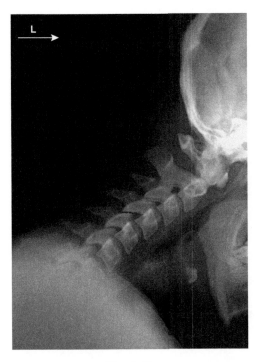

Fig. 9.73

18. Fig. 9.73: _____

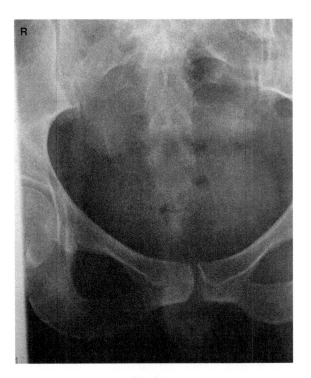

Fig. 9.74

19. Fig. 9.74: _____

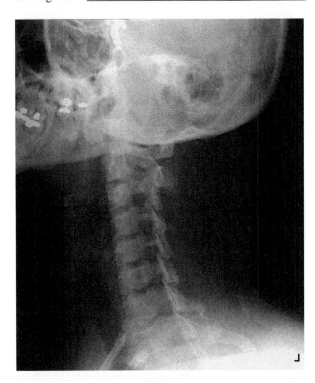

Fig. 9.75

20. Fig. 9.75, LAO position: _____

297

Section 2: Exercise 8: Evaluating Images of the Vertebral Column

This exercise presents images of the vertebral column to give you practice evaluating vertebral column positioning. These images are not from Merrill's Atlas. Each image shows at least one positioning error. Examine each image and answer the questions that follow by providing a short answer.

1. Fig. 9.76 shows an image of the AP projection (open mouth) with the patient incorrectly positioned. State the positioning error that produced this image.

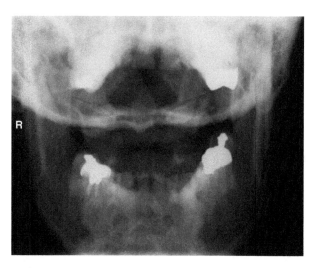

Fig. 9.76 AP (open mouth) C1-C2 image with error.

2. Fig. 9.77 shows an image of the AP projection (open mouth) with the patient incorrectly positioned. State the positioning error that produced this image.

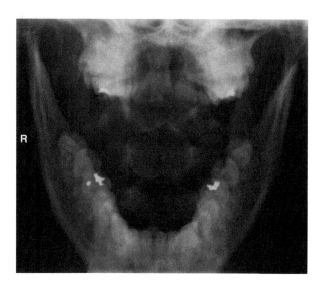

Fig. 9.77 AP (open mouth) C1-C2 image with error.

3. Fig. 9.78 shows an image of a lateral projection that does not meet all evaluation criteria for this projection. What evaluation criterion for this projection is not met?

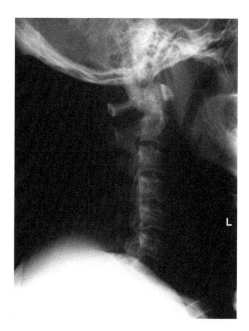

Fig. 9.78 Lateral cervical spine image with error.

4. Fig. 9.79 shows an AP axial oblique projection image. Examine the image and answer the questions that follow.

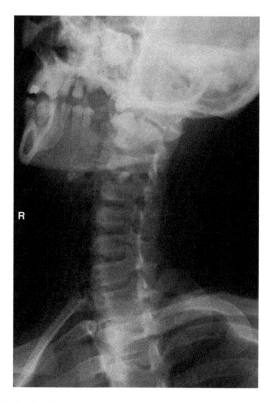

Fig. 9.79 AP axial oblique cervical spine image with errors.

a. In what body position was the patient placed?

b. List two evaluation criteria that this image does not meet.

c. List two ways the positioning of the patient could be improved to correct the errors seen in this image.

5. Fig. 9.80 shows a PA axial oblique projection image of the left cervical intervertebral foramina demonstrated with the patient in the right anterior oblique (RAO) position. Examine the image and state why it is unacceptable.

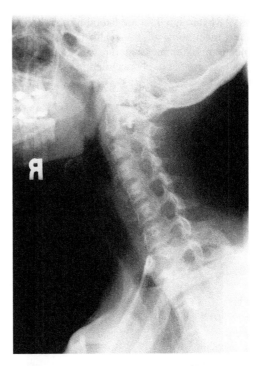

Fig. 9.80 PA axial oblique cervical spine image with error.

6. Figs. 9.81 through 9.84 are lateral lumbar images that do not meet some of the evaluation criteria for the projection. Examine each image and describe what type of error most likely occurred in the production of the image.

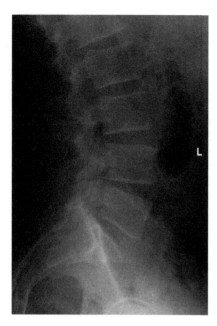

Fig. 9.81 Rejected lateral lumbar image.

a. Fig. 9.81: _____

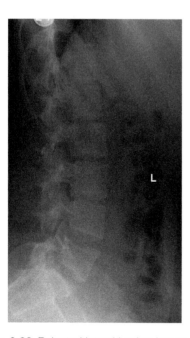

Fig. 9.82 Rejected lateral lumbar image.

b. Fig. 9.82: _____

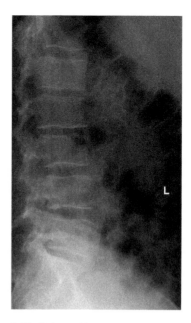

Fig. 9.83 Rejected lateral lumbar image.

c. Fig. 9.83: _____

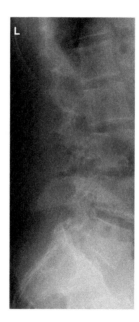

Fig. 9.84 Rejected lateral lumbar image.

d. Fig. 9.84: _____

7. Fig. 9.85 shows an image of an AP oblique projection (posterior oblique position) with incorrect positioning of the patient. Examine the image and answer the questions that follow.

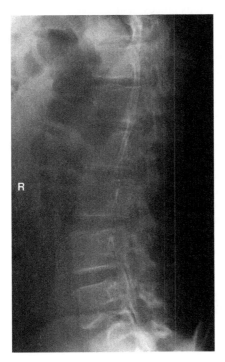

Fig. 9.85 AP oblique lumbar image with positioning error.

a. What posterior oblique position does the image represent?

b. Which side of the lumbar zygapophyseal joints should be best demonstrated?

c. Are the lumbar zygapophyseal joints well demonstrated?

d. Are the pedicles properly located within the "Scottie dog"? Explain.

e. What positioning error most likely caused the image to appear this way?

8. Fig. 9.86 shows an image of an AP oblique projection (posterior oblique position) with the patient incorrectly positioned. Examine the image and answer the questions that follow.

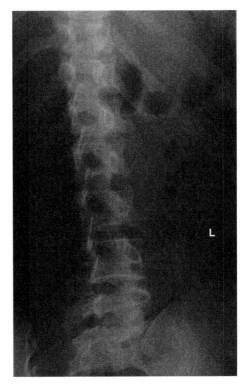

Fig. 9.86 AP oblique lumbar image with positioning error.

a. Which posterior oblique position does the image represent?

b. Which side of the lumbar zygapophyseal joints should be best demonstrated?

c. Are the lumbar zygapophyseal joints well demonstrated?

d. Are the pedicles properly located within the "Scottie dog"? Explain.

e. What positioning error most likely caused the image to appear this way?

Answer the following questions by selecting the best choice.

1. Which two vertebral curvatures are anteriorly concave?
   a. Cervical and lumbar
   b. Cervical and pelvic
   c. Thoracic and lumbar
   d. Thoracic and pelvic

2. Which two vertebral curves are kyphotic curves?
   a. Cervical and lumbar
   b. Cervical and pelvic
   c. Thoracic and lumbar
   d. Thoracic and pelvic

3. Which two vertebral curves are lordotic curves?
   a. Cervical and lumbar
   b. Cervical and pelvic
   c. Thoracic and lumbar
   d. Thoracic and pelvic

4. Which two vertebral curves are primary curves?
   a. Cervical and lumbar
   b. Cervical and pelvic
   c. Thoracic and lumbar
   d. Thoracic and pelvic

5. Which spinal condition involves abnormally increased anterior concavity (posterior convexity) of the thoracic vertebral column?
   a. Lordosis
   b. Scoliosis
   c. Kyphosis
   d. Spina bifida

6. Which abnormal spinal condition involves any lateral curvature of the vertebral column?
   a. Lordosis
   b. Scoliosis
   c. Kyphosis
   d. Spondylolisthesis

7. What is the name of the short, thick bony processes that project posteriorly from the lateral and superior aspects of vertebral bodies of typical vertebrae?
   a. Laminae
   b. Pedicles
   c. Spinous processes
   d. Transverse processes

8. From the junction of which two vertebral structures do transverse processes originate in typical vertebrae?
   a. Pedicle and body
   b. Pedicle and lamina
   c. Spinous process and body
   d. Spinous process and lamina

9. Which vertebral structures unite at the origin of the spinous process of a typical vertebra?
   a. Both laminae
   b. Both pedicles
   c. Pedicle and body
   d. Pedicle and transverse process

10. Which structures of a typical vertebra are the zygapophyses?
    a. Vertebral foramen
    b. Articular processes
    c. Transverse processes
    d. Intervertebral foramina

11. On which structure is the dens located?
    a. C1
    b. C2
    c. Spinous process
    d. Transverse process

12. Which structure is known as the "atlas"?
    a. C1
    b. C2
    c. Dens
    d. Vertebra prominens

13. Which structure is known as the "axis"?
    a. C1
    b. C2
    c. Dens
    d. Vertebra prominens

14. On which structure is the dens located?
    a. Body of C1
    b. Body of C2
    c. Transverse process of C1
    d. Transverse process of C2

15. Which cervical vertebral structures are perforated with a foramen for the passage of the vertebral artery and vein?
    a. Body
    b. Pedicles
    c. Spinous processes
    d. Transverse processes

16. Which vertebral structures have bifid tips?
    a. Spinous processes of cervical vertebrae
    b. Spinous processes of thoracic vertebrae
    c. Transverse processes of cervical vertebrae
    d. Transverse processes of thoracic vertebrae

17. With reference to the midsagittal plane, how do zyg-apophyseal joints open in cervical vertebrae?
    a. 20 degrees anteriorly
    b. 25 degrees posteriorly
    c. 45 degrees posteriorly
    d. 90 degrees laterally

18. With reference to the midsagittal plane, how do zyg-apophyseal joints open in thoracic vertebrae?
    a. 15 to 20 degrees anteriorly
    b. 30 to 45 degrees posteriorly
    c. 70 to 75 degrees anteriorly
    d. 90 degrees laterally

19. Thoracic vertebrae differ from cervical and lumbar vertebrae because thoracic vertebrae have:
    a. demifacets.
    b. no transverse processes.
    c. the largest spinous processes.
    d. bifid tips on the spinous processes.

20. Which structures articulate with vertebral demifacets?
    a. Heads of ribs
    b. Tubercles of ribs
    c. Transverse processes
    d. Zygapophyseal joints

21. With reference to the midsagittal plane, how do zyg-apophyseal joints open in lumbar vertebrae?
    a. 15 to 20 degrees anteriorly
    b. 30 to 60 degrees anteriorly
    c. 30 to 60 degrees posteriorly
    d. 90 degrees laterally

22. Lumbar vertebrae differ from cervical and thoracic vertebrae because lumbar vertebrae have:
    a. Demifacets
    b. Bifid spinous process tips
    c. Broad, large spinous processes
    d. Foramina through the transverse processes

23. Which parts of the sacrum form the joints with the ilia of the pelvis?
    a. Sacral cornua
    b. Auricular surfaces
    c. Sacral promontory
    d. Median sacral crest

24. The AP projection that demonstrates the dens using the Fuchs method differs from the AP projection (open mouth) because the Fuchs method:
    a. directs the central ray to C4.
    b. angles the central ray 15 degrees cephalad.
    c. extends the chin and keeps the mouth closed.
    d. demonstrates intervertebral foramina of the upper vertebrae.

25. The radiographer should not use the Fuchs method to obtain the AP projection of the dens if the patient is:
    a. intoxicated.
    b. unable to suspend respiration.
    c. unable to depress both shoulders.
    d. suspected to have a fracture or degenerative disease.

26. Which projection of the cervical vertebrae demonstrates the dens imaged within the foramen magnum?
    a. Lateral projection
    b. AP axial oblique projection
    c. AP projection (open mouth)
    d. AP projection (Fuchs method)

27. Which cervical structures are best demonstrated with the AP projection (open mouth)?
    a. C1 and C2
    b. Spinous processes
    c. Intervertebral disks
    d. Intervertebral foramina

28. How should the central ray be directed for the AP projection (open mouth)?
    a. Perpendicularly
    b. 15 degrees caudally
    c. 15 degrees cephalically
    d. 20 degrees cephalically

29. How and where should the central ray be directed for the AP axial projection of the cervical vertebral column?
    a. Perpendicular to C4
    b. Perpendicular to C7
    c. 15 to 20 degrees cephalad to C4
    d. 15 to 20 degrees cephalad to C7

30. How should the IR be positioned for the AP axial projection of the cervical vertebral column?
    a. Centered to C4
    b. Centered to mastoid tips
    c. With the top border at the level of C4
    d. With the top border at the level of mastoid tips

31. For which projection of the cervical vertebrae should the central ray be angled 15 to 20 degrees cephalad?
    a. AP axial projection
    b. PA axial oblique projection
    c. AP projection (open mouth)
    d. AP projection (Fuchs method)

32. Which evaluation criterion does not apply to the AP axial projection of the cervical vertebral column?
    a. The intervertebral disk spaces should be open.
    b. The spinous processes should be equidistant to the pedicles.
    c. The mandibular angles should be equidistant to the vertebrae.
    d. C1 and C2 should be seen without mandibular superimposition.

33. Which projection of the cervical vertebral column requires an SID of 40 to 48 inches?
    a. AP projection
    b. Lateral projection
    c. PA axial oblique projection
    d. AP axial oblique projection

34. Which maneuver should be used to help obtain maximum depression of the shoulders in the lateral projection of the cervical vertebral column?
    a. Direct the central ray 15 degrees caudad.
    b. Direct the central ray 15 degrees cephalad.
    c. Suspend respiration after full inhalation.
    d. Suspend respiration after full expiration.

35. What should be done so that the magnified shoulder farthest from the IR is projected below the lower cervical vertebrae for the lateral projection of the cervical vertebrae?
    a. Direct a horizontal central ray to C4.
    b. Direct a horizontal central ray to C7.
    c. Angle the central ray 15 degrees caudad.
    d. Angle the central ray 15 degrees cephalad.

36. What should be done to prevent mandibular rami from superimposing cervical vertebrae in the lateral projection of the cervical vertebral column?
    a. Elevate the chin.
    b. Direct a horizontal central ray to C4.
    c. Angle the central ray 15 degrees cephalad.
    d. Instruct the patient to hold weights in each hand.

37. What should be done to reduce the magnification caused by the increased object-to-image distance in the lateral projection of the cervical vertebrae?
    a. Angle the central ray 15 degrees cephalad.
    b. Instruct the patient to hold weights in each hand.
    c. Take the exposure on suspended full expiration.
    d. Use a 72-inch (183-cm) SID.

38. What is the recommended size of the collimated radiation field for the lateral projection of the cervical vertebrae?
    a. 5 × 5 inches (13 × 13 cm)
    b. 8 × 10 inches (20 × 24 cm)
    c. 10 × 12 inches (24 × 30 cm)
    d. 14 × 17 inches (35 × 43 cm)

39. Which projection of the cervical vertebrae demonstrates the spinous processes elevated and widely separated?
    a. AP axial projection
    b. AP axial oblique projection
    c. Hyperflexion lateral projection
    d. Hyperextension lateral projection

40. Which projection of the cervical vertebrae demonstrates the spinous processes depressed and in close approximation?
    a. AP axial projection
    b. AP axial oblique projection
    c. Hyperflexion lateral projection
    d. Hyperextension lateral projection

41. Which projection for cervical vertebrae must be exposed with a horizontal and perpendicular central ray?
    a. Lateral
    b. AP axial
    c. AP open mouth
    d. AP axial oblique

42. How should the central ray be directed for an AP axial oblique projection of the cervical vertebral column?
    a. Horizontally
    b. Perpendicularly
    c. 15 to 20 degrees caudad
    d. 15 to 20 degrees cephalad

43. How should the central ray be directed for the PA axial oblique projection of the cervical vertebral column?
    a. Vertically
    b. Perpendicularly
    c. 15 to 20 degrees caudad
    d. 15 to 20 degrees cephalad

44. Which projection of the cervical vertebral column best demonstrates the intervertebral foramina?
    a. Lateral projection
    b. AP axial projection
    c. AP axial oblique projection
    d. AP projection (open mouth)

45. Which position of the cervical vertebral column best demonstrates the left intervertebral foramina when the central ray is angled 15 to 20 degrees cephalad?
    a. LAO
    b. LPO
    c. RAO
    d. RPO

46. Which position of the cervical vertebral column best demonstrates the right intervertebral foramina when the central ray is angled 15 to 20 degrees caudad?
    a. LAO
    b. LPO
    c. RAO
    d. RPO

47. How many degrees from supine or the anatomic position should the entire body be rotated for the AP axial oblique projection of the cervical vertebrae?
    a. 15 degrees
    b. 20 degrees
    c. 45 degrees
    d. 90 degrees

48. What is the proper amount of head and body rotation for the PA axial oblique projection of the cervical vertebrae?
    a. 15 degrees
    b. 20 degrees
    c. 35 degrees
    d. 45 degrees

49. Which evaluation criterion pertains to the AP projection (Fuchs method) of the cervical vertebrae?
    a. The mandible rami should be superimposed.
    b. All seven cervical vertebrae should be demonstrated.
    c. The intervertebral foramina and disk spaces should be open.
    d. The entire dens should be seen through the foramen magnum.

50. Which evaluation criterion pertains to the AP axial projection of the cervical vertebral column?
    a. All seven cervical vertebrae should be demonstrated.
    b. The spinous processes should be equidistant to the pedicles.
    c. The intervertebral foramina should be open with foramina closest to the IR well demonstrated.
    d. The intervertebral foramina should be open with foramina farthest from the IR well demonstrated.

51. Which evaluation criterion pertains to the lateral projection of the cervical vertebral column?
    a. All seven cervical vertebrae should be demonstrated.
    b. The spinous processes should be equidistant to the pedicles.
    c. The intervertebral foramina should be open with foramina closest to the IR well demonstrated.
    d. The intervertebral foramina should be open with foramina farthest from the IR well demonstrated.

52. Which evaluation criterion pertains to the AP axial oblique projection of the cervical vertebral column?
    a. The rami of the mandible should be superimposed.
    b. The spinous processes should be equidistant to the pedicles.
    c. The intervertebral foramina should be open with foramina closest to the IR well demonstrated.
    d. The intervertebral foramina should be open with foramina farthest from the IR well demonstrated.

53. Which evaluation criterion pertains to PA axial oblique projections of the cervical vertebral column?
    a. The rami of the mandible should be superimposed.
    b. The spinous processes should be equidistant to the pedicles.
    c. The intervertebral foramina should be open with foramina closest to the IR well demonstrated.
    d. The intervertebral foramina should be open with foramina farthest from the IR well demonstrated.

54. Which projection should be included in a cervical series if the lateral projection does not demonstrate the C7 vertebra?
    a. AP axial oblique projection
    b. Lateral projection (swimmer's technique)
    c. Lateral projection (dorsal decubitus position)
    d. AP projection with a perpendicular central ray

55. For the lateral projection (swimmer's technique) of the cervical vertebrae, how and where should the central ray be directed?
    a. Perpendicular to C4
    b. Perpendicular to the intervertebral disk space of C7 and T1
    c. Angled 15 degrees cephalad to C4
    d. Angled 15 degrees cephalad to the intervertebral disk space of C7 and T1

56. Which of the following structures are best demonstrated with the lateral projection (swimmer's technique)?
    a. Lower cervical and upper thoracic vertebrae
    b. Lower thoracic and upper cervical vertebrae
    c. Thoracic zygapophyseal joints
    d. Cervical intervertebral foramina

57. For the AP projection of the thoracic vertebral column, where should the central ray be centered on the anterior chest wall?
    a. At the sternal angle
    b. At the jugular notch
    c. At the level of the inferior angles of the scapulae
    d. At a point halfway between the jugular notch and the xiphoid process

58. With reference to the patient, where should the top border of the IR or collimated field be positioned for the AP projection of the thoracic vertebrae?
    a. To the level of T7
    b. To the level of the jugular notch
    c. 1½ to 2 inches (3.8 to 5 cm) above the sternal angle
    d. 1½ to 2 inches (3.8 to 5 cm) above the top of the shoulders

59. For the AP projection of the thoracic vertebral column with the patient in the supine position, why should the patient's hips and knees be flexed?
    a. To reduce kyphosis
    b. To decrease lordosis
    c. To depress the diaphragm to its lowest level
    d. To raise the diaphragm to its highest level

60. Which projection most requires usage of the anode heel effect to improve its image quality?
    a. AP projection of the lumbar vertebral column
    b. AP projection of the thoracic vertebral column
    c. AP axial projection of the cervical vertebral column
    d. AP projection of the cervical vertebrae (open mouth)

61. Which projection best demonstrates the intervertebral foramina of the thoracic vertebral column?
    a. AP projection
    b. Lateral projection
    c. From true lateral, patient rotated 20 degrees anteriorly
    d. From true lateral, patient rotated 20 degrees posteriorly

62. What structures are not well visualized on a lateral projection of the thoracic vertebrae?
    a. T1 to T3
    b. T1 to T5
    c. Intervertebral disk spaces
    d. Intervertebral foramina

63. To what level of the body should the central ray be directed for the lateral projection of the thoracic vertebrae?
    a. Sternal angle
    b. Manubrial notch
    c. Xiphoid process
    d. Inferior angle of the scapula

64. What compensation should be made in the lateral projection of the thoracic vertebral column on a recumbent patient when the lower thoracic region is not parallel with the table?
    a. Place cushions under the patient's head.
    b. Direct the perpendicular central ray to T10.
    c. Angle the central ray 10 to 15 degrees caudad.
    d. Angle the central ray 10 to 15 degrees cephalad.

65. Which of the following would improve visualization of the spinous processes and overall image quality on the lateral projection of the thoracic vertebrae?
    a. Activation of the center detector on the automatic exposure control
    b. Placing lead rubber on the table behind the patient
    c. Use of a breathing technique (low milliamperage with a long exposure time)
    d. Use of a bow-tie–type compensating filter

66. Which projection of the vertebral column best demonstrates kyphosis?
    a. AP projection of the lumbar vertebral column
    b. AP projection of the thoracic vertebral column
    c. Lateral projection of the lumbar vertebral column
    d. Lateral projection of the thoracic vertebral column

67. Which projection of the vertebral column best demonstrates scoliosis?
    a. PA projection of the thoracolumbar vertebral column
    b. Lateral projection of the lumbosacral vertebral column
    c. Lateral projection of the cervicothoracic vertebral column
    d. AP projection of the cervicothoracic vertebral column

68. Which projection of the vertebral column best demonstrates lordosis?
    a. AP projection of the lumbar vertebral column
    b. AP projection of the thoracic vertebral column
    c. Lateral projection of the lumbar vertebral column
    d. Lateral projection of the thoracic vertebral column

69. Why should the patient flex the hips and knees for the AP projection of the lumbar vertebrae?
    a. To reduce lumbar lordosis
    b. To increase lumbar lordosis
    c. To raise the diaphragm to its highest level
    d. To depress the diaphragm to its lowest level

70. Where should the central ray be centered on the patient for the AP projection of the lumbosacral vertebrae?
    a. On the xiphoid process
    b. On MSP at the level of the iliac crests
    c. On MSP at the level of the greater trochanters
    d. On MSP 1½ inches (3.8 cm) above the iliac crests

71. When is it recommended that the collimated field size for an AP projection of the lumbar vertebrae be open to 14 × 17 inches (35 × 43 cm)?
    a. When demonstration of only the lumbar vertebrae is needed
    b. For trauma patients for visualization of the liver, kidney, spleen, and psoas muscle margins along with air or gas patterns
    c. When the patient is positioned prone or upright
    d. When the patient has extreme kyphosis

72. Which plane or line of the patient should be centered on the midline of the table for the AP projection of the lumbar vertebral column?
    a. Oblique
    b. Horizontal
    c. Midsagittal
    d. Midcoronal

73. Where should the central ray be directed for the AP projection of only the lumbar vertebrae?
    a. L4
    b. 1.5 inches (3.8 cm) above the iliac crests
    c. 3 inches (7.6 cm) above the iliac crests
    d. 2 inches (5 cm) above the symphysis pubis

74. Which plane or line of the patient should be centered on the midline of the table for the lateral projection of the lumbar vertebral column?
    a. Oblique
    b. Horizontal
    c. Midsagittal
    d. Midcoronal

75. Which projection of the lumbar vertebrae best demonstrates intervertebral foramina?
    a. AP projection
    b. Lateral projection
    c. PA oblique projection
    d. AP oblique projection

76. How many degrees and in which direction should the central ray be directed for the lateral projection of the lumbar vertebrae when the vertebral column is positioned parallel with the table?
    a. Perpendicular
    b. 5 to 8 degrees caudad
    c. 5 to 8 degrees cephalad
    d. 15 to 20 degrees caudad

77. How many degrees and in which direction should the central ray be directed for the lateral projection of the lumbar vertebrae when the vertebral column is *not* parallel with the table?
    a. Perpendicular for males, 8 degrees caudad for females
    b. Perpendicular for females, 5 degrees caudad for males
    c. 5 degrees caudad for males, 8 degrees caudad for females
    d. 5 degrees caudad for females, 8 degrees caudad for males

78. How many degrees and in which direction should the central ray be directed for the lateral projection of L5-S1 when the vertebral column is positioned parallel with the table?
    a. Perpendicular
    b. 5 to 8 degrees caudad
    c. 5 to 8 degrees cephalad
    d. 10 to 15 degrees caudad

79. Which projection of the lumbar vertebrae best demonstrates the zygapophyseal joints?
    a. AP projection
    b. Lateral projection
    c. AP oblique projection
    d. AP axial oblique projection

80. Which vertebral structures are best demonstrated if a supine patient is rotated 45 degrees with the right side elevated and a perpendicular central ray is directed at the third lumbar vertebra?
    a. Intervertebral foramina on the left side
    b. Intervertebral foramina on the right side
    c. Zygapophyseal joints on the left side
    d. Zygapophyseal joints on the right side

81. Which vertebral structures are best demonstrated with the AP oblique projection of the lumbar vertebral column with the patient positioned in a 45-degree RPO?
    a. Intervertebral foramina of the right side
    b. Intervertebral foramina of the left side
    c. Zygapophyseal joints of the left side
    d. Zygapophyseal joints of the right side

82. Which vertebral structures are best demonstrated with the AP oblique projection of the lumbar vertebral column with the patient positioned in a 45-degree LPO?
    a. Intervertebral foramina
    b. Lumbar vertebral bodies in profile
    c. Zygapophyseal joints of the left side
    d. Zygapophyseal joints of the right side

83. Which positioning error most likely occurred if the zygapophyseal joints were not well demonstrated and the pedicle was quite anterior on the vertebral body in an image of an AP oblique projection of the lumbar vertebrae?
    a. The patient was rotated too much.
    b. The patient was not rotated enough.
    c. The spine was not parallel with the table.
    d. The central ray was not perpendicular to the IR.

84. Which positioning error most likely occurred if the zygapophyseal joints were not well demonstrated and the pedicle was quite posterior on the vertebral body in an image of an AP oblique projection of the lumbar vertebrae?
    a. The patient was rotated too much.
    b. The patient was not rotated enough.
    c. The spine was not parallel with the table.
    d. The central ray was not perpendicular to the IR.

85. Which projection of the vertebral column demonstrates the "Scottie dog"?
    a. Lateral projection of the lumbar vertebral column
    b. Lateral projection of the thoracic vertebral column
    c. Oblique projection of the lumbar vertebral column
    d. Oblique projection of the cervical vertebral column

86. What is demonstrated if the "Scottie dog" is well visualized?
    a. Zygapophyseal joints of the lumbar vertebrae
    b. Zygapophyseal joints of the thoracic vertebrae
    c. Intervertebral foramina of the lumbar vertebrae
    d. Intervertebral foramina of the thoracic vertebrae

87. How many degrees of body rotation are necessary for the AP oblique projection of the lumbar vertebrae?
    a. 15 to 20 degrees
    b. 25 to 30 degrees
    c. 45 degrees
    d. 70 degrees

88. Which projection of the lumbar vertebrae requires MSP to be positioned perpendicular to the IR?
    a. AP projection
    b. Lateral projection
    c. AP oblique projection
    d. Lateral projection, L5-S1

89. Which projection of the lumbar vertebrae requires MSP to be positioned parallel with the IR?
    a. AP projection
    b. Lateral projection
    c. AP oblique projection
    d. PA oblique projection

90. How many degrees and in which direction should the central ray be directed for an AP axial projection of the lumbosacral junction and SI joints?
    a. 5 to 8 degrees caudad
    b. 5 to 8 degrees cephalad
    c. 30 to 35 degrees caudad
    d. 30 to 35 degrees cephalad

91. Which projection best demonstrates the right SI joint?
    a. Lateral projection with the patient in right lateral recumbent position
    b. PA oblique projection with the patient in the LAO position
    c. AP oblique projection with the patient in the LPO position
    d. AP oblique projection with the patient in the RPO position

92. Which projection best demonstrates the left SI joint?
    a. Lateral projection with the patient in left lateral recumbent position
    b. AP oblique projection with the patient in the LPO position
    c. PA oblique projection with the patient in the RAO position
    d. AP oblique projection with the patient in the RPO position

93. How many degrees of body rotation from the supine position are required for an AP oblique projection of the SI joints?
    a. 15 to 20 degrees
    b. 25 to 30 degrees
    c. 35 to 45 degrees
    d. 45 to 55 degrees

94. How many degrees and in which direction should the central ray be directed for AP axial projections of the sacrum?
    a. 10 degrees caudad
    b. 10 degrees cephalad
    c. 15 degrees caudad
    d. 15 degrees cephalad

95. How many degrees and in which direction should the central ray be directed if it is necessary to have the patient prone for a PA axial projection of the sacrum?
    a. 10 degrees caudad
    b. 10 degrees cephalad
    c. 15 degrees caudad
    d. 15 degrees cephalad

96. How many degrees and in which direction should the central ray be directed for an AP axial projection of the coccyx?
    a. Perpendicular
    b. 10 degrees caudad
    c. 10 degrees cephalad
    d. 15 degrees cephalad

97. How many degrees and in which direction should the central ray be directed if it is necessary to have the patient prone for a PA axial projection of the coccyx?
    a. 10 degrees caudad
    b. 10 degrees cephalad
    c. 15 degrees caudad
    d. 15 degrees cephalad

98. How many degrees and in which direction should the central ray be directed for the lateral projection of the sacrum?
    a. Perpendicular
    b. 10 degrees caudad
    c. 15 degrees cephalad
    d. 15 degrees caudad

99. How many degrees and in which direction should the central ray be directed for the lateral projection of the coccyx?
    a. Perpendicular
    b. 10 degrees caudad
    c. 10 degrees cephalad
    d. 15 degrees caudad

100. Which projection of the Ferguson method should be performed to evaluate scoliosis best?
    a. Upright PA
    b. Upright AP
    c. Recumbent PA
    d. Recumbent AP

10 Bony Thorax

OSTEOLOGY AND ARTHROLOGY OF THE BONY THORAX

Section 1: Exercise 1

This exercise pertains to the bony thorax. Identify structures for each question.

1. Identify each lettered structure shown in Fig. 10.1.

A. _____

B. _____

C. _____

D. _____

E. _____

F. _____

G. _____

H. _____

I. _____

J. _____

K. _____

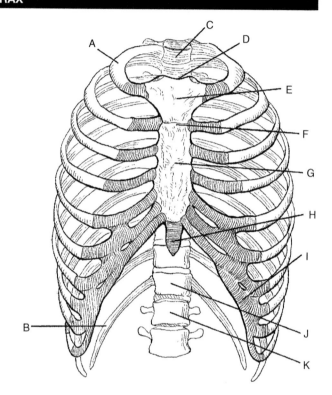

Fig. 10.1 Anterior aspect of the bony thorax.

2. Identify each lettered structure of the sternum and the three types or groups of ribs shown in Fig. 10.2.

A. _____

B. _____

C. _____

D. _____

E. _____

F. _____

G. _____

3. Identify each lettered structure shown in Fig. 10.3.

A. _____

B. _____

C. _____

D. _____

E. _____

F. _____

G. _____

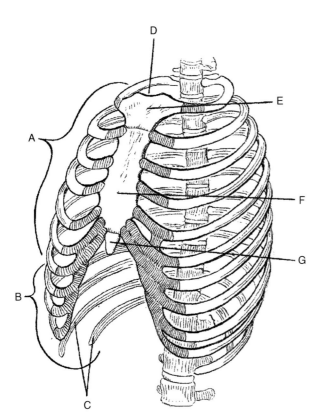

Fig. 10.2 Oblique aspect of the bony thorax.

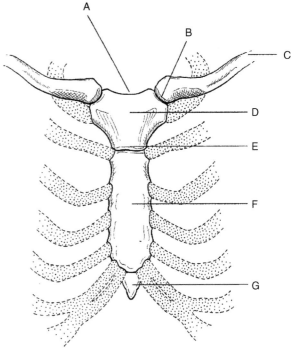

Fig. 10.3 Anterior aspect of the sternum and sternoclavicular joints.

4. Identify each lettered rib or vertebra shown in Fig. 10.4.

   A. _____

   B. _____

   C. _____

   D. _____

   E. _____

   F. _____

5. Identify each lettered structure shown in Fig. 10.5.

   A. _____

   B. _____

   C. _____

   D. _____

   E. _____

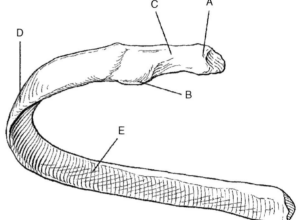

Fig. 10.5 A typical rib viewed from the back.

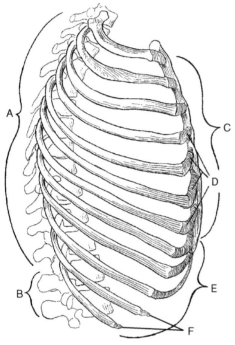

Fig. 10.4 Lateral aspect of the bony thorax.

6. Identify each lettered structure or articulation shown in Fig. 10.6.

A. _____

B. _____

C. _____

D. _____

E. _____

F. _____

G. _____

H. _____

I. _____

J. _____

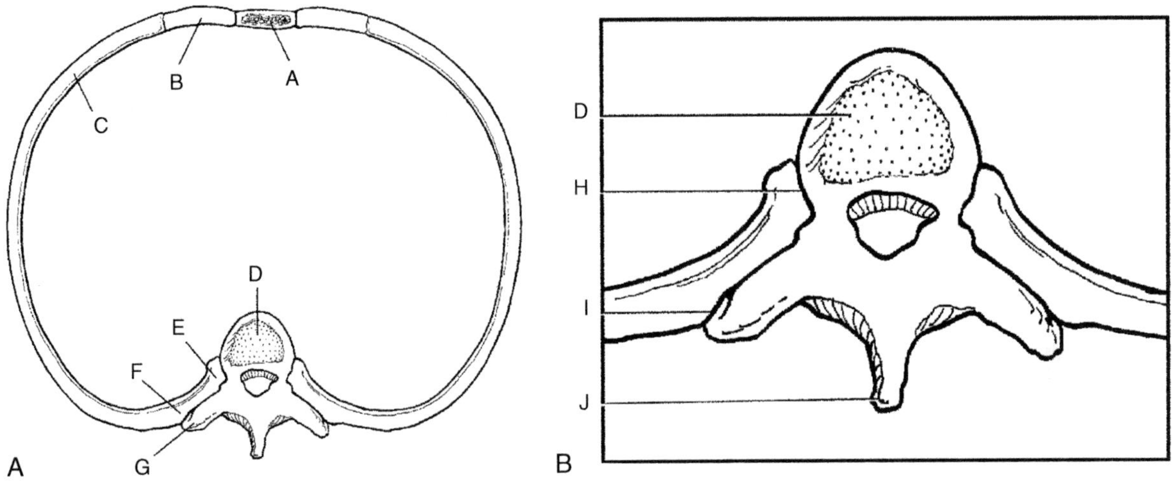

Fig. 10.6 (A) Superior aspect of ribs articulating with thoracic vertebra and sternum. (B) Enlarged image of costovertebral articulations.

Section 1: Exercise 2

Use the clues to fill in the crossword puzzle on bony thorax anatomy and pathology.

Across

3. Superior part of sternum
5. The breastbone
8. Classification of first seven rib pairs
12. Increased density of atypically soft bone
13. Inferior part of sternum
14. Classification of rib pairs 11 and 12
15. Only articulation between the upper limbs and the trunk

Down

1. Pathologic condition in which new tissue growth is uncontrolled
2. Palpable concavity at superior manubrial border (two words)
4. Pathologic condition in which there is a loss of bone density
6. Transfer of a cancerous lesion from one area to another
7. A malignant cartilaginous tumor
9. Pyogenic inflammatory bone infection
10. Portion of rib that articulates with transverse process of thoracic vertebrae
11. Classification of rib pairs that do not articulate directly with sternum

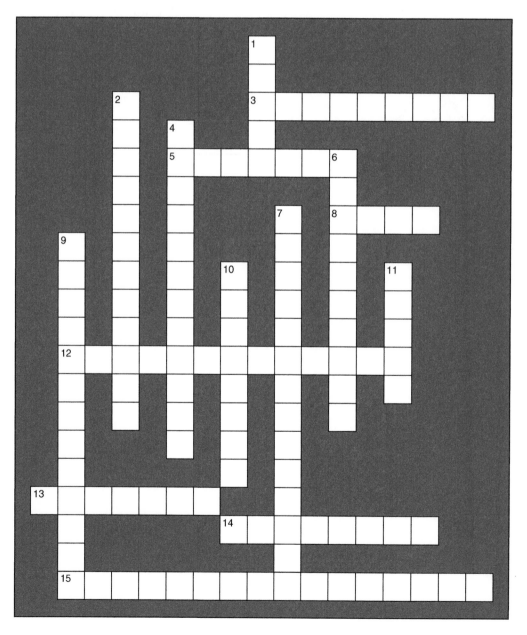

Section 1: Exercise 3

This exercise is a comprehensive review of the osteology and arthrology of the bony thorax. Provide a short answer, select the correct answer from a list, or choose true or false (explain any statement you believe to be false) for each item.

1. List the names and quantity of the structures that form the bony thorax.

2. What is the purpose of the bony thorax?

3. What is the formal name for the breastbone?

4. Name the parts of the sternum.

5. What is the approximate length of the sternum for the average adult?
   a. 2 inches (5 cm)
   b. 4 inches (10 cm)
   c. 6 inches (15 cm)
   d. 8 inches (20.3 cm)

6. How many parts comprise the sternum?
   a. Two
   b. Three
   c. Four
   d. Five

7. Which pairs of ribs attach their costal cartilage to the lateral borders of the sternum?
   a. The first seven pairs
   b. Pairs 8, 9, and 10
   c. Pairs 8, 9, 10, 11, and 12
   d. The last two pairs

8. Which part of the sternum supports the sternal ends of the clavicles?
   a. Body
   b. Manubrium
   c. Xiphoid process
   d. Jugular notch

9. What is the name for the most superior part of the sternum?
   a. Body
   b. Manubrium
   c. Xiphoid process
   d. Sternal angle

10. What is the name for the middle part of the sternum?
    a. Body
    b. Manubrium
    c. Xiphoid process
    d. Costal facet

11. Which is the distal part of the sternum?
    a. Body
    b. Manubrium
    c. Xiphoid process
    d. Sternal angle

12. What is the name of the notch found on the superior border of the sternum?
    a. Sternal notch
    b. Jugular notch
    c. Manubrial notch
    d. Clavicular notch

13. The jugular notch is found anterior to which precise location of the thoracic vertebral column?
    a. The disk space between C6 and C7
    b. The disk space between T2 and T3
    c. The disk space between T6 and T7
    d. The pedicles of T7

14. Where is the sternal angle located?
    a. At the junction of clavicles and manubrium
    b. At the junction of manubrium and sternal body
    c. At the junction of manubrium and xiphoid process
    d. At the junction of the body and xiphoid process

15. To which location of the thoracic column does the sternal angle correspond?
    a. The disk space between C7 and T1
    b. The disk space between T2 and T3
    c. The disk space between T4 and T5
    d. The body of T6

16. To which location of the thoracic column does the xiphoid process correspond?

17. What determines whether a particular rib is a true rib or a false rib?

18. What pairs of ribs are classified as true ribs?

19. What pairs of ribs are classified as false ribs?

20. What pairs of ribs are referred to as "floating" ribs?

21. What structures form costovertebral joints?

22. With which structures do costal tubercles articulate?

23. What part of the sternum articulates with the anterior ends of the first pair of ribs to form the first sterno-costal joints?

24. True or false. The anterior end of a rib generally is located 3 to 5 inches (7.6 to 12.5 cm) below the level of its head.

25. True or false. Ribs increase in thickness the closer they are to the lumbar column.

316

Chapter **10** **Bony Thorax**

POSITIONING OF THE BONY THORAX

Section 2: Exercise 1: Positioning for the Sternum

This exercise pertains to the two essential projections of the sternum. Identify structures, select the correct answer from a list, or choose true or false (explaining any statement you believe to be false) for each item.

1. List the essential projections for the sternum, and describe the positioning steps used for each, as follows:

   Essential projection: _____
   - Size of collimated field:

   - Key patient/part positioning points:

   - Anatomic landmarks and relation to IR:

   - CR orientation and entrance point:

   Essential projection: _____
   - Size of collimated field:

   - Key patient/part positioning points:

   - Anatomic landmarks and relation to IR:

   - CR orientation and entrance point:

Items 2 to 13 pertain to the *PA oblique projection, RAO position.* Examine Fig. 10.7, which shows a patient positioned for the right PA oblique projection, as you answer the following questions.

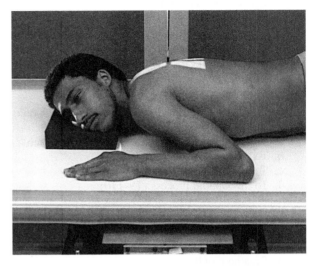

Fig. 10.7 PA oblique sternum, RAO position.

2. Why should the patient be rotated into an oblique position instead of the positions used for AP or PA projections?
   a. To position the sternum parallel with the IR
   b. To prevent superimposition of the sternum with the heart
   c. To prevent superimposition of the sternum with the vertebral column
   d. To demonstrate the costochondral joints

3. Why is an anterior oblique position preferred to a posterior oblique position?
   a. To reduce object-to-image receptor distance (OID) of the sternum
   b. To increase OID of the sternum
   c. To prevent superimposition of the sternum with the vertebral column
   d. To increase patient comfort

317

4. Why is the PA oblique projection, RAO position, preferred to the PA oblique projection, left anterior oblique (LAO) position?
   a. To use the background density of the heart for visualization of the sternum
   b. To increase source-to-image receptor distance (SID) of the sternum
   c. To prevent superimposition of the sternum with the vertebral column
   d. To demonstrate the costochondral joints

5. Which patient characteristic requires a greater amount of patient rotation to the RAO position?

6. With reference to the patient, to what level should the top of the IR or collimated field be placed?
   a. To 1½ inches (3.8 cm) above the jugular notch
   b. To the jugular notch (T2-T3)
   c. To the midsternal area (T7)
   d. To the xiphoid process (T9-T10)

7. From the following list, circle the two ways the patient's breathing should be controlled for the exposure.
   a. Breathe rapidly.
   b. Breathe shallowly.
   c. Suspend respiration after expiration.
   d. Suspend respiration after inspiration.

8. If a short exposure time is preferred, what breathing instructions should be given to the patient?
   a. Breathe rapidly.
   b. Breathe shallowly.
   c. Suspend respiration after expiration.
   d. Suspend respiration after inspiration.

9. When the image made with the patient in the RAO position is properly viewed, where will the sternum appear with reference to the vertebral column?
   a. Toward the viewer's left and on the right side of the patient's thorax without vertebral superimposition
   b. Toward the viewer's right and on the left side of the patient's thorax without vertebral superimposition

10. True or false. The entire sternum should be seen without superimposition with thoracic vertebrae.

11. True or false. Pulmonary marking should be blurred when the patient is instructed to breathe slowly during the exposure.

12. True or false. The right sternoclavicular (SC) joint should be demonstrated superimposed with the vertebral column.

13. Identify each lettered structure shown in Fig. 10.8.

   A. _____

   B. _____

   C. _____

   D. _____

   E. _____

   F. _____

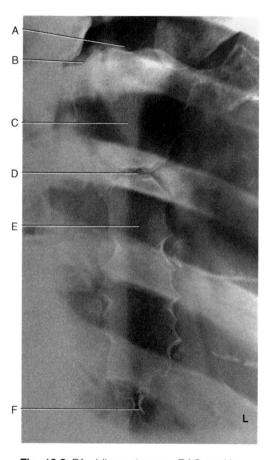

Fig. 10.8 PA oblique sternum, RAO position.

Items 14 to 25 pertain to the *lateral projection*. Examine Fig. 10.9 as you answer the following questions.

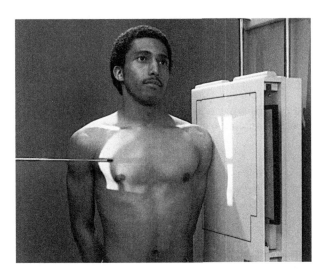

Fig. 10.9 Lateral sternum.

14. How much SID is recommended for the lateral projection and why?
    a. 40 inches (102 cm); to blur overlying ribs
    b. 40 inches (102 cm); to reduce magnification of the sternum
    c. 72 inches (183 cm); to blur overlying ribs
    d. 72 inches (183 cm); to reduce magnification of the sternum

15. With reference to the patient, where exactly should the top of the IR or collimated field be placed?
    a. At the level of the jugular notch
    b. At the level of the sternal angle
    c. 1½ inches (3.8 cm) above the jugular notch
    d. At the level of the thyroid cartilage

16. Describe how the patient's shoulders, arms, and hands should be positioned when the patient is in the upright position.

17. Describe how the patient's arms should be positioned when the patient is in the recumbent position.

18. For female patients with large breasts, what procedure should be done to prevent breast shadows from superimposing the sternum?

19. What breathing instructions should be given to the patient?

20. Why should the exposure be made with the patient following the required breathing instructions?

21. When the patient is in the lateral recumbent position, why should a support be placed under the lower thoracic region?

22. True or false. The patient should breathe slowly during the exposure in an effort to blur lung markings that may superimpose the sternum.

23. True or false. The sternum should be demonstrated in its entirety.

24. True or false. Patients who have experienced severe trauma should be examined in the dorsal decubitus position.

319

25. Identify each lettered structure shown in Fig. 10.10.

A. _____

B. _____

C. _____

D. _____

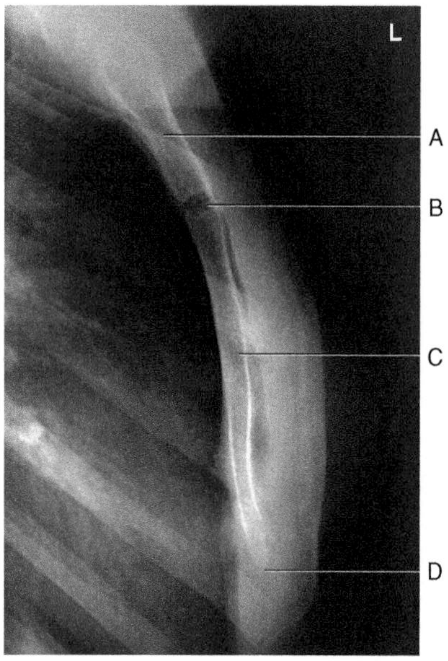

Fig. 10.10 Lateral sternum.

Section 2: Exercise 2: Positioning for Sternoclavicular Articulations

This exercise reviews the essential projections used to demonstrate the SC joints. Provide a short answer, select the correct answer from a list, or choose true or false (explaining any statement you believe to be false) for each item.

1. List the essential projections for the SC joints, and describe the positioning steps used for each, as follows:

Essential projection: _____
- Size of collimated field:

- Key patient/part positioning points:

- Anatomic landmarks and relation to IR:

- CR orientation and entrance point:

Essential projection: _____ (_____ method)
- Size of collimated field:

- Key patient/part positioning points:

- Anatomic landmarks and relation to IR:

- CR orientation and entrance point:

Essential projection: _____ (method)
- Size of collimated field:

- Key patient/part positioning points:

- Anatomic landmarks and relation to IR:

- CR orientation and entrance point:

Items 2 to 7 pertain to the *PA projection*. Examine Fig. 10.11 as you answer the following questions.

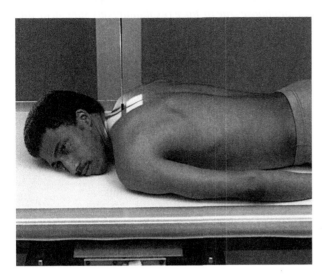

Fig. 10.11 PA projection of left sternoclavicular articulation.

2. Describe how the patient's arms should be positioned when the patient is in the prone position.

3. For the bilateral procedure, how should the patient's head be positioned?

4. How does rotation of the patient's head to one side improve the demonstration of the affected SC joint?

5. Which breathing instructions should be given to the patient?
   a. Breathe rapidly.
   b. Breathe shallowly.
   c. Suspend respiration after expiration.
   d. Suspend respiration after inspiration.

6. True or false. The clavicles should be demonstrated in their entirety.

7. True or false. Slight rotation of the vertebral column is permitted for the PA projection in bilateral examinations.

Items 8 to 13 pertain to the *PA oblique projection*. Examine Fig. 10.12 as you answer the following questions.

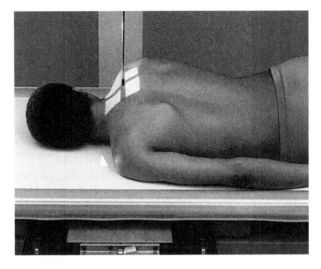

Fig. 10.12 PA oblique projection of sternoclavicular articulation, LAO position.

8. Which SC joint (the affected side or the unaffected side) should be positioned closer to the IR for the body rotation method?

9. How many degrees should the patient be rotated for the body rotation method?

10. Describe how the central ray should be directed for the central ray angulation method.

Fig. 10.13 shows an image produced by the body rotation method. Examine the image and answer the questions that follow.

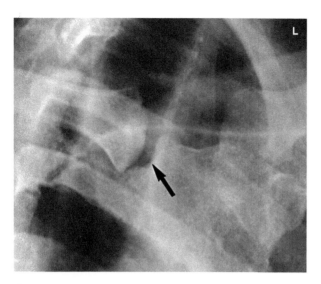

Fig. 10.13 Body rotation showing the sternoclavicular joint *(arrow)*.

11. How should the central ray be directed—angled or perpendicularly?

12. Which body position (RAO or LAO) is represented in the image?

13. Which SC joint (right or left) is of primary interest?

Section 2: Exercise 3: Positioning for the Ribs

This exercise pertains to the essential projections used to demonstrate ribs. Provide a short answer, select from a list, or choose true or false (explaining any statement you believe to be false) for each question.

1. List the essential projections for the ribs, and describe the positioning steps used for each, as follows:

Essential projection: _____
- Size of collimated field:

- Key patient/part positioning points:

- Anatomic landmarks and relation to IR:

- CR orientation and entrance point:

Essential projection: _____
- Size of collimated field:

- Key patient/part positioning points:

- Anatomic landmarks and relation to IR:

- CR orientation and entrance point:

Essential projection: _____
- Size of collimated field:

- Key patient/part positioning points:

- Anatomic landmarks and relation to IR:

- CR orientation and entrance point:

Essential projection: _____
- Size of collimated field:

- Key patient/part positioning points:

- Anatomic landmarks and relation to IR:

- CR orientation and entrance point:

Items 2 to 9 pertain to the *PA projection*. Examine Fig. 10.14 as you answer the following questions.

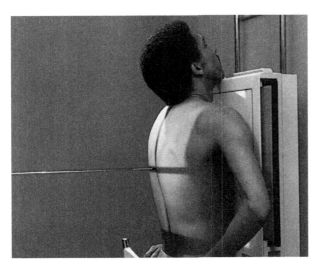

Fig. 10.14 PA ribs.

2. Which ribs are best demonstrated with the PA projection?

3. How should the patient be positioned (recumbent or upright) for the best demonstration of the ribs with the PA projection? Explain why.

4. With reference to the patient, where should the top of the IR or collimated field be positioned?

5. How should the patient's upper limbs (extremities) be placed to cause the scapulae to rotate laterally?

6. How should the patient's head be positioned if the patient is in the prone position?

7. What breathing instructions should be given to the patient? Explain why.

8. Describe how the PA projection can be adjusted to demonstrate the seventh, eighth, and ninth ribs better when the diaphragm is in the way.

9. What pairs of ribs should be demonstrated in their entirety?

Items 10 to 16 pertain to AP projections for *demonstrating ribs above the diaphragm.* Examine Fig. 10.15 as you answer the following questions.

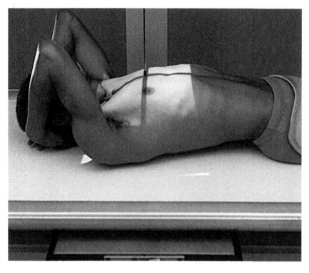

Fig. 10.15 AP ribs above the diaphragm.

10. What is the preferred body position (supine or upright) for the patient? Explain why.

11. With reference to the patient, where should the top of the IR or collimated field be positioned?

12. Why should a patient's shoulders be rotated forward?

13. What breathing instructions should be given to the patient? Explain why.

14. Which ribs (anterior or posterior) are presented in best recorded detail?

15. What ribs should be demonstrated on the image?

16. A patient with injured posterior ribs Nos. 5 and 6 needs proper images. List (a) the body position in which the patient should be placed and (b) the recommended breathing instructions.

   a. _____

   b. _____

Items 17 to 25 pertain to *AP projections for demonstrating ribs below the diaphragm.* Examine Fig. 10.16 as you answer the following questions.

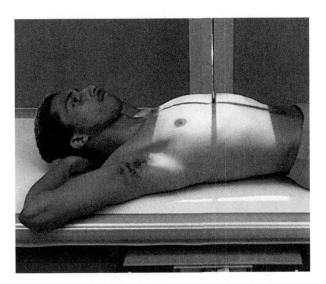

Fig. 10.16 AP ribs below the diaphragm.

17. What is the preferred body position (supine or upright) for the patient? Explain why.

18. The lower edge of the collimated field should extend to _____.

19. What breathing instructions should be given to the patient? Explain why.

20. How and where should the central ray be directed?

21. What pairs of ribs should be demonstrated on the image?

22. A patient with injured posterior ribs Nos. 10 and 11 needs proper images. List (a) the body position in which the patient should be placed and (b) the recommended breathing instructions.

a. _____

b. _____

Items 23 to 32 pertain to *AP oblique projections, right posterior oblique (RPO) and left posterior oblique (LPO) positions.* Examine Fig. 10.17 and answer the following questions.

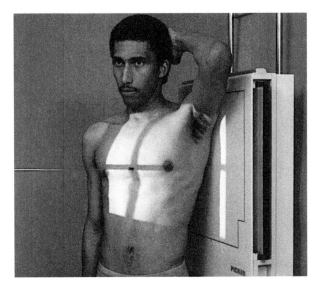

Fig. 10.17 AP oblique ribs, LPO position.

23. True or false. AP oblique projections demonstrate posterior ribs better than anterior ribs.

24. True or false. The AP oblique projection with the patient LPO best demonstrates the posterior and axillary portions of the left ribs.

325

25. Which ribs (the affected side or the unaffected side) should be placed closer to the IR for the best imaging with AP oblique projections?

26. How many degrees of body rotation are required to image the axillary portion of the ribs without self-superimposition?

27. What factor determines the breathing instructions that should be given to the patient?

28. What pairs of ribs above the diaphragm should be demonstrated on AP oblique images?

29. What pairs of ribs below the diaphragm should be demonstrated on AP oblique images?

Examine Fig. 10.18 and answer the following questions.

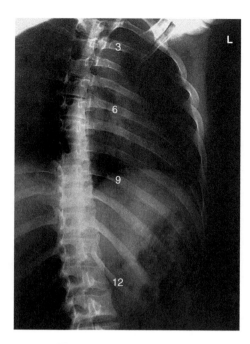

Fig. 10.18 AP oblique ribs.

30. What radiographic position is represented in the image?

31. The ribs of which side are best demonstrated?

32. Which side of the patient is closest to the IR?

Questions 33 to 40 pertain to *PA oblique projections, RAO and LAO positions*. Examine Fig. 10.19 and answer the following questions.

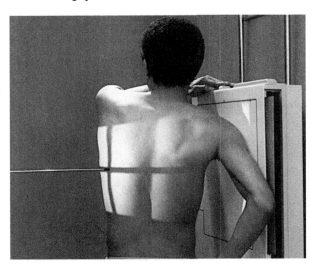

Fig. 10.19 PA oblique ribs, RAO position.

33. With a patient in the upright position, which shoulder should be elevated if the axillary portion of the right ribs needs to be examined?

34. Which PA oblique position (RAO or LAO) should be used for the best demonstration of the axillary portion of the left ribs?

35. The RAO position best demonstrates the _____ portion of the _____ ribs.

Examine Fig. 10.20 and answer the following questions.

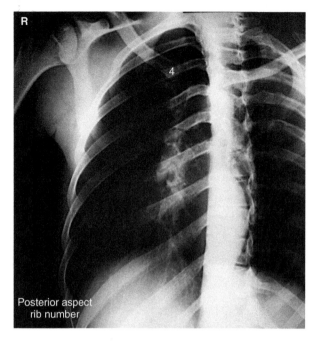

Fig. 10.20 PA oblique ribs.

36. Which body position is represented in the image?

37. Which ribs are best demonstrated?

38. Which side of the patient is closest to the IR?

39. What breathing instructions should be given to the patient?

40. From the following list, circle the five evaluation criteria indicating that the patient was properly positioned and imaged for AP oblique and PA oblique projections.
    a. The trachea should be visible in the midline.
    b. The first through tenth ribs should be seen above the diaphragm for upper ribs.
    c. The axillary portion of the ribs should be demonstrated free of superimposition.
    d. The eighth through twelfth ribs should be seen below the diaphragm for lower ribs.
    e. Both clavicles should be seen in a horizontal placement superior to the apices.
    f. The ribs should be demonstrated clearly through the lungs or abdomen according to the region examined.
    g. The distance from the vertebral column to the lateral border of the ribs should be equidistant on each side.
    h. The distance between the vertebral column and the outer border of the ribs on the affected side should be approximately twice that of the unaffected side.

Answer the following questions by selecting the best choice.

1. All of the following comprise the bony thorax *except for*:
   a. the sternum.
   b. the 12 pairs of ribs.
   c. the 12 thoracic vertebrae.
   d. the scapulae.

2. What is the proper name for that structure commonly called the "breastbone"?
   a. Scapula
   b. Sternum
   c. Manubrium
   d. Xiphoid process

3. Which bone classification is the sternum?
   a. Flat
   b. Long
   c. Short
   d. Irregular

4. Which three bony parts compose the sternum?
   a. Head, body, and xiphoid process
   b. Head, body, and odontoid process
   c. Manubrium, body and xiphoid process
   d. Manubrium, body and odontoid process

5. Which part of the sternum is most superior?
   a. Head
   b. Body
   c. Manubrium
   d. Xiphoid process

6. Which of the following articulates with the articular facets located just lateral to the jugular notch?
   a. Ribs
   b. Clavicles
   c. Sternal body
   d. Xiphoid process

7. The junction of which structures creates the sternal angle?
   a. Ribs and sternal body
   b. Clavicles and manubrium
   c. Manubrium and sternal body
   d. Manubrium and xiphoid process

8. Which part of the sternum is the elongated central portion?
   a. Head
   b. Body
   c. Sternal angle
   d. Xiphoid process

9. Where on the sternum is the jugular notch located?
   a. Lateral border of the body
   b. Lateral border of the manubrium
   c. Superior border of the body
   d. Superior border of the manubrium

10. What is the smallest part of the sternum?
    a. Body
    b. Manubrium
    c. Xiphoid process

11. Which part of the sternum is located at the level of T10?
    a. Body
    b. Angle
    c. Manubrium
    d. Xiphoid process

12. With which part of the sternum does the first pair of ribs articulate?
    a. Lateral border of the manubrium
    b. Lateral border of the body
    c. Superior border of the manubrium
    d. Superior border of the body

13. Which classification refers to ribs that attach their costal cartilages directly to the sternum?
    a. True
    b. False
    c. Primary
    d. Floating

14. Which classification refers to ribs that have no anterior attachments?
    a. True
    b. Primary
    c. Floating
    d. Secondary

15. Which classification refers to the eighth through twelfth pairs of ribs?
    a. True
    b. False
    c. Primary
    d. Secondary

329

16. Which pairs of ribs are classified as true ribs?
    a. First seven pairs
    b. Pairs 8, 9, and 10
    c. Pairs 8, 9, 10, 11, and 12
    d. Last two pairs

17. How many pairs of ribs are classified as floating ribs?
    a. One
    b. Two
    c. Seven
    d. Ten

18. Which articulation is formed in part with the head of a rib?
    a. Costosternal
    b. Costovertebral
    c. Costotransverse
    d. Sternoclavicular

19. With which structures do heads of ribs articulate?
    a. Cartilage of adjacent ribs
    b. Lateral borders of the sternum
    c. Demifacets of thoracic vertebrae
    d. Transverse processes of thoracic vertebrae

20. Which articulation involves the tubercle of a rib?
    a. Costosternal
    b. Costovertebral
    c. Costotransverse
    d. Sternoclavicular

21. Which radiographic position best demonstrates the sternum projected within the heart shadow?
    a. LAO
    b. LPO
    c. RAO
    d. RPO

22. For the oblique position that best demonstrates the sternum, how many degrees should the patient be rotated?
    a. 15 to 20 degrees
    b. 25 to 30 degrees
    c. 30 to 40 degrees
    d. 35 to 45 degrees

23. Which two projections generally comprise the typical series demonstrating the sternum?
    a. PA and lateral
    b. PA and PA oblique, RAO position
    c. Lateral and PA oblique, LAO position
    d. Lateral and PA oblique, RAO position

24. How should the central ray be directed for the oblique position to best demonstrate the sternum?
    a. Perpendicularly
    b. Caudally 15 degrees
    c. Cephalically 15 degrees
    d. Caudally 20 degrees

25. To demonstrate the sternum best, the patient should be rotated into the _____ position to image the sternum _____.
    a. LAO; within the heart shadow
    b. RAO; within the heart shadow
    c. LAO; without superimposing with the vertebral column
    d. RAO; without superimposing with the vertebral column

26. With reference to the patient, where should the top border of the IR be positioned for the lateral projection of the sternum?
    a. At the level of the clavicles
    b. At the level of the sternal angle
    c. 1½ inches (3.8 cm) above the jugular notch
    d. 1½ inches (3.8 cm) above the top of the shoulders

27. Which procedure should be performed for the lateral projection of the sternum?
    a. Rotate the shoulders forward.
    b. Ask the patient to take slow, shallow breaths.
    c. Raise both arms and rest forearms on top of the head.
    d. Increase the SID to 72 inches (183 cm).

28. Which procedure should be performed to demonstrate only one SC joint with the PA projection?
    a. Rest the patient's head on the chin.
    b. Direct the central ray 15 degrees medially.
    c. Turn the patient's head to face the affected side.
    d. Elevate the shoulder of the affected side 15 degrees.

29. Which procedure should be performed to demonstrate both SC joints with the PA projection?
    a. Rest the patient's head on the chin.
    b. Direct the central ray 15 degrees medially.
    c. Have the patient breathe slowly with shallow breaths.
    d. Direct the central ray to enter the patient's back at T7.

30. How should the central ray be directed and centered for the PA projection for bilateral SC joints?
    a. Perpendicular to T3
    b. Perpendicular to T7
    c. Angled medially 15 degrees, entering at T3
    d. Angled cephalically 15 degrees, entering at T7

31. To demonstrate bilateral SC joints, which evaluation criterion indicates that the patient was properly positioned?
    a. Slight rotation of the affected side should be seen.
    b. The sternum should be demonstrated in its entirety.
    c. No rotation of the SC joints should be demonstrated.
    d. Both clavicles should be demonstrated in their entirety.

32. To demonstrate injured anterior ribs Nos. 5 and 6 on the right side most effectively, which two projections should be included as part of the series?
    a. PA and PA oblique with the patient LAO
    b. PA and PA oblique with the patient RAO
    c. AP and AP oblique with the patient LPO
    d. AP and AP oblique with the patient RPO

33. To demonstrate injured anterior ribs Nos. 6 and 7 on the left side most effectively, which two projections should be included as part of the series?
    a. PA and PA oblique with the patient LAO
    b. PA and PA oblique with the patient RAO
    c. AP and AP oblique with the patient LPO
    d. AP and AP oblique with the patient RPO

34. To demonstrate injured posterior ribs Nos. 5 and 6 on the left side most effectively, which two projections should be included as part of the series?
    a. PA and PA oblique with the patient LAO
    b. PA and PA oblique with the patient RAO
    c. AP and AP oblique with the patient LPO
    d. AP and AP oblique with the patient RPO

35. To demonstrate injured posterior ribs Nos. 6 and 7 on the right side most effectively, which two projections should be included as part of the series?
    a. PA and PA oblique with the patient LAO
    b. PA and PA oblique with the patient RAO
    c. AP and AP oblique with the patient LPO
    d. AP and AP oblique with the patient RPO

36. Which procedure should be used to obtain images of injured anterior ribs Nos. 5 and 6?
    a. Patient upright; exposure taken on suspended expiration
    b. Patient upright; exposure taken on suspended inspiration
    c. Patient recumbent; exposure taken on suspended expiration
    d. Patient recumbent; exposure taken on suspended inspiration

37. If the patient's condition permits, which procedure should be used to demonstrate injured posterior ribs Nos. 10, 11, and 12 best?
    a. Patient prone; exposure taken on suspended expiration
    b. Patient prone; exposure taken on suspended inspiration
    c. Patient supine; exposure taken on suspended expiration
    d. Patient supine; exposure taken on suspended inspiration

38. Which two projections best demonstrate injured posterior ribs Nos. 10, 11, and 12 on the right side?
    a. AP and AP oblique with the patient LPO
    b. AP and AP oblique with the patient RPO
    c. PA and AP oblique with the patient LPO
    d. PA and AP oblique with the patient RPO

39. Which two projections best demonstrate injured posterior ribs Nos. 10, 11, and 12 on the left side?
    a. PA and AP oblique with the patient LPO
    b. PA and AP oblique with the patient RPO
    c. AP and AP oblique with the patient LPO
    d. AP and AP oblique with the patient RPO

40. Which radiographic position best demonstrates the posterior eleventh rib on the right side without vertebral superimposition?
    a. LAO
    b. LPO
    c. RAO
    d. RPO

41. Which radiographic position best demonstrates the posterior tenth rib on the left side without vertebral superimposition?
    a. LAO
    b. LPO
    c. RAO
    d. RPO

42. Which radiographic position best demonstrates the anterior sixth rib on the left side without vertebral superimposition?
    a. LAO
    b. LPO
    c. RAO
    d. RPO

43. Which radiographic position best demonstrates the anterior fifth rib on the right side without vertebral superimposition?
    a. LAO
    b. LPO
    c. RAO
    d. RPO

44. With reference to the patient, where should the top border of the IR/collimated field be positioned for the PA projection to demonstrate ribs above the diaphragm?
    a. At the level of T7
    b. At the level of the clavicles
    c. 1½ inches (3.8 cm) above the shoulders
    d. 1½ inches (3.8 cm) above the sternal angle

45. For the AP projection demonstrating ribs above the diaphragm, when should respiration be suspended, and what effect will that have on the diaphragm?
    a. On full inspiration; will depress the diaphragm
    b. On full inspiration; will elevate the diaphragm
    c. On full expiration; will depress the diaphragm
    d. On full expiration; will elevate the diaphragm

46. For the AP projection demonstrating ribs below the diaphragm, when should respiration be suspended, and what effect will that have on the diaphragm?
    a. On full inspiration; will depress the diaphragm
    b. On full inspiration; will elevate the diaphragm
    c. On full expiration; will depress the diaphragm
    d. On full expiration; will elevate the diaphragm

47. When performing the AP projection to demonstrate ribs below the diaphragm, with reference to the patient, how should the IR/collimated field be positioned?
    a. Center IR/collimated field at the level of L3
    b. Center IR/collimated field at the level of iliac crests
    c. Lower border of the IR/collimated field at the level of L3
    d. Lower border of the IR/collimated field at the level of iliac crests

48. Which projection best demonstrates the axillary portion of ribs?
    a. AP projection
    b. PA projection
    c. Lateral projection
    d. AP oblique projection

49. Which procedure can be performed to demonstrate the seventh, eighth, and ninth ribs better away from the shadow of the diaphragm?
    a. Central ray directed perpendicular to T7
    b. Rapid breathing to blur the diaphragm shadow
    c. Higher centering and caudal angulation of the central ray
    d. Higher centering and cephalad angulation of the central ray

50. Which of the following evaluation criteria pertains to the AP oblique projection for ribs?
    a. Trachea should be seen in the midline of the thorax.
    b. Heart and mediastinum should be seen in the center of the image.
    c. Axillary portion of the ribs of interest should be free of superimposition.
    d. Sternal ends of the clavicles should be equidistant from the vertebral column.

11 Cranium

OSTEOLOGY OF THE SKULL

Section 1: Exercise 1

This exercise pertains to the osteology of the skull. Identify structures for each illustration.

1. Identify each lettered structure shown in Fig. 11.1.

A. _____

B. _____

C. _____

D. _____

E. _____

F. _____

G. _____

H. _____

I. _____

J. _____

K. _____

L. _____

M. _____

N. _____

O. _____

P. _____

Q. _____

R. _____

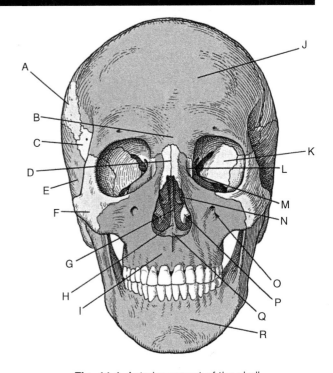

Fig. 11.1 Anterior aspect of the skull.

2. Identify each lettered structure shown in Fig. 11.2.

A. _____

B. _____

C. _____

D. _____

E. _____

F. _____

G. _____

H. _____

I. _____

J. _____

K. _____

L. _____

M. _____ (fontanelle)

N. _____ (suture)

O. _____

P. _____ (suture)

Q. _____ (fontanelle)

R. _____ (suture)

S. _____

T. _____

U. _____

V. _____

W. _____

X. _____

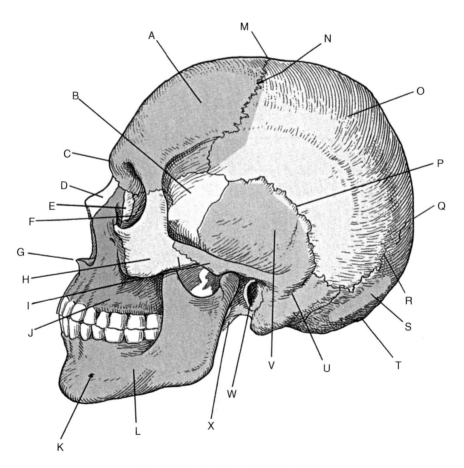

Fig. 11.2 Lateral aspect of the skull.

3. Identify each lettered structure shown in Fig. 11.3.

A. _____

B. _____

C. _____

D. _____

E. _____

F. _____

G. _____

H. _____

I. _____

J. _____

K. _____

L. _____

M. _____

N. _____

O. _____

P. _____

Q. _____

R. _____

S. _____

T. _____

U. _____

V. _____

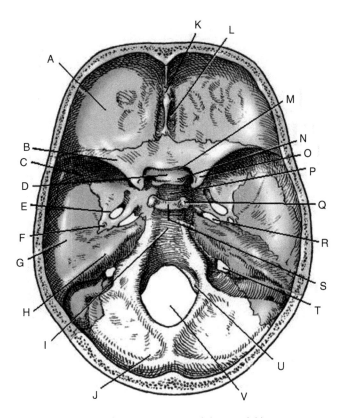

Fig. 11.3 Superior aspect of the cranial base.

4. Identify each lettered structure shown in Fig. 11.4.

A. _____   I. _____

B. _____   J. _____

C. _____   K. _____

D. _____   L. _____

E. _____   M. _____

F. _____   N. _____

G. _____   O. _____

H. _____   P. _____

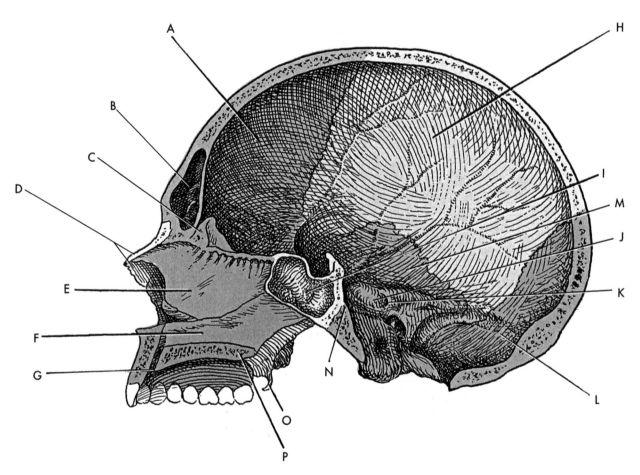

Fig. 11.4 Lateral aspect of the interior of the cranium.

5. Identify each lettered structure shown in Fig. 11.5.

   A. _____

   B. _____

   C. _____

   D. _____

   E. _____

   F. _____

   G. _____

6. Identify each lettered structure shown in Fig. 11.6.

   A. _____

   B. _____

   C. _____

   D. _____

   E. _____

   F. _____

   G. _____

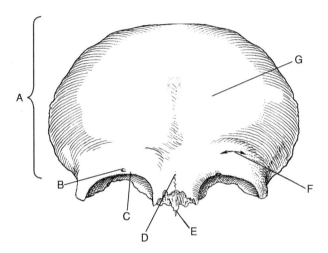

Fig. 11.5 Anterior aspect of the frontal bone.

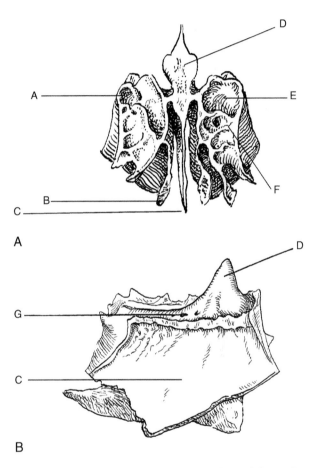

Fig. 11.6 Two illustrations of the ethmoid bone. (A) Anterior aspect. (B) Lateral aspect with the labyrinth removed.

7. Identify the four angles and the four articulating borders of the left parietal bone shown in Fig. 11.7.

A. Articulates with the _____ bone

B. _____ angle

C. Articulates with the _____ bone

D. _____ angle

E. _____ angle

F. Articulates with the _____ bone

G. _____ angle

H. Articulates with the _____ bone

8. Identify each lettered structure shown in Fig. 11.8.

A. _____

B. _____

C. _____

D. _____

E. _____

F. _____

G. _____

H. _____

I. _____

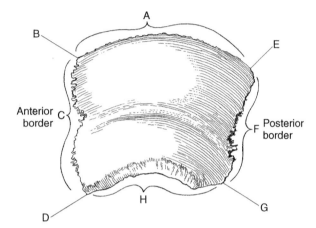

Fig. 11.7 External surface of the left parietal bone.

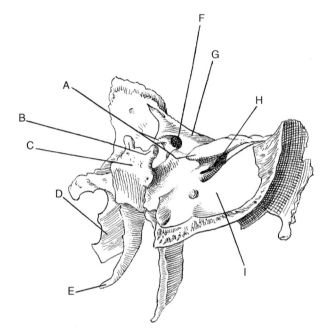

Fig. 11.8 Oblique view of the upper and lateroposterior aspects of the sphenoid bone.

9. Identify each lettered structure shown in Fig. 11.9.

A. _____   D. _____

B. _____   E. _____

C. _____

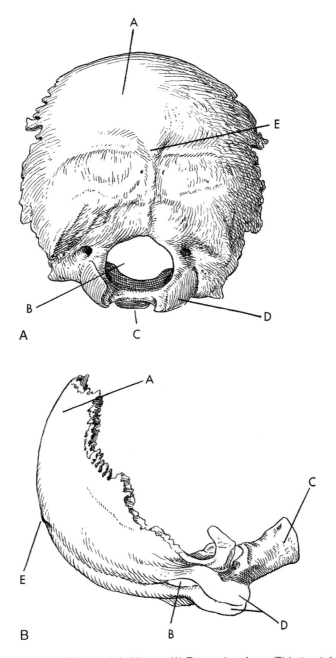

Fig. 11.9 Two illustrations of the occipital bone. (A) External surface. (B) Lateroinferior surface.

10. Identify each lettered structure shown in Fig. 11.10.

A. _____

B. _____

C. _____

D. _____

E. _____

F. _____

G. _____

H. _____

I. _____

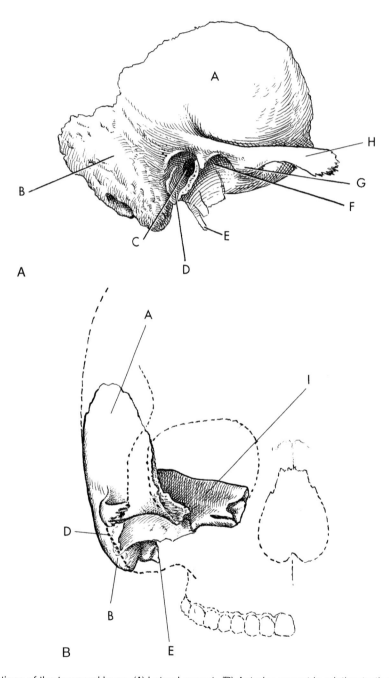

Fig. 11.10 Two illustrations of the temporal bone. (A) Lateral aspect. (B) Anterior aspect in relation to the surrounding structures.

11. Identify each lettered structure shown in Fig. 11.11.

A. _____

B. _____

C. _____

D. _____

E. _____

F. _____

G. _____

H. _____

I. _____

J. _____

K. _____

L. _____

M. _____

N. _____

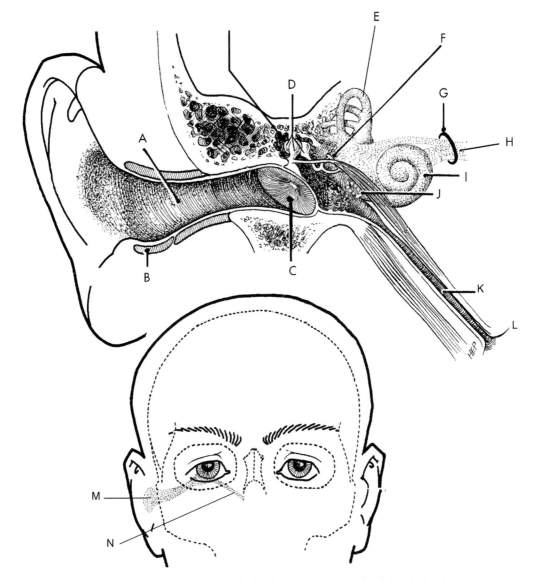

Fig. 11.11 Frontal section through the right ear showing the internal structures.

12. Identify each lettered structure shown in Fig. 11.12.

A. _____

B. _____

C. _____

D. _____

E. _____

F. _____

G. _____

H. _____

I. _____

J. _____

K. _____

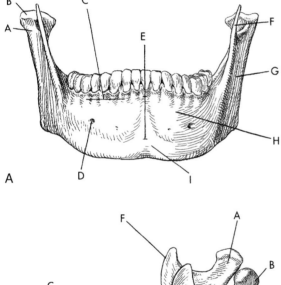

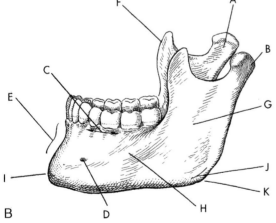

Fig. 11.12 Two illustrations of the mandible. (A) Anterior aspect. (B) Lateral aspect.

13. Identify each lettered structure shown in Fig. 11.13.

A. _____

B. _____

C. _____

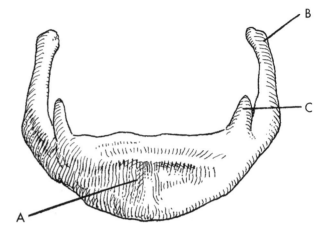

Fig. 11.13 Anterior aspect of the hyoid.

14. Identify each lettered structure shown in Fig. 11.14.

A. _____

B. _____

C. _____

D. _____

E. _____

F. _____

G. _____

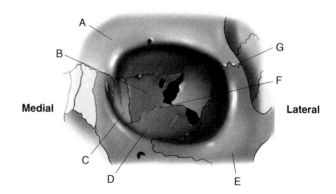

Fig. 11.14 Anterior view of the orbit.

Section 1: Exercise 2

Use the following clues to complete the crossword puzzle. All answers refer to the skull.

Across
1. Perpendicular _____
4. Midpoint of the frontonasal sutures
5. This bone has wings
7. Vertical part of the frontal bone
8. _____ galli
9. Number of cranial bones
12. Densest part of the cranial floor
13. Articulates frontal bone with parietals
16. Fibrous cranial joint
19. Anterior fontanelle
20. Posterior fontanelle
21. Forms top of the cranium
22. Posterior part of the skull
23. Eyebrow arches

Down
1. Inferior sphenoidal process
2. Sphenoidal endocrine
3. _____ turcica
5. Lateral suture
6. Long and narrow skull
10. Average skull
11. Smooth frontal elevation
14. Posterior to the nasal bones
15. Ear bone
17. Where occipital bone joins parietals
18. Forehead bone
19. Anteroinferior occipital part

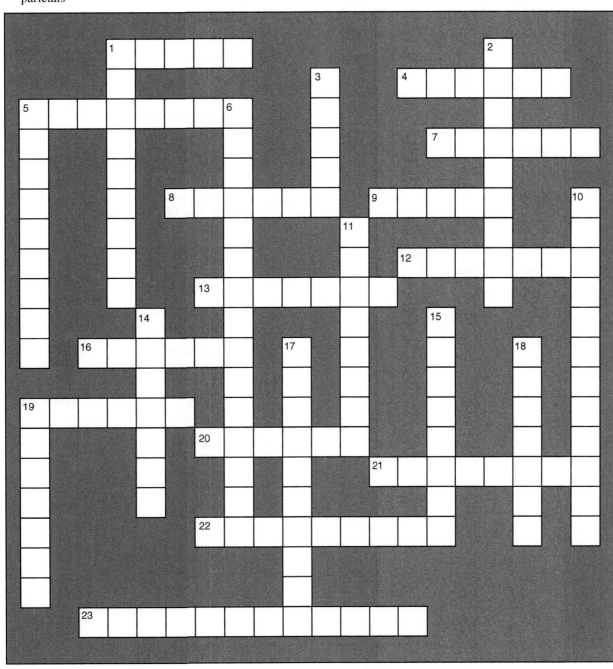

Section 1: Exercise 3

Match the structures (Column A) with the cranial bones on which they are found (Column B).

Column A

_____ 1. Nasion

_____ 2. Glabella

_____ 3. Four angles

_____ 4. Lesser wing

_____ 5. Greater wing

_____ 6. Two condyles

_____ 7. Crista galli

_____ 8. Sella turcica

_____ 9. Foramen magnum

_____ 10. Cribriform plate

_____ 11. Mastoid process

_____ 12. Basilar portion

_____ 13. Petrous portion

_____ 14. Pterygoid hamulus

_____ 15. Zygomatic process

_____ 16. Supraorbital margin

_____ 17. Perpendicular plate

_____ 18. Lateral pterygoid process

_____ 19. Anterior clinoid processes

_____ 20. Posterior clinoid processes

Column B

a. Frontal

b. Ethmoid

c. Parietal

d. Sphenoid

e. Temporal

f. Occipital

Section 1: Exercise 4

Match the statements (Column A) with the facial bone terms to which they refer (Column B). Only one selection from Column B applies to each statement in Column A. Not all terms from Column B should be used.

Column A

_____ 1. Cheekbone

_____ 2. Largest facial bone

_____ 3. Number of facial bones

_____ 4. Forms bridge of the nose

_____ 5. Vertical mandibular portion

_____ 6. Found in the roof of the mouth

_____ 7. Midpoint of the anterior nasal spine

_____ 8. Articulating process of the mandible

_____ 9. Spongy processes that hold the teeth

_____ 10. Anterior part of the mandibular ramus

_____ 11. Landmark at the angle of the mandible

_____ 12. Found in the medial walls of the orbits

_____ 13. Forms inferior portion of the nasal septum

_____ 14. Horseshoe-shaped mandibular portion

_____ 15. Thin, scroll-like bones that extend horizontally inside the nasal cavity

Column B

a. Head

b. Body

c. Nasal

d. Hyoid

e. Ramus

f. Vomer

g. Gonion

h. Twelve

i. Fourteen

j. Lacrimal

k. Alveolar

l. Condyle

m. Zygoma

n. Palatine

o. Maxillae

p. Coronoid

q. Mandible

r. Acanthion

s. Inferior conchae

t. Mental protuberance

Section 1: Exercise 5

Items 1 to 10 pertain to the paranasal sinuses. Identify structures, provide short answers, select from a list, or choose true or false (explain any item you believe to be false).

1. Name the four groups of sinuses.

2. Identify the sinus groups shown in Fig. 11.15.

   A. _____

   B. _____

   C. _____

   D. _____

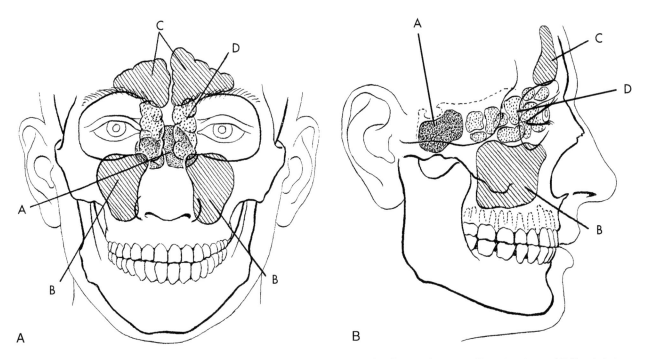

Fig. 11.15 Two diagrams showing paranasal sinuses in relation to each other and surrounding structures. (A) Frontal view. (B) Lateral view.

3. Which paranasal sinus group is superior to the other sinus groups?
   a. Frontal
   b. Maxillary
   c. Ethmoidal
   d. Sphenoidal

4. Which paranasal sinuses are mostly located inferior to the orbits?
   a. Frontal
   b. Maxillary
   c. Ethmoidal
   d. Sphenoidal

5. Which paranasal sinuses are located directly below the sella turcica?
   a. Frontal
   b. Maxillary
   c. Ethmoidal
   d. Sphenoidal

6. Which paranasal sinus group is posterior to the ethmoidal sinuses?
   a. Frontal
   b. Maxillary
   c. Ethmoidal
   d. Sphenoidal

7. Which sinus group is subdivided into three main groups?
   a. Frontal
   b. Maxillary
   c. Ethmoidal
   d. Sphenoidal

8. List five functions of the sinus cavities.

9. Which sinus group is well developed and aerated at birth?
   a. Frontal
   b. Maxillary
   c. Ethmoidal
   d. Sphenoidal

10. True or false. At age 15 or 16 years, the sinuses are fully developed and communicate with each other.

Section 1: Exercise 6

Match the pathology terms in Column A with the appropriate definition in Column B. Not all choices from Column B should be selected.

Column A

_____ 1. Sinusitis

_____ 2. Mastoiditis

_____ 3. TMJ syndrome

_____ 4. Basal fracture

_____ 5. Linear fracture

_____ 6. Tripod fracture

_____ 7. LeFort fracture

_____ 8. Blowout fracture

_____ 9. Depressed fracture

_____ 10. Contrecoup fracture

_____ 11. Osteoma

_____ 12. Metastases

_____ 13. Acoustic neuroma

_____ 14. Pituitary adenoma

_____ 15. Multiple myeloma

Column B

a. Tumor composed of bony tissue

b. Fracture of the floor of the orbit

c. Irregular or jagged fracture of the skull

d. Fracture located at the base of the skull

e. Dysfunction of the temporomandibular joint (TMJ)

f. Bilateral horizontal fractures of the maxillae

g. Inflammation of the mastoid antrum and air cells

h. Inflammation of the bone resulting from a pyogenic infection

i. Inflammation of one or more of the paranasal sinuses

j. Transfer of a cancerous lesion from one area to another

k. Tumor arising from the pituitary gland, usually in the anterior lobe

l. Benign tumor arising from Schwann cells of the eighth cranial nerve

m. Fracture to one side of a structure caused by trauma to the other side

n. Fracture causing a portion of the skull to be pushed into the cranial cavity

o. Fracture of the zygomatic arch and orbital floor or rim and dislocation of the frontozygomatic suture

p. Malignant neoplasm of plasma cells involving the bone marrow and causing destruction of the bone

Section 1: Exercise 7

This exercise is a comprehensive review of the osteology and arthrology of the skull and facial bones. Fill in missing words or provide a short answer for each item.

1. The bones of the skull are divided into two major groups, the _____ bones and the _____ bones.

2. List the cranial bones by name and quantity.

3. List the facial bones by name and quantity.

4. List the three classifications of fundamental skull shapes, and indicate the number of degrees of angulation (formed by the petrous pyramids and the midsagittal plane) for each classification.

5. The bones of the cranial vault are classified as _____ bones.

6. The inner layer of spongy tissue found inside cranial bones is called _____.

7. The two fontanelles located on the midsagittal plane of the skull are the _____ and the _____.

8. The fontanelle located at the junction of the coronal and sagittal sutures is the _____.

9. The fontanelle located at the junction of the lambdoidal and sagittal sutures is the _____.

10. The bone that forms the anterior portion of the cranium is the _____ bone.

11. The cranial bone located between the orbits and posterior to the nasal bones is the _____ bone.

12. The cranial bones that form the vertex and most of the sides of the cranium are the _____ bones.

13. The prominent bulge of a parietal bone is called the parietal _____.

14. The two parietal bones join together to form the _____ suture.

15. The two parietal bones articulate with the frontal _____ bone to form the _____ suture.

16. The two parietal bones articulate posteriorly with the _____ bone.

17. The two parietal bones and the occipital bone join together to form the _____ suture.

18. The cranial bone that provides a depression to house the pituitary gland is the _____ bone.

19. The cranial bone that forms the posteroinferior portion of the cranium is the _____ bone.

20. The portion of the occipital bone that projects anteriorly from the foramen magnum is the _____ _____ portion.

21. The large opening of the occipital bone through which part of the medulla oblongata passes is the _____.

22. The basilar portion of the occipital bone fuses anteriorly with the body of the _____ bone.

23. The structure that articulates with the occipital condyles is the _____.

24. The middle portion of the cranial base is formed by the _____ bone.

25. The organs of hearing are located in the _____ bone.

26. The structure that separates the external acoustic meatus (EAM) from the auditory ossicles is the _____ membrane.

27. The process of the temporal bone that encloses radiographically significant air cells is the _____ process.

28. The thickest and densest portion of bone in the cranium is the _____.

29. The petrous portion is a part of the _____ bone.

30. The fibrocartilaginous, oval-shaped portion of the external ear is the _____.

31. The three auditory ossicles are the _____, the _____, and the _____.

32. The zygomatic process projects anteriorly from the _____ bone.

33. The bone that forms part of the cranial base between the greater wings of the sphenoid bone and the occipital bone is the _____ bone.

34. The facial bones that form the bridge of the nose are the _____ bones.

35. The anterior portion of the medial walls of the orbits is formed by the _____ bones.

36. The largest of the immovable bones of the face is the _____ bone.

37. The body of each maxilla contains a large, pyramidal cavity called the _____.

38. The thick ridge on the inferior border of the maxillary bone that supports the teeth is the _____.

39. The anterior nasal spine projects superiorly from the _____.

40. The radiographically significant landmark that is the midpoint of the anterior nasal spine is the _____.

41. The facial bones that form the inferolateral portion of the orbital margin are the _____ bones.

42. The facial bones that form the prominence of the cheeks are the _____ bones.

43. The facial bones that form the posterior one fourth of the roof of the mouth are the _____ bones.

44. The scroll-like bony tissues that extend along the lateral walls of the nasal cavity are the _____.

45. The facial bone forming the inferior part of the nasal septum is the _____.

46. The largest and densest bone of the face is the

_____.

47. The portion of the mandible that extends superiorly from the posterior aspect of the mandibular body is

the _____.

48. The U-shaped bone located at the base of the tongue

is the _____ bone.

49. The two processes that extend superiorly from a

mandibular ramus are the _____ and the

_____ process.

50. The part of the mandible that articulates with the mandibular fossa of the temporal bone to form the

TMJ is the _____.

51. The orbit consists of _____ cranial

bones and _____ facial bones.

52. The lateral wall of the orbit comprises the

_____ and _____ bones.

53. The inferior border of the orbit consists of the

_____ and _____ bones.

54. The _____ facial bone is located at the apex of the orbit.

55. The _____ facial bone is located on the interior medial wall of the orbit.

Section 1: Exercise 8: Abbreviations

This exercise provides practice in the use of common abbreviations used in skull procedures. Write out the words beside each abbreviation.

1. AML: _____

2. TEA: _____

3. IAM: _____

4. IPL: _____

5. GML: _____

6. OML: _____

7. IOML: _____

8. MML: _____

RADIOGRAPHY OF THE SKULL

Section 2: Exercise 1: Skull Topography

This exercise pertains to positioning landmarks used in skull radiography. Identify landmarks or provide a short answer for each item.

1. Identify each lettered positioning landmark shown in Fig. 11.16.

   A. _____

   B. _____

   C. _____

   D. _____

   E. _____

   F. _____

   G. _____

   H. _____

   I. _____

   J. _____

2. Identify each lettered positioning landmark shown in Fig. 11.17.

   A. _____

   B. _____

   C. _____

   D. _____

   E. _____

   F. _____

   G. _____

   H. _____

   I. _____

   J. _____

   K. _____

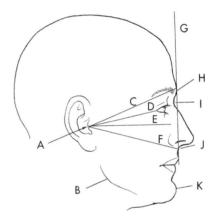

Fig. 11.17 Lateral aspect landmarks.

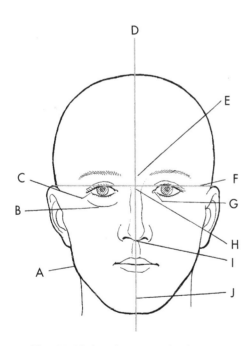

Fig. 11.16 Anterior aspect landmarks.

3. Match the definitions in Column A with the appropriate term from Column B. Each term may be used only once.

Column A

_____ 1. Midpoint of the frontonasal suture

_____ 2. Midpoint of the anterior nasal spine

_____ 3. Posterior surface of the occipital bone

_____ 4. Smooth elevation between the superciliary arches

_____ 5. Lateral aspect of each orbit; where the two eyelids originate

_____ 6. Angle of the mandible; lateroposterior aspect of the mandible

_____ 7. Superior aspect of the cranium; where the parietal bones join together

_____ 8. Raised prominence just above each orbit on the frontal bone; coincides with the eyebrows

_____ 9. Midpoint of the mental protuberance; anterior aspect of the mandible; where the two mandibular bodies join together

Column B

a. Inion

b. Vertex

c. Nasion

d. Gonion

e. Glabella

f. Acanthion

g. Mental point

h. Outer canthus

i. Superciliary arch

4. Match the definitions in Column A with the appropriate terms in Column B. The terms represent skull topography lines or planes. Each term may be used once, more than once, or not at all.

Column A

_____ 1. Line extending across the front through both eyes

_____ 2. Plane dividing the skull into equal right and left halves

_____ 3. Line extending from the glabella to the anterior aspect of the maxilla

_____ 4. Line extending from the EAM to the outer canthus

_____ 5. Line extending from the EAM to the inferior margin of the orbit

_____ 6. Line extending from the EAM to the midpoint of the anterior nasal spine

_____ 7. Line extending from the EAM to the smooth elevation between the superciliary arches

Column B

a. Sagittal

b. Midsagittal

c. Midcoronal

d. Orbitomeatal

e. Interpupillary

f. Glabellomeatal

g. Acanthiomeatal

h. Glabelloalveolar

i. Infraorbitomeatal

5. How many degrees exist in the angles formed by the following lines?

a. Orbitomeatal and infraorbitomeatal lines: _____

b. Orbitomeatal and glabellomeatal lines: _____

Section 2: Exercise 2: Positioning for the Cranium

The typical radiographic evaluation of the skull, usually referred to as a skull series, involves a series of images that may include a posteroanterior (PA) or anteroposterior (AP) projection, an AP axial projection, a full basal view, and one or two lateral views. This exercise pertains to those projections. Identify structures, fill in missing words, provide a short answer, select from a list, or choose true or false (explaining any statement you believe to be false) for each item.

Items 1 to 12 pertain to the *lateral projection*. Examine Fig. 11.18 as you answer the following questions.

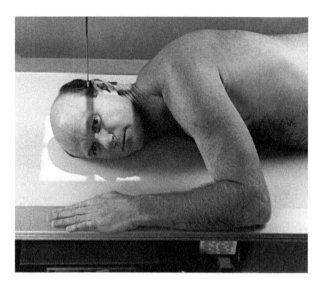

Fig. 11.18 Lateral skull.

1. Which size exposure field or CR plate should be used for average-sized adult skulls, and how should it be placed in the IR holder?
   a. 14 × 17 inches (35 × 43 cm); crosswise
   b. 14 × 17 inches (35 × 43 cm); lengthwise
   c. 10 × 12 inches (24 × 30 cm); crosswise
   d. 10 × 12 inches (23 × 30 cm); lengthwise

2. Indicate how the midsagittal plane and the interpupillary line should be positioned (perpendicular or parallel) with reference to the plane of the IR.

   a. Midsagittal plane: _____

   b. Interpupillary line: _____

3. Which positioning line of the head should be parallel with the transverse plane of the IR?
   a. Interpupillary line
   b. Glabelloalveolar line
   c. Infraorbitomeatal line (IOML)

4. Which structure should be nearest to the center of the midline of the grid?
   a. Acanthion
   b. Zygomatic bone
   c. Outer canthus
   d. EAM

5. To what level of the patient should the IR be centered?

6. Describe how and where the central ray should be directed.

7. Which positioning line of the head should be perpendicular to the IR?
   a. Interpupillary line
   b. Glabelloalveolar line
   c. IOML

8. True or false. The unaffected side of the skull is positioned closest to the IR.

9. True or false. The radiation field should be adjusted to extend ½ to 1 inch (1.3 to 2.5 cm) beyond the skin line of the skull.

10. From the following list, circle the eight evaluation criteria that indicate the patient was properly positioned for a lateral projection.
    a. The petrous ridges should be symmetric.
    b. The sella turcica should be seen in profile.
    c. The orbital roofs should be superimposed.
    d. The mastoid regions should be superimposed.
    e. The mandible should not overlap the cervical vertebrae.
    f. The greater wings of sphenoid should be superimposed.
    g. The TMJs should be superimposed.
    h. The EAMs should be superimposed.
    i. The dorsum sellae should be within the foramen magnum.
    j. The entire cranium should be demonstrated without rotation or tilt.
    k. The mental protuberance should be superimposed over the anterior frontal bone.
    l. The distance from the lateral border of the skull to the lateral border of the orbit should be equal on both sides.

11. Fig. 11.19 shows two diagrams of a recumbent patient with the midsagittal plane improperly aligned. Examine the diagrams and explain how the position of the patient in each should be adjusted to align the midsagittal plane with the IR properly.
    a. Diagram A:

    b. Diagram B:

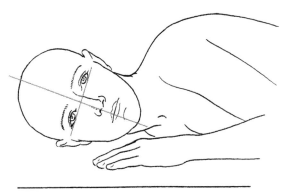

A   Asthenic or hyposthenic patient

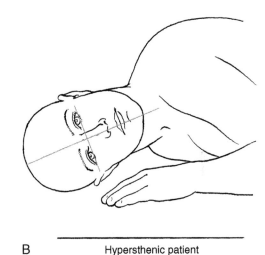

B   Hypersthenic patient

Fig. 11.19 Adjusting the midsagittal plane with the patient in the recumbent position. (A) Asthenic or hyposthenic patient. (B) Hypersthenic patient.

12. Identify each lettered structure shown in Fig. 11.20.

A. _____

B. _____

C. _____

D. _____

E. _____

F. _____

G. _____

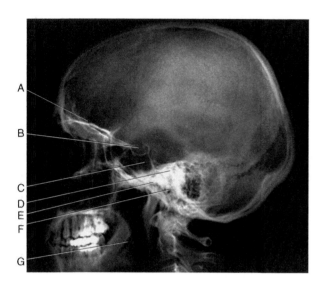

Fig. 11.20 Lateral skull image.

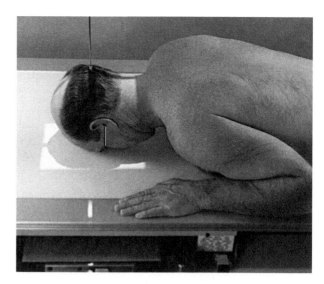

Fig. 11.21 PA skull.

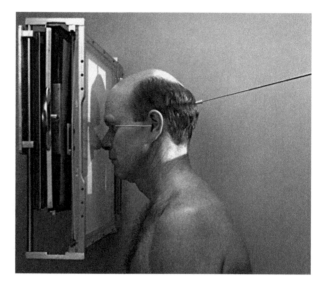

Fig. 11.22 PA axial skull.

Items 13 to 20 pertain to PA and PA *axial projections.* Examine Figs. 11.21 and 11.22 as you answer the following questions.

13. Indicate how the midsagittal plane and the orbitomeatal line (OML) should be positioned (perpendicular or parallel) with reference to the plane of the IR.

a. Midsagittal plane: _____

b. OML: _____

14. Which parts of the patient's facial area should be in contact with the table or vertical grid device?
a. Chin and nose
b. Chin and cheek
c. Forehead and nose
d. Forehead and cheek

15. To demonstrate each of the following structures (Column A), identify how the central ray should be directed (Column B) with the patient positioned for a PA projection of the skull.

Column A

_____ 1. Frontal bone

_____ 2. General survey

_____ 3. Rotundum foramina

_____ 4. Superior orbital fissures

Column B

a. Perpendicular

b. 15 degrees caudad

c. 20 to 25 degrees caudad

d. 25 to 30 degrees caudad

16. The central ray should exit the skull at the

_____.

17. The IR should be centered to the skull at the level of

the _____.

18. What breathing instructions should be given to the patient?

19. From the following list, circle the five evaluation criteria that indicate the patient was properly positioned for either PA or PA axial projections.
    a. The petrous ridges should be symmetric.
    b. The orbital roofs should be superimposed.
    c. The entire cranial perimeter should be included.
    d. The mandible should not overlap the cervical vertebrae.
    e. The dorsum sellae should be within the foramen magnum.
    f. The mental protuberance should be superimposed over the anterior frontal bone.
    g. The frontal bone should be penetrated.
    h. The distance from the lateral border of the skull to the lateral border of the orbit should be equal on both sides.
    i. The petrous pyramids should lie in the lower third of the orbit with a central ray angulation of 15 degrees caudad and should fill the orbits with no central ray angulation.

20. Identify each lettered structure shown in Fig. 11.23.

A. _____

B. _____

C. _____

D. _____

E. _____

F. _____

G. _____

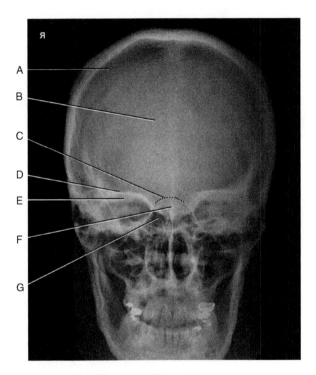

Fig. 11.23 PA skull image.

Items 21 to 27 pertain to AP and AP *axial projections.* Examine Figs. 11.24 and 11.25 as you answer the following questions.

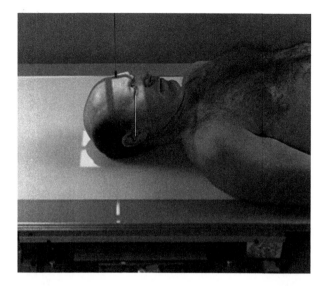

Fig. 11.24 AP skull.

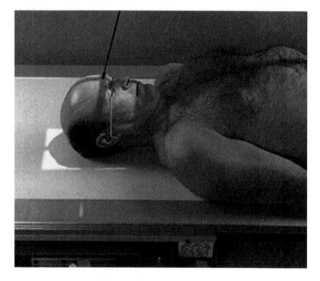

Fig. 11.25 AP axial skull.

21. Indicate how the midsagittal plane and the OML should be positioned (perpendicular or parallel) with reference to the plane of the IR.

    a. Midsagittal plane: _____

    b. OML: _____

22. For the AP projection, the central ray should be directed _____ (caudally, cephalically, or perpendicularly).

23. For the AP axial projection, the central ray should be directed _____ (caudally, cephalically, or perpendicularly).

24. When performing either the AP or the AP axial projection for general surveys of the skull, where on the skull should the central ray be directed?
    a. Nasion
    b. Acanthion
    c. Tip of the nose

25. Which of the following image characteristics indicates that a general survey image of the skull is an AP projection instead of a PA projection?
    a. The petrous ridges are symmetric.
    b. The petrous pyramids fill the orbits.
    c. The orbits are considerably magnified.
    d. The entire cranial perimeter is demonstrated.

26. From the following list, circle the five evaluation criteria that indicate the patient was properly positioned for either the AP or the AP axial projection.
    a. The petrous ridges should be symmetric.
    b. The orbital roofs should be superimposed.
    c. The entire cranial perimeter should be included.
    d. The mandible should not overlap the cervical vertebrae.
    e. The dorsum sellae should be within the foramen magnum.
    f. The mental protuberance should be superimposed over the anterior frontal bone.
    g. The frontal bone should be penetrated.
    h. The distance from the lateral border of the skull to the lateral border of the orbit should be equal on both sides.
    i. The petrous pyramids should lie in the lower third of the orbit, with a central ray angulation of 15 degrees caudad, and should fill the orbits with no central ray angulation.
    j. The petrous pyramids should lie in the lower third of the orbit, with a central ray angulation of 15 degrees cephalically, and should fill the orbits with no central ray angulation.

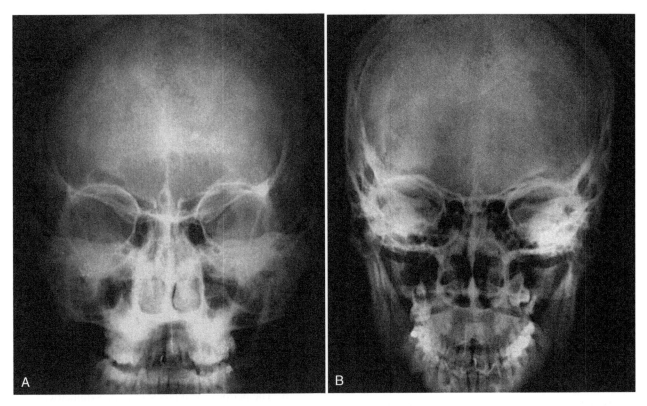

Fig. 11.26 Two images of the skull.

27. Fig. 11.26 shows two skull images: one AP and one AP axial. Examine each image and state how the central ray was directed by indicating how specific structures appear in relation to the surrounding structures.

   a. Figure A: _____

   b. Figure B: _____

Items 28 to 35 pertain to the AP axial projection, *Towne method*. Examine Fig. 11.27 as you answer the following questions.

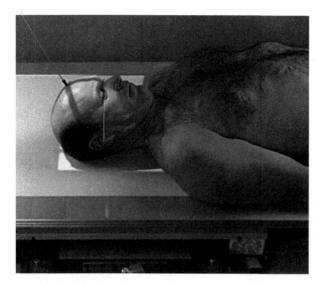

Fig. 11.27 AP axial skull, Towne method.

28. Which size exposure field or CR plate should be used for average-sized adult skulls, and how should it be placed in the IR holder?
    a. 14 × 17 inches (35 × 43 cm); crosswise
    b. 14 × 17 inches (35 × 43 cm); lengthwise
    c. 10 × 12 inches (24 × 30 cm); crosswise
    d. 10 × 12 inches (24 × 30 cm); lengthwise

29. To what level of the patient should the upper border of the IR be aligned?
    a. Nasion
    b. Glabella
    c. Highest point of the vertex

30. In addition to the midsagittal plane, either the _____

    _____ line or the

    _____

    line must be perpendicular to the plane of the IR.

31. Which two central ray angulations could be used to perform the AP axial projection properly?
    a. 30 degrees caudad and 37 degrees caudad
    b. 30 degrees caudad and 37 degrees cephalad
    c. 30 degrees cephalad and 37 degrees caudad
    d. 30 degrees cephalad and 37 degrees cephalad

32. Which positioning factor determines the number of degrees that the central ray should be angled?
    a. The type of skull being positioned
    b. Whether the patient is supine or seated upright
    c. How much SID is used
    d. Which positioning line is perpendicular to the IR

33. Where exactly on the patient's head should the central ray enter?
    a. 1 inch (2.5 cm) above the nasion
    b. 1 inch (2.5 cm) below the nasion
    c. 2 to 2½ inches (5 to 6.25 cm) above the glabella
    d. 2 to 2½ inches (5 to 6.25 cm) below the glabella

34. From the following list, circle the four evaluation criteria that indicate the patient was properly positioned for the AP axial projection, Towne method.
    a. The orbital roofs should be superimposed.
    b. The petrous pyramids should be symmetric.
    c. The mandible should not overlap the cervical vertebrae.
    d. The petrous pyramids should lie in the lower third of the orbits.
    e. The mental protuberance should be superimposed over the anterior frontal bone.
    f. The occipital bone should be penetrated.
    g. The dorsum sellae and posterior clinoid processes should be visualized within the foramen magnum.
    h. The distance from the lateral border of the skull to the lateral border of the orbit should be equal on both sides.
    i. The distance from the lateral border of the skull to the lateral margin of the foramen magnum should be equal on both sides.

35. Identify each lettered structure shown in Fig. 11.28.

A. _____

B. _____

C. _____

D. _____

E. _____

F. _____

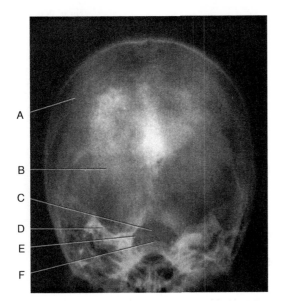

Fig. 11.28 AP axial skull, Towne method image.

Items 36 to 43 pertain to the PA *axial projection, Haas method*. Examine Fig. 11.29 as you answer the following questions.

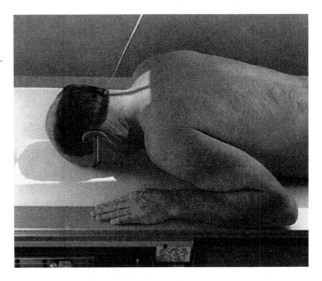

Fig. 11.29 PA axial skull, Haas method.

36. True or false. The PA axial projection, Haas method, demonstrates the occipital region of the cranium.

37. True or false. Hypersthenic patients should be positioned while recumbent in the supine position.

38. Which parts of the patient's head should be in contact with the table or vertical grid device?
    a. Chin and nose
    b. Chin and cheek
    c. Forehead and nose
    d. Forehead and cheek

39. In addition to the midsagittal plane, which positioning line of the skull should be perpendicular to the plane of the IR?
    a. Orbitomeatal
    b. Glabellomeatal
    c. Acanthiomeatal
    d. Infraorbitomeatal

40. How many degrees and in which direction should the central ray be directed?
   a. 25 degrees caudad
   b. 25 degrees cephalad
   c. 30 degrees caudad
   d. 30 degrees cephalad

41. Where on the midsagittal plane of the patient's skull should the central ray enter?
   a. At the vertex of the skull
   b. At a point approximately 1½ inches (3.8 cm) above the external occipital protuberance
   c. At a point approximately 1½ inches (3.8 cm) below the external occipital protuberance
   d. At a point approximately 3 inches (7.6 cm) below the external occipital protuberance

42. From the following list, circle the four evaluation criteria that indicate the patient was properly positioned for the PA axial projection, Haas method.
   a. The entire cranium should be included.
   b. The orbital roofs should be superimposed.
   c. The petrous pyramids should be symmetric.
   d. The mandible should not overlap the cervical vertebrae.
   e. The petrous pyramids should lie in the lower third of the orbits.
   f. The mental protuberance should be superimposed over the anterior frontal bone.
   g. The dorsum sellae and posterior clinoid processes should be seen within the foramen magnum.
   h. The distance from the lateral border of the skull to the lateral border of the orbit should be equal on both sides.
   i. The distance from the lateral border of the skull to the lateral border of the foramen magnum should be equal on both sides.

43. Identify each lettered structure shown in Fig. 11.30.

A. _____

B. _____

C. _____

D. _____

E. _____

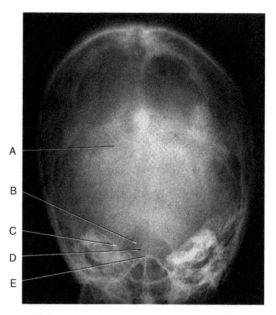

Fig. 11.30 PA axial skull, Haas method image.

362

Items 44 to 50 pertain to the *submentovertical (SMV) projection, Schüller method*. Examine Fig. 11.31 as you answer the following questions.

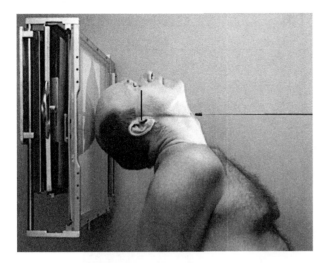

Fig. 11.31 Submentovertical cranial base.

44. Indicate how the midsagittal plane and the IOML should be positioned (perpendicular or parallel) with reference to the plane of the IR.

    a. Midsagittal plane: _____

    b. Infraorbitomeatal: _____

45. To what positioning line of the skull should the perpendicular central ray be directed?

46. Describe where the central ray should enter the patient.

47. Through which cranial structure should the central ray pass?
    a. Sella turcica
    b. Ethmoidal air cells
    c. EAM

48. From the following list, select the two positioning factors on which the success of SMV projections most depend.
    a. Directing the central ray perpendicular to the OML
    b. Directing the central ray perpendicular to the IOML
    c. Directing the central ray perpendicular to the midsagittal plane
    d. Placing the OML as near as possible to parallel with the plane of the IR
    e. Placing the IOML as near as possible to parallel with the plane of the IR
    f. Placing the midsagittal plane as near as possible to parallel with the plane of the IR

49. From the following list, circle the five evaluation criteria that indicate the patient was properly positioned for an SMV projection.
    a. The petrosae should be symmetric.
    b. The orbital roofs should be superimposed.
    c. The mandibular rami should be superimposed.
    d. The mental protuberance should superimpose the anterior frontal bone.
    e. The petrous pyramids should lie in the lower third of the orbits.
    f. The mandibular condyles should be anterior to the petrous pyramids.
    g. The dorsum sellae should be seen and projected within the foramen magnum.
    h. Exposure factors should be sufficient to penetrate the cranial base.
    i. The distance from the lateral border of the skull to the mandibular condyles should be equal on both sides.

50. Identify each lettered structure shown in Fig. 11.32.

A. _____   F. _____

B. _____   G. _____

C. _____   H. _____

D. _____   I. _____

E. _____

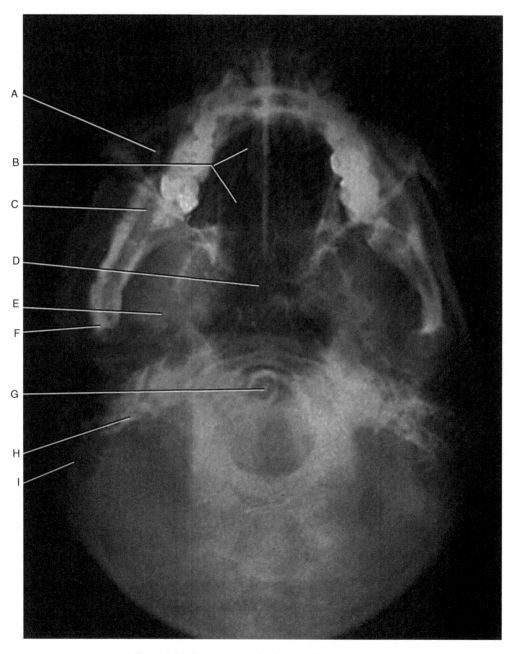

Fig. 11.32 Submentovertical cranial base image.

Section 2: Exercise 3: Evaluating Radiographic Images of the Skull

This exercise consists of images of the skull, most of which show at least one positioning error, to give you practice evaluating skull positioning. These images are not from Merrill's Atlas. Examine each image and answer the questions that follow by providing a short answer.

Figs. 11.33 through 11.35 are lateral projection images of a phantom skull. Only one image demonstrates acceptable positioning. Examine the images and answer questions 1 to 4. Refer to specific evaluation criteria for this projection when explaining your answers.

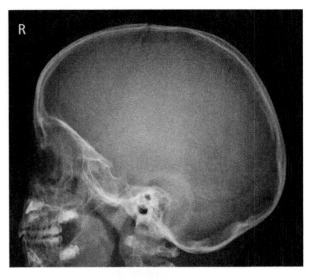

Fig. 11.35 Lateral skull image.

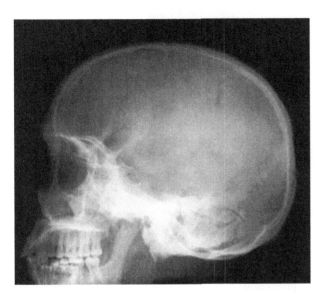

Fig. 11.33 Lateral skull image.

1. Which image best demonstrates an optimally positioned skull? Explain.

2. Which image shows the skull incorrectly positioned because the vertex and midsagittal plane are tilted toward the plane of the IR? Explain.

3. Which image shows the skull incorrectly positioned because the face and midsagittal plane are rotated toward the x-ray table and IR? Explain.

4. Which image shows the skull positioned similarly to that seen in Fig. 11.19B?

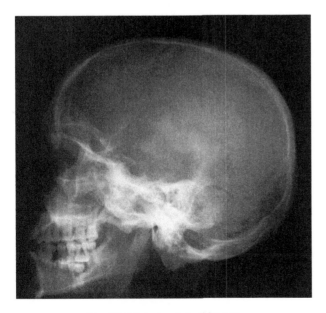

Fig. 11.34 Lateral skull image.

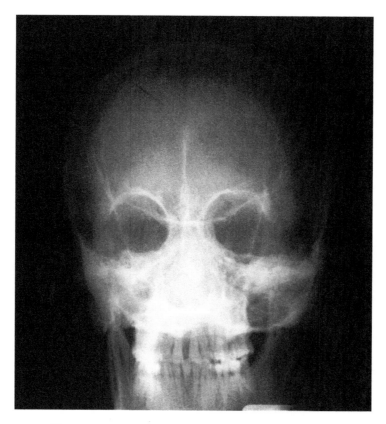

Fig. 11.36 PA skull image showing incorrect positioning.

Fig. 11.36 shows a PA projection image of a phantom skull with incorrect positioning. Examine the image and answer questions 5 to 8.

5. Assuming that the OML was perpendicular to the plane of the IR, describe how the central ray most likely was directed.

6. Describe where the petrous ridges should appear in the image when the central ray is directed caudally 15 degrees.

7. What image characteristic most likely prevents this image from meeting all the evaluation criteria for this projection?

8. Describe the positioning error that most likely caused the image to appear as it does.

366

Fig. 11.37 shows a PA projection radiograph of a phantom skull with incorrect positioning. Examine the image and answer questions 9 to 13.

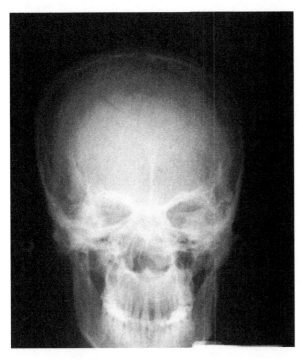

Fig. 11.37 PA skull image showing incorrect positioning.

9. Assuming that the OML was perpendicular to the plane of the IR, describe how the central ray most likely was directed.

10. Describe where the petrous ridges should appear in the image when the central ray is directed perpendicularly.

11. Do the petrous ridges nearly fill the orbits?

12. What image characteristic most likely prevents this image from meeting all evaluation criteria for this projection?

13. Describe the positioning error that most likely caused the image to appear as it does.

Figs. 11.38 and 11.39 show AP projection images of a phantom skull. Only one image demonstrates acceptable positioning. Examine the images and answer questions 14 to 17.

14. Is the positioning quality for Fig. 11.38 acceptable or unacceptable?

15. Is the positioning quality for Fig. 11.39 acceptable or unacceptable?

16. Describe the positioning error that probably caused the unacceptable image.

17. Assuming that the OML was perpendicular for both images, in which way does the central ray appear to have been directed?

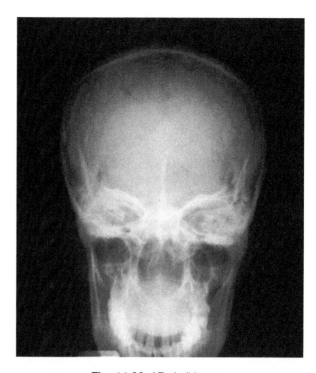

Fig. 11.38 AP skull image.

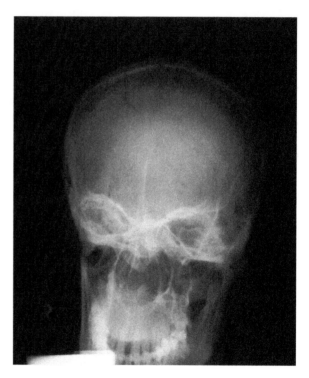

Fig. 11.39 AP skull image.

18. Examine Fig. 11.40 and state why it does not meet the evaluation criteria for this type of projection.

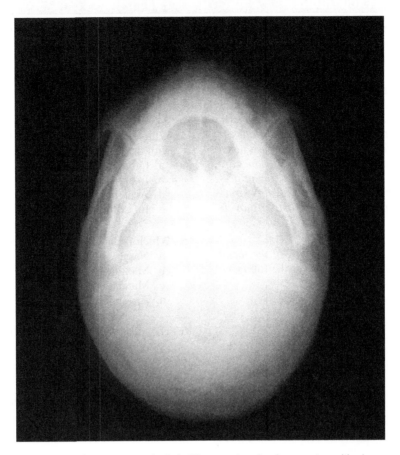

Fig. 11.40 Submentovertical skull image showing incorrect positioning.

RADIOGRAPHY OF THE FACIAL BONES

Section 3: Exercise 1: Positioning for Facial Bones and Nasal Bones

A standard radiographic series to demonstrate facial bones includes various projections that examine facial structures from different perspectives. Some projections commonly used are the lateral, parietoacanthial (Waters method), and acanthioparietal (reverse Waters method). Additionally, a lateral projection of the nasal bones is sometimes added to a facial bone series because nasal bones are sometimes affected when other facial bones are damaged by trauma. This exercise pertains to the projections of the facial bones and nasal bones. Identify structures, fill in missing words, select from a list, or provide a short answer for each item.

Items 1 to 9 pertain to *lateral projections of the facial bones*. Examine Fig. 11.41 as you answer the following questions.

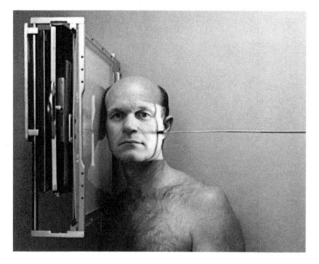

Fig. 11.41 Lateral facial bones.

1. The IR should be placed in the IR holder _____ (crosswise or lengthwise).

2. The plane of the head that should be parallel with the plane of the IR is the _____ (midsagittal or midcoronal) plane.

3. Which positioning line of the head should be perpendicular to the IR?
   a. Orbitomeatal
   b. Interpupillary
   c. Acanthiomeatal
   d. Infraorbitomeatal

4. Which positioning line of the head should be parallel with the transverse axis of the IR?
   a. Orbitomeatal
   b. Interpupillary
   c. Acanthiomeatal
   d. Infraorbitomeatal

5. Which facial bone should be centered to the IR?
   a. Nasal
   b. Maxilla
   c. Mandible
   d. Zygomatic

6. The central ray should be directed to the patient _____ (perpendicularly, angled cephalically, or angled caudally)?

7. Where on the patient's face should the central ray be directed?

8. From the following list, circle the four evaluation criteria that indicate the patient was properly positioned for a lateral projection of the facial bones.
   a. The sella turcica should not be rotated.
   b. The orbital roofs should be superimposed.
   c. The sella turcica should be seen within the foramen magnum.
   d. The mandibular rami should be almost perfectly superimposed.
   e. The petrous bones should lie in the lower third of the orbit.
   f. The mental protuberance should be superimposed over the anterior frontal bone.
   g. All facial bones should be completely included with the zygomatic bone in the center.
   h. The distance from the lateral border of the skull to the lateral border of the orbit should be equal on both sides.

9. Identify each lettered structure shown in Fig. 11.42.

A. _____

B. _____

C. _____

D. _____

E. _____

F. _____

G. _____

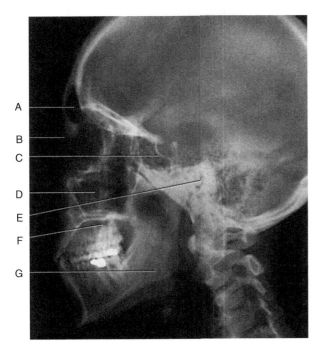

Fig. 11.42 Lateral facial bones.

Items 10 to 15 pertain to the *parietoacanthial projection, Waters method*. Examine Fig. 11.43 as you answer the following questions.

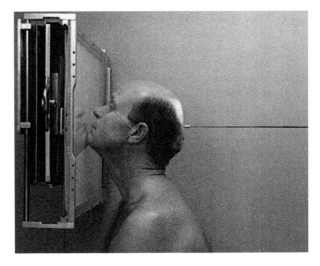

Fig. 11.43 Parietoacanthial facial bones, Waters method.

10. Indicate how the OML and the midsagittal plane should be positioned with reference to the IR.

a. OML: _____

b. Midsagittal plane: _____

11. To which landmark of the head should the IR be centered?
a. Nasion
b. Acanthion
c. Mental point
d. Outer canthus

12. How should the central ray be directed relative to the IR?
a. Perpendicularly
b. 37 degrees caudally
c. 37 degrees cephalically

13. Describe where the petrous ridges most likely will appear in the image if the OML creates the following angles with the IR:

a. 25 degrees: _____

b. 37 degrees: _____

c. 55 degrees: _____

Chapter **11 Cranium**

14. From the following list, circle the two evaluation criteria that indicate the patient was properly positioned for a parietoacanthial projection.
    a. The orbital roofs should be superimposed.
    b. The petrous ridges should nearly fill the orbits.
    c. The entire cranium should be demonstrated without rotation or tilt.
    d. The petrous ridges should be projected immediately below the maxillary sinuses.
    e. The distance between the lateral border of the skull and orbit should be equal on both sides.

15. Identify each lettered structure shown in Fig. 11.44.

    A. _____

    B. _____

    C. _____

    D. _____

    E. _____

    F. _____

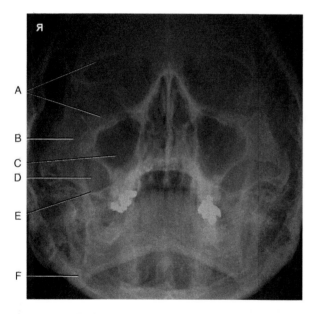

Fig. 11.44 Parietoacanthial facial bones, Waters method.

Items 16 to 24 pertain to the *acanthioparietal projection, reverse Waters method.* Examine Fig. 11.45 as you answer the following questions.

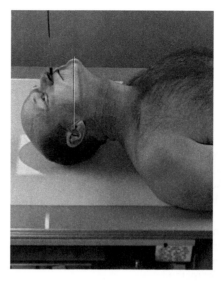

Fig. 11.45 Acanthioparietal facial bones, reverse Waters method.

16. The acanthioparietal projection can be used to demonstrate facial bones when the patient is lying in the

    _____ (prone or supine) position.

17. The image of the acanthioparietal projection is

    similar to the image of the _____ projection

    (_____ method).

18. Which plane and positioning line of the head should be perpendicular to the IR?
    a. Midsagittal plane and OML
    b. Midsagittal plane and mentomeatal line
    c. Midcoronal plane and OML
    d. Midcoronal plane and mentomeatal line

19. Where should the midpoint of the IR be centered to the patient?
    a. Nasion
    b. Glabella
    c. Acanthion
    d. 1 inch (2.5 cm) inferior to the acanthion

20. Which breathing instructions should be given to the patient?
    a. Stop breathing.
    b. Breathe slowly.
    c. Breathe rapidly.

21. How should the central ray be directed?
    a. Perpendicularly
    b. 15 degrees caudally
    c. 15 degrees cephalically
    d. 30 degrees cephalically

22. To which positioning landmark should the central ray be directed?
    a. Nasion
    b. Glabella
    c. Acanthion
    d. Mental point

23. From the following list, circle the two evaluation criteria that indicate the patient was properly positioned for an acanthioparietal projection, reverse Waters method.
    a. The orbital roofs should be superimposed.
    b. The petrous ridges should nearly fill the orbits.
    c. The petrous ridges should be projected in the maxillary sinuses.
    d. The petrous ridges should be projected immediately below the maxillary sinuses.
    e. The distance between the lateral border of the skull and orbit should be equal on both sides.

24. Identify each lettered structure shown in Fig. 11.46.

    A. _____

    B. _____

    C. _____

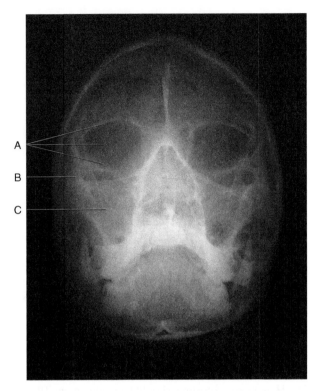

Fig. 11.46 Acanthioparietal facial bones, reverse Waters method.

Items 25 to 30 pertain to the *lateral projection of the nasal bones*. Examine Fig. 11.47 as you answer the following questions.

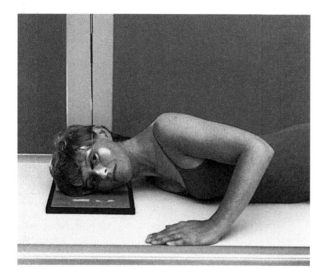

Fig. 11.47 Lateral nasal bones.

25. Indicate how the interpupillary line and midsagittal plane should be positioned with reference to the IR-perpendicular or parallel.

    a. Interpupillary line: _____

    b. Midsagittal plane: _____

26. How many exposures should be made on one IR?

27. To which facial landmark (the nasion or acanthion) should the unmasked portion of the IR be centered?

28. Describe how and where the central ray should be directed.

29. From the following list, circle the two evaluation criteria that indicate the patient was properly positioned for a lateral projection.
    a. All facial bones should be demonstrated.
    b. The zygomatic processes should be seen superimposed.
    c. The anterior nasal spine and frontonasal suture should be visualized.
    d. The nasal bone and soft tissue should be demonstrated without rotation.

30. Identify each lettered structure shown in Fig. 11.48.

    A. _____ (suture)

    B. _____

    C. _____

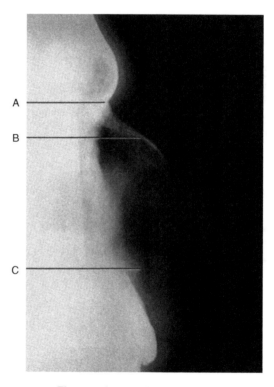

Fig. 11.48 Lateral nasal bones.

Section 3: Exercise 2: Positioning for Zygomatic Arches

Zygomatic arches are commonly demonstrated with three projections: SMV projection, tangential projection, and AP axial projection. This exercise pertains to those projections. Identify structures, fill in missing words, provide a short answer, select from a list, or choose true or false (explaining any statement you believe to be false) for each item.

Items 1 to 9 pertain to the SMV *projection for bilateral zygomatic arches*. Examine Fig. 11.49 as you answer the following questions.

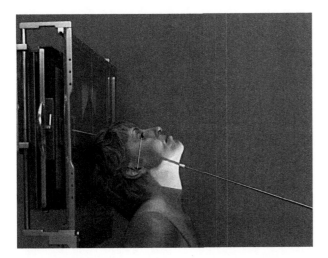

Fig. 11.49 Submentovertical zygomatic arches.

1. True or false. The SMV projection should demonstrate both zygomatic arches with one exposure.

2. True or false. Zygomatic arches should be demonstrated superimposed with the anterior frontal bone.

3. True or false. The entire cranial base should be demonstrated.

4. True or false. The midsagittal plane should be parallel with the IR.

5. Which positioning line of the head should be parallel with the IR?
   a. Orbitomeatal
   b. Acanthiomeatal
   c. Infraorbitomeatal

6. Which part of the patient should be in contact with the grid device?
   a. Forehead
   b. Mandible
   c. Vertex of the skull

7. Which statement best describes how the central ray should be directed?
   a. Angled cephalically and centered to the glabella
   b. Angled caudally and centered to the zygomatic arch of interest
   c. Perpendicular to the IOML and centered on the midsagittal plane of the throat

8. For the SMV projection, what causes the zygomatic arches to be projected beyond the parietal eminences?
   a. The divergent x-ray beam
   b. The head tilted 15 degrees
   c. The head rotated 15 degrees

9. From the following list, circle the three evaluation criteria that indicate the patient was properly positioned for the SMV projection.
   a. No rotation of the head should occur.
   b. The zygomatic arches should be free from overlying structures.
   c. The entire cranium should be demonstrated without rotation or tilt.
   d. The zygomatic arches should be symmetric and without foreshortening.
   e. Exposure factors should be sufficient to penetrate the cranial base.
   f. The distance from the lateral border of the skull to the lateral border of the orbit should be equal on both sides.

375

Items 10 to 14 pertain to the *tangential projection*. Examine Fig. 11.50 as you answer the following questions.

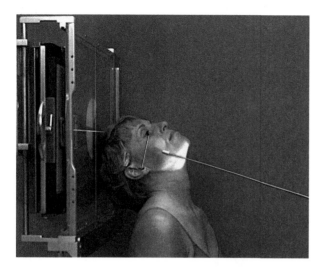

Fig. 11.50 Tangential zygomatic arch.

10. True or false. The patient should hyperextend the neck and rest the head on the vertex.

11. True or false. The midsagittal plane should be perpendicular to the IR.

12. What positioning line of the head should be as parallel as possible with the IR?

13. Describe how the central ray should be directed.

14. From the following list, circle the evaluation criterion that indicates the patient was properly positioned for a tangential projection.
    a. No rotation of the head should occur.
    b. The zygomatic arch should be free from overlying structures.
    c. The entire cranium should be demonstrated without rotation or tilt.

Items 15 to 20 pertain to the AP *axial projection, modified Towne method*. Examine Fig. 11.51 as you answer the following questions.

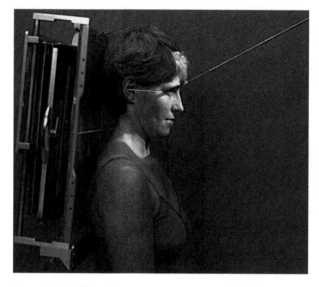

Fig. 11.51 AP axial zygomatic arches, modified Towne method.

15. Indicate how the OML and midsagittal plane should be positioned with reference to the IR—perpendicular or parallel.

    a. OML: _____

    b. Midsagittal plane: _____

16. How many degrees and in which direction should the central ray be directed when each of the following positioning lines is placed perpendicular to the plane of the IR?

    a. OML: _____

    b. IOML: _____

17. The central ray should enter 1 inch (2.5 cm) above

the landmark _____.

18. True or false. Both zygomatic arches should be demonstrated on the image with a single exposure.

19. True or false. The entire vertex should be included on the image.

20. Identify each lettered structure shown in Fig. 11.52.

A. _____

B. _____

C. _____

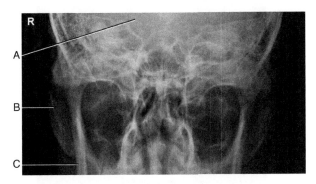

Fig. 11.52 AP axial zygomatic arches, modified Towne method.

Section 3: Exercise 3: Positioning for the Mandible

Usually three or four projections are needed to demonstrate the mandible. PA, PA axial, and axiolateral or axiolateral oblique projections are often included in the typical mandible examination. This exercise pertains to those projections. Identify structures, provide a short answer, select from a list, or choose true or false (explaining any statement you believe to be false) for each item.

Items 1 to 10 pertain to the PA *projection demonstrating the mandibular rami.* Examine Fig. 11.53 as you answer the following questions.

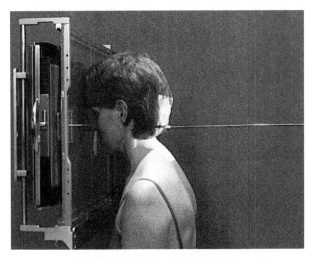

Fig. 11.53 PA mandibular rami.

1. To demonstrate the mandibular rami with the PA projection, which two facial structures should be touching the vertical grid device?
   a. Nose and chin
   b. Forehead and nose
   c. Forehead and cheek

2. Which positioning line should be perpendicular to the plane of the IR?
   a. Orbitomeatal
   b. Glabellomeatal
   c. Acanthiomeatal
   d. Infraorbitomeatal

3. How should the midsagittal plane be positioned with reference to the IR—parallel or perpendicular?

4. What breathing instructions should be given to the patient?

5. Through which positioning landmark of the face should the central ray exit?
   a. Nasion
   b. Acanthion
   c. Mental point

6. How does the vertebral column affect the image?
   a. It superimposes mandibular rami.
   b. It superimposes the central part of the mandibular body.
   c. It increases the object-to-image receptor distance (OID) of the mandible.

7. True or false. The central ray should be directed perpendicularly to the midpoint of the IR.

8. True or false. The PA projection demonstrates the mandibular body without bony superimpositioning.

9. From the following list, circle the two evaluation criteria that indicate the patient was properly positioned for the PA projection of the mandibular rami.
   a. The entire mandible should be included.
   b. The mandibular rami should be superimposed.
   c. The mandibular body and rami should be symmetric on both sides.
   d. The temporomandibular articulation should be seen lying anterior to the EAM.

10. Identify each lettered structure and fracture shown in Fig. 11.54.

    A. _____

    B. _____

    C. _____

    D. _____

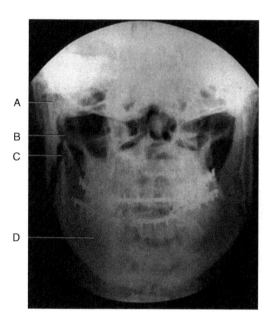

Fig. 11.54 PA mandibular rami.

Items 11 to 17 pertain to the *PA axial projection of the mandibular rami*. Examine Fig. 11.55 as you answer the following questions.

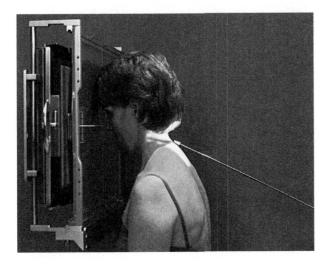

Fig. 11.55 PA axial mandibular rami.

11. Which two facial structures should be touching the vertical grid device?
    a. Nose and chin
    b. Forehead and nose
    c. Forehead and cheek

12. Which body plane and positioning line should be perpendicular to the plane of the IR?
    a. Midcoronal plane and OML
    b. Midcoronal plane and acanthiomeatal line
    c. Midsagittal plane and OML
    d. Midsagittal plane and acanthiomeatal line

13. Which breathing instructions should be given to the patient?
    a. Stop breathing.
    b. Breathe slowly.
    c. Breathe rapidly.

14. Which positioning landmark should be centered to the IR?
    a. Nasion
    b. Glabella
    c. Acanthion
    d. Mental point

15. How many degrees and in which direction should the central ray be directed?
    a. 10 to 15 degrees caudad
    b. 10 to 15 degrees cephalad
    c. 20 to 25 degrees caudad
    d. 20 to 25 degrees cephalad

16. What prevents the central part of the mandibular body from being clearly demonstrated?
    a. Superimposition with the spine
    b. Caudal angulation of the central ray
    c. Increased OID

17. From the following list, circle the three evaluation criteria that indicate the patient was properly positioned for a PA axial projection.
    a. The entire mandible should be demonstrated.
    b. The mandibular rami should be superimposed.
    c. The condylar processes should be clearly demonstrated.
    d. The mandibular body and rami should be symmetric on both sides.
    e. The temporomandibular articulation should be seen lying anterior to the EAM.

Items 18 to 31 pertain to the axiolateral and axiolateral oblique projections of the mandible (with the patient either prone or upright). Figs. 11.56 to 11.58 represent three positions that demonstrate parts of the mandible. Match each of the following positioning statements to one or more of these figures by writing the appropriate figure number in the space provided. Some statements may have more than one figure (projection) associated with them. Some statements do not relate to any of the three projections; answer "NA" for "not applicable" for these items.

_____ 18. Keep the head in a true lateral position.

_____ 19. Used for demonstrating the mandibular body

_____ 20. Used for demonstrating the mandibular ramus

_____ 21. Used for demonstrating the mental protuberance

_____ 22. Rotate the head 30 degrees toward the IR.

_____ 23. Rotate the head 45 degrees toward the IR.

_____ 24. The central ray should exit the mental protuberance.

_____ 25. The central ray should be directed 15 degrees cephalad.

_____ 26. The central ray should be directed 25 degrees.

_____ 27. The central ray should be directed perpendicular to the IR.

_____ 28. The OML should be perpendicular to the plane of the IR.

_____ 29. The interpupillary line should be perpendicular to the plane of the IR.

_____ 30. The broad surface of the ramus should be parallel with the plane of the IR.

_____ 31. The broad surface of the mandibular body should be parallel with the plane of the IR.

32. True or false. The mouth should be closed with the teeth held together.

33. True or false. The neck should be flexed to pull the chin downward.

34. True or false. The area of interest should be parallel with the IR.

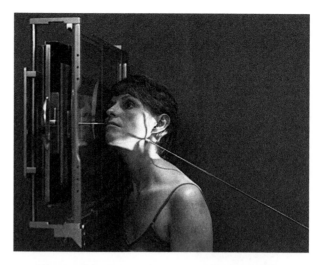

Fig. 11.56 Upright axiolateral oblique projection.

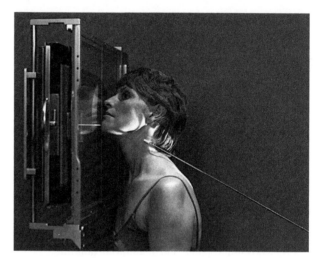

Fig. 11.57 Upright axiolateral oblique projection.

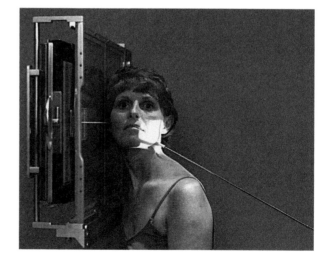

Fig. 11.58 Upright axiolateral projection.

35. Identify each lettered structure shown in Fig. 11.59.

A. _____

B. _____

C. _____

D. _____

E. _____

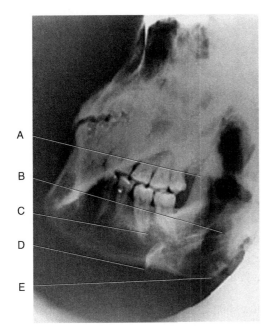

Fig. 11.59 Axiolateral oblique mandibular body.

Section 3: Exercise 4: Positioning for the Temporomandibular Joints

Two projections often performed to demonstrate TMJs are the AP axial projection and the axiolateral oblique projection. This exercise pertains to those projections. Identify structures, provide a short answer, select from a list, or choose true or false (explaining any statement you believe to be false) for each question.

Items 1 to 10 pertain to the AP *axial projection*. Examine Fig. 11.60 as you answer the following questions.

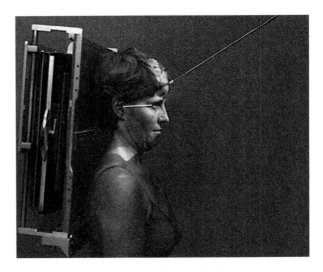

Fig. 11.60 AP axial TMJs.

1. True or false. For the AP axial projection in the closed-mouth position, the upper posterior teeth should be in contact with the lower posterior teeth.

2. True or false. The long axis of the mandibular body should be parallel with the transverse axis of the IR.

3. Why should the incisors not contact when the patient is positioned for the closed-mouth AP axial projection?

4. Identify a typical situation in which the patient should not be asked to open his or her mouth wide for an AP axial projection. Explain why.

5. Which plane and positioning line of the head should be perpendicular to the IR?
   a. Midcoronal plane and OML
   b. Midcoronal plane and IOML
   c. Midsagittal plane and OML
   d. Midsagittal plane and IOML

6. How many degrees and in which direction should the central ray be directed?
   a. 25 degrees caudad
   b. 25 degrees cephalad
   c. 35 degrees caudad
   d. 35 degrees cephalad

7. Where should the central ray enter the patient?
   a. Glabella
   b. Acanthion
   c. 3 inches (7.6 cm) above the nasion
   d. 3 inches (7.6 cm) below the nasion

8. To which landmark should the IR be centered?
   a. Nasion
   b. Glabella
   c. Central ray
   d. Mental protuberance

9. From the following list, circle the two evaluation criteria that indicate the patient was properly positioned for an AP axial projection with the mouth closed.
   a. The head should not be rotated.
   b. The condyle should be seen anterior to the EAM.
   c. Only minimal superimposition by the petrosa on the condyle should be seen.
   d. The condyle and temporomandibular articulation should be seen below the pars petrosa.

10. From the following list, circle the two evaluation criteria that indicate the patient was properly positioned for an AP axial projection with the mouth open.
    a. The head should not be rotated.
    b. The condyle should be seen anterior to the EAM.
    c. Only minimal superimposition by the petrosa on the condyle should be seen.
    d. The condyle and temporomandibular articulation should be demonstrated below the petrosa.

Items 11 to 20 pertain to *axiolateral oblique projections*. Examine Fig. 11.61 as you answer the following questions.

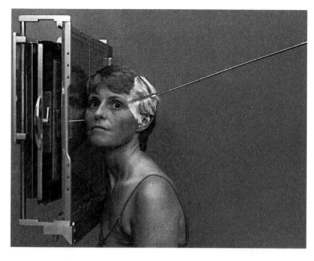

Fig. 11.61 Axiolateral oblique temporomandibular joint.

11. Where on the patient should the IR be centered?
    a. 2 inches (5 cm) inferior to the TMJs
    b. 2 inches (5 cm) superior to the TMJs
    c. ½ inch (1.2 cm) anterior to the EAM
    d. ½ inch (1.2 cm) posterior to the EAM

12. How should the midsagittal plane be positioned with reference to the IR?
    a. Parallel
    b. Perpendicular
    c. Form an angle of 15 degrees
    d. Form an angle of 37 degrees

13. Which positioning line of the head should be parallel with the transverse axis of the IR?
    a. Orbitomeatal
    b. Interpupillary
    c. Acanthiomeatal
    d. Infraorbitomeatal

14. How many degrees and in what direction should the central ray be directed?

15. Through what structure should the central ray exit the patient?

16. In relation to surrounding structures, where in the image should the mandibular condyle be seen for axiolateral oblique projections with the patient holding the mouth closed?

17. True or false. The central ray should enter the patient at the TMJ farther from the IR.

18. True or false. Both open-mouth and closed-mouth positions should be performed with the axiolateral oblique projection unless contraindicated.

19. True or false. The entire side of the mandible from the condyle to the symphysis should be demonstrated.

20. Identify each lettered structure shown in Fig. 11.62.

A. _____

B. _____

C. _____

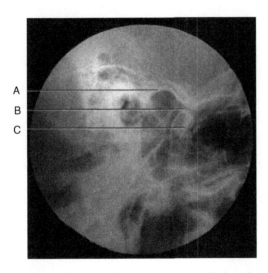

Fig. 11.62 Axiolateral oblique temporomandibular joint with the patient's mouth open.

Section 3: Exercise 5: Evaluating Radiographic Images of Facial Bones

This exercise consists of facial bone images to give you practice evaluating facial bone positioning. These images are not from Merrill's Atlas. Most images show at least one positioning error. Examine each image and answer the questions that follow by providing a short answer.

1. Fig. 11.63 shows a lateral projection image of the facial bones with incorrect positioning of a phantom skull. Examine the image and state why it does not meet the evaluation criteria for this type of projection.

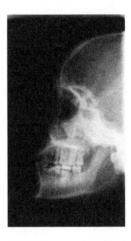

Fig. 11.63 Lateral facial bones showing incorrect positioning of a phantom skull.

2. Figs. 11.64 through 11.66 show parietoacanthial projection images of the facial bones of a phantom skull. Only one image demonstrates acceptable positioning. Examine the images and answer the questions that follow.

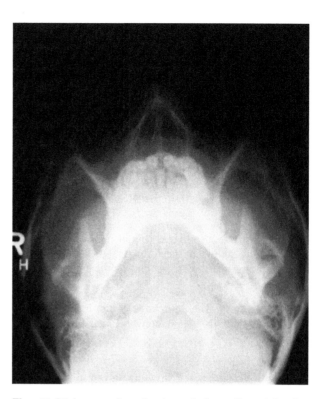

Fig. 11.65 Image of a phantom skull positioned for the parietoacanthial projection.

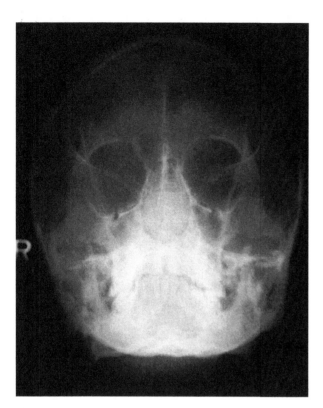

Fig. 11.64 Image of a phantom skull positioned for the parietoacanthial projection.

a. Which image demonstrates acceptable positioning?

b. In which image does the phantom skull appear to be incorrectly positioned because the angle between the OML and the IR is greater than the required amount? (This error results when the patient is unable to extend the neck far enough.)

c. In which image does the phantom skull appear to be incorrectly positioned because the angle between the OML and the IR is less than the required amount? (This error results when the patient extends the neck too much.)

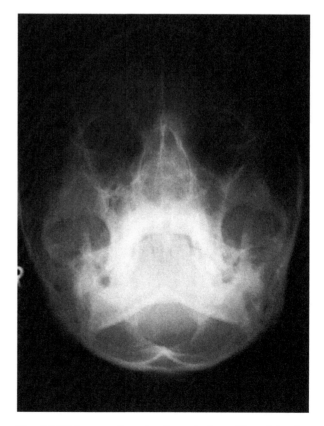

Fig. 11.66 Image of a phantom skull positioned for the parietoacanthial projection.

3. Fig. 11.67 shows an SMV projection image of the zygomatic arches with incorrect positioning of a phantom skull. Examine the image and answer the questions that follow.

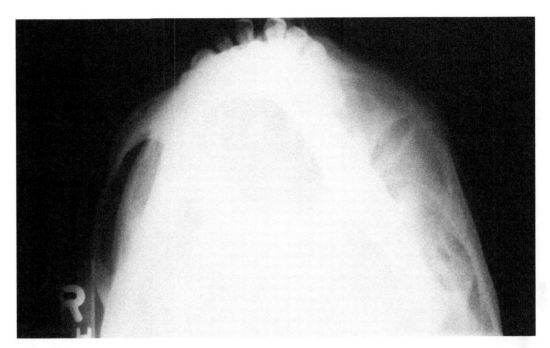

Fig. 11.67 Submentovertical projection of a phantom skull for zygomatic arches.

a. What image characteristics prevent the image from meeting all evaluation criteria for this projection?

b. What positioning error most likely resulted in this unacceptable image?

4. Fig. 11.68 shows a PA projection image demonstrating the mandibular rami with incorrect positioning of a phantom skull. Examine the image and answer the questions that follow.

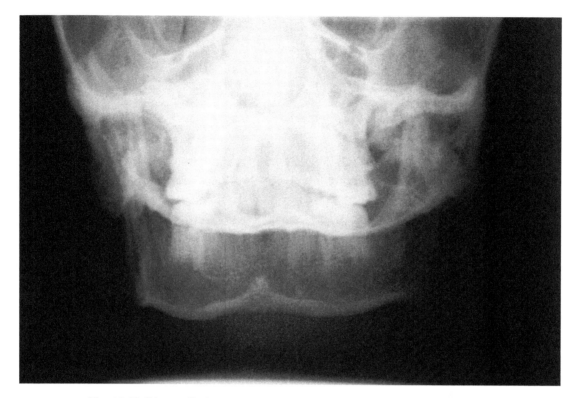

Fig. 11.68 PA mandibular rami showing incorrect positioning of a phantom skull.

a. What image characteristic prevents this image from being of acceptable quality?

b. To comply with the evaluation criteria for this projection, how should the position of the phantom skull be adjusted for a subsequent image?

5. Fig. 11.69 shows an axiolateral oblique projection image of the mandibular body with incorrect positioning of a phantom skull. Examine the image and answer the questions that follow.

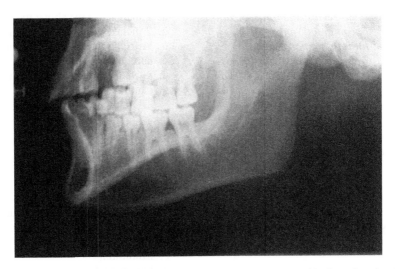

Fig. 11.69 Axiolateral oblique mandibular body showing incorrect positioning of a phantom skull.

a. What image characteristic prevents the image from meeting all evaluation criteria for this type of projection?

b. How should the position of the phantom skull be adjusted for a subsequent image?

387

RADIOGRAPHY OF THE PARANASAL SINUSES

Section 4: Exercise 1

Usually three or four of the following projections comprise the typical paranasal sinus series: lateral, PA axial (Caldwell method), parietoacanthial (Waters method), and SMV. This exercise pertains to the paranasal sinuses and the projections used to demonstrate them. Identify structures, provide a short answer, select from a list, or choose true or false (explaining any statement you believe to be false) for each item.

1. In which body position should the patient be placed for images of the paranasal sinuses?
   a. Prone
   b. Supine
   c. Upright

2. Give two reasons why the patient should be positioned as indicated in question 1.

3. Why should the radiographer ensure that the exposure factors used do not cause the paranasal sinuses to appear underpenetrated?

Items 4 to 10 pertain to the *lateral projection*. Examine Fig. 11.70 as you answer the following questions.

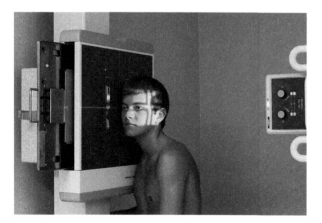

Fig. 11.70 Lateral sinuses.

4. State how the midsagittal plane and the interpupillary line should be placed with reference to the plane of the IR (perpendicular or parallel).

   a. Midsagittal plane: _____

   b. Interpupillary line: _____

5. Where on the patient's head should the central ray be directed?
   a. 2 inches (5 cm) above the EAM
   b. 2 inches (5 cm) below the EAM
   c. ½ to 1 inch (1.2 to 2.5 cm) anterior to the outer canthus
   d. ½ to 1 inch (1.2 to 2.5 cm) posterior to the outer canthus

6. How should the central ray be directed relative to the patient's head?
   a. Perpendicular
   b. 15 degrees caudad
   c. 15 degrees cephalad

7. Which sinus group is of primary importance?
   a. Frontal
   b. Maxillary
   c. Ethmoidal
   d. Sphenoidal

8. How many sinus groups should be clearly demonstrated with the lateral projection image?
   a. One
   b. Two
   c. Three
   d. Four

9. From the following list, circle the six evaluation criteria that indicate the patient was properly positioned for a lateral projection.
   a. The sella turcica should not be rotated.
   b. The sinuses should be visualized clearly.
   c. The orbital roofs should be superimposed.
   d. All four sinus groups should be included.
   e. The mandibular rami should be superimposed.
   f. Close beam restriction of the sinus area is needed.
   g. The petrous ridges should be lying in the lower third of the orbits.
   h. The anterior frontal bone should be superimposed by the mental protuberance.
   i. The petrous ridges should be lying just below the floor of the maxillary sinuses.
   j. The distance between the lateral border of the skull and the lateral border of the orbits should be equal.
   k. The distance from the lateral border of the skull to the mandibular condyles should be equal on both sides

388

10. Identify each lettered structure shown in Fig. 11.71.

A. _____   D. _____

B. _____   E. _____

C. _____   F. _____

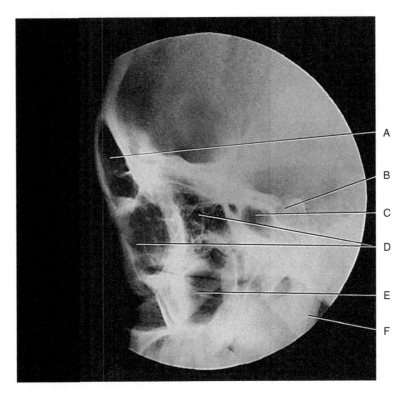

Fig. 11.71 Lateral sinuses.

Items 11 to 18 pertain to the PA *axial projection, Caldwell method.* Examine Fig. 11.72 as you answer the following questions.

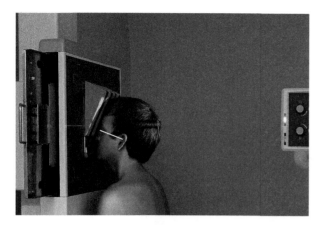

Fig. 11.72 PA axial sinuses, Caldwell method, vertical IR method.

11. Which two practices can be used for performing PA axial projection, Caldwell method for sinuses? (select two)
    a. CR 15 degrees caudad, IR vertical, OML perpendicular to IR
    b. CR horizontal, IR angled 15 degrees, OML perpendicular to IR
    c. CR horizontal, IR vertical, OML 15 degrees to CR
    d. CR 15 degrees cephalad, IR vertical, OML perpendicular to IR

12. Regardless of which technique is used for performing the PA axial projection, Caldwell method, which of the following procedures is common for both techniques?
    a. Directing the central ray caudally
    b. Using a vertically placed IR
    c. Using a horizontally directed central ray
    d. Centering the acanthion to the IR

13. How should the patient's head be positioned when the IR is *not* vertical?
    a. With the OML parallel with the central ray
    b. With the IOML parallel with the central ray
    c. With the OML perpendicular to the IR
    d. With the IOML perpendicular to the IR

14. To which positioning landmark of the skull should the IR be centered?
    a. Nasion
    b. Glabella
    c. Acanthion

15. Which sinus structures are primarily demonstrated?
    a. Frontal sinuses and anterior ethmoidal air cells
    b. Frontal sinuses and posterior ethmoidal air cells
    c. Maxillary sinuses and anterior ethmoidal air cells
    d. Maxillary sinuses and posterior ethmoidal air cells

16. Where should the petrous ridges be demonstrated in the image?
    a. Completely filling the orbits
    b. In the lower third of the orbits
    c. Just below the floor of the maxillary sinuses

17. From the following list, circle the eight evaluation criteria that indicate the patient was properly positioned for a PA axial projection, Caldwell method.
    a. The orbital roofs should be superimposed.
    b. The mandibular rami should be superimposed.
    c. The air-fluid levels, if present, are clearly visible.
    d. Close beam restriction of the sinus area is needed.
    e. The petrous ridges should be symmetric on both sides.
    f. All four sinus groups should be clearly demonstrated.
    g. The petrous ridges should lie in the lower one third of the orbits.
    h. The frontal and anterior ethmoidal sinuses should be visualized clearly.
    i. The anterior frontal bone should be superimposed by the mental protuberance.
    j. The petrous ridges should be lying just below the floor of the maxillary sinuses.
    k. The frontal sinuses should lie above the frontonasal suture and be clearly demonstrated.
    l. The anterior ethmoidal air cells above the petrous ridges should be clearly demonstrated.
    m. The distance between the lateral border of the skull and the lateral border of the orbits should be equal.

18. Identify each lettered structure shown in Fig. 11.73.

A. _____

B. _____

C. _____

D. _____

E. _____

F. _____

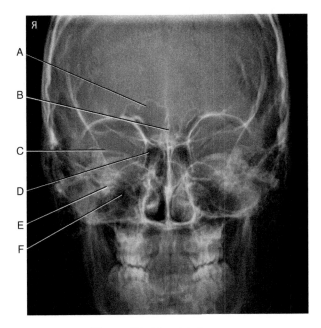

Fig. 11.73 PA axial sinuses.

Items 19 to 30 pertain to the *parietoacanthial projection, Waters method*. Examine Fig. 11.74 as you answer the following questions.

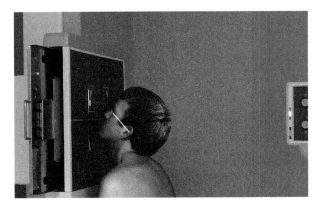

Fig. 11.74 Parietoacanthial sinuses, Waters method.

19. Which paranasal sinuses are best demonstrated with the parietoacanthial projection, Waters method?

20. Where will the petrous ridges probably be demonstrated in the image if the patient does not extend the neck sufficiently?

21. How will the maxillary sinuses appear in the image (elongated or foreshortened) if the patient extends the neck too much?

22. What positioning line of the head should form an angle of 37 degrees with the plane of the IR?

23. What positioning line of the head should be approximately perpendicular to the plane of the IR?

24. To what facial landmark should the IR be centered?

25. With reference to the surrounding structures, where should petrous ridges be demonstrated in the image?

26. Where on the image should the rotundum foramina be demonstrated?

27. True or false. The patient's nose and forehead should touch the vertical grid device.

28. True or false. The midsagittal plane should be perpendicular to the IR.

29. From the following list, circle the five evaluation criteria that indicate the patient was properly positioned for a parietoacanthial projection, Waters method.
    a. The orbital roofs should be superimposed.
    b. The mandibular rami should be superimposed.
    c. The maxillary sinuses should be visualized clearly.
    d. The petrous ridges should completely fill the orbits.
    e. Close beam restriction of the sinus area is needed.
    f. The petrous ridges should be lying in the lower third of the orbits.
    g. The orbits and maxillary sinuses should be symmetric on both sides.
    h. The sphenoidal sinuses should be seen projected through the open mouth.
    i. The anterior frontal bone should be superimposed by the mental protuberance.
    j. The petrous pyramids should lie immediately inferior to the floor of the maxillary sinuses.
    k. The distance from the lateral border of the skull to the lateral border of the orbit should be equal on both sides.

30. Identify each lettered structure shown in Fig. 11.75.

A. _____

B. _____

C. _____

D. _____

E. _____

F. _____

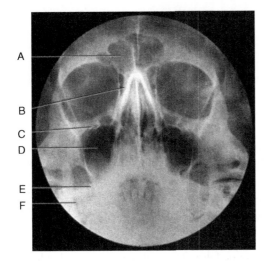

Fig. 11.75 Parietoacanthial sinuses, Waters method.

Items 31 to 35 pertain to the *parietoacanthial projection, open-mouth Waters method*. Examine Fig. 11.76 as you answer the following questions.

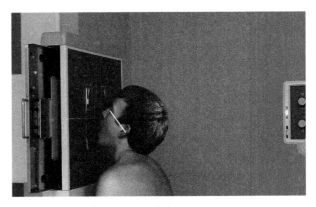

Fig. 11.76 Parietoacanthial sinuses, open-mouth Waters method.

31. To which landmark should the IR be centered?

32. What part of the patient's head should be resting on the vertical grid device?

33. What positioning line of the skull should form an angle of 37 degrees with the plane of the IR?

34. Which of the sinuses should be demonstrated in the image through the patient's open mouth?

35. From the following list, circle the six evaluation criteria that indicate the patient was properly positioned for a parietoacanthial projection, open-mouth Waters method.
   a. The orbital roofs should be superimposed.
   b. The mandibular rami should be superimposed.
   c. The maxillary sinuses should be visualized clearly.
   d. The petrous ridges should completely fill the orbits.
   e. Close beam restriction of the sinus area is needed.
   f. The petrous ridges should be lying in the lower third of the orbits.
   g. The orbits and maxillary sinuses should be symmetric on both sides.
   h. The sphenoidal sinuses should be seen projected through the open mouth.
   i. The anterior frontal bone should be superimposed by the mental protuberance.
   j. The petrous pyramids should lie immediately inferior to the floor of the maxillary sinuses.
   k. The distance from the lateral border of the skull to the lateral border of the orbit should be equal on both sides.

Items 36 to 48 pertain to the *SMV projection*. Examine Fig. 11.77 as you answer the following questions.

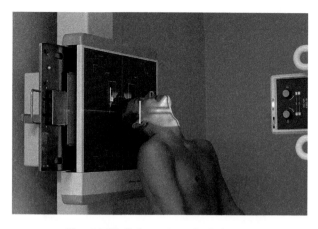

Fig. 11.77 Submentovertical sinuses

36. True or false. The patient should rest his or her head with the chin contacting the vertical grid device.

37. True or false. The OML should be as close to parallel with the IR as possible.

38. True or false. The midsagittal plane should be perpendicular to the IR.

39. True or false. The central ray should be directed perpendicular to the IOML, entering the midline of the base of the skull so that it passes through the sella turcica.

40. True or false. The distance from the lateral border of the skull to the lateral border of the mandibular condyles should be the same on both sides.

41. True or false. The entire occipital bone should be included in the image of the SMV projection to demonstrate paranasal sinuses.

42. What two sinus groups should be well demonstrated with the SMV projection?

43. Where in the image should the mental protuberance appear in relation to the frontal bone?

44. Where in the image should the mandibular condyles appear in relation to the surrounding structures?

45. What positioning error is most likely to occur if the mental protuberance is imaged posterior to, and separated from, the anterior frontal bone?

46. What positioning error most likely occurred if the mental protuberance is imaged superior to the anterior frontal bone?

47. From the following list, circle the three evaluation criteria that indicate the patient was properly positioned for an SMV projection.
    a. The orbital roofs should be superimposed.
    b. The mandibular rami should be superimposed.
    c. The maxillary sinuses should be visualized clearly.
    d. The mental protuberance should superimpose the anterior frontal bone.
    e. The mandibular condyles should be anterior to the petrous pyramids.
    f. The distance from the lateral border of the skull to the mandibular condyles should be equal on both sides.

48. Identify each lettered structure shown in Fig. 11.78.

A. _____

B. _____

C. _____

D. _____

E. _____

F. _____

G. _____

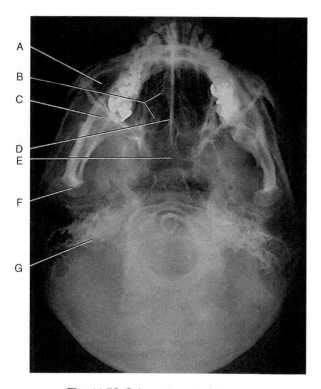

Fig. 11.78 Submentovertical sinuses.

Section 4: Exercise 2: Evaluating Images of the Paranasal Sinuses

This exercise presents sinus images to provide practice evaluating sinus positioning. These images are not from Merrill's Atlas. Each image shows at least one positioning error. Examine each image and answer the questions that follow by providing a short answer.

Examine Fig. 11.79 and answer the questions that follow.

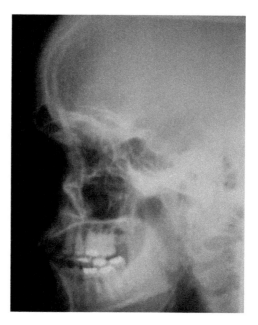

Fig. 11.79 Lateral sinus image with error.

1. State why this image does not meet the evaluation criteria for this projection.

2. List the specific radiographic baselines that were mispositioned in Fig. 11.79.

Examine Fig. 11.80 and answer the questions that follow.

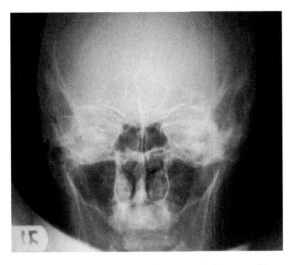

Fig. 11.80 PA axial (Caldwell) image of sinuses with error.

Examine Fig. 11.81 and answer the questions that follow.

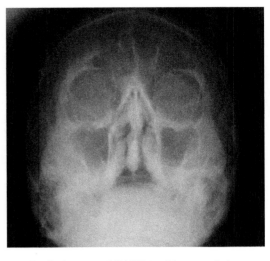

Fig. 11.81 Parietoacanthial (Waters) image of sinuses with error.

3. Which paranasal sinuses are not well demonstrated in Fig. 11.80? Explain why.

5. What primary positioning error is demonstrated in Fig. 11.81?

4. If you were to repeat Fig. 11.80 using a vertical IR, how would you correct the positioning error?

6. What positioning maneuver would be needed to correct the above-mentioned error?

Examine Fig. 11.82 and answer the questions that follow.

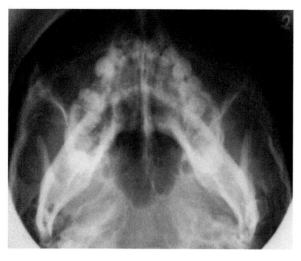

Fig. 11.82 Submentovertical image of sinuses with error.

7. What error is evident in Fig. 11.82?

8. Which paranasal sinuses are not well demonstrated in Fig. 11.82?

CHAPTER 11: SELF-TEST: OSTEOLOGY OF THE CRANIUM AND RADIOGRAPHY OF THE SKULL, FACIAL BONES, AND PARANASAL SINUSES

Answer the following questions by selecting the best choice.

1. Which positioning line extends from the EAM to the outer canthus?
   a. Orbitomeatal
   b. Glabellomeatal
   c. Acanthiomeatal
   d. Infraorbitomeatal

2. Which positioning landmark is located at the base of the nasal spine?
   a. Nasion
   b. Gonion
   c. Glabella
   d. Acanthion

3. Which positioning landmark is located at the superiormost point of the nasal bones?
   a. Nasion
   b. Canthus
   c. Glabella
   d. Acanthion

4. Which positioning landmark is the smooth elevation that is located between the superciliary arches?
   a. Nasion
   b. Glabella
   c. Acanthion
   d. Mental point

5. Which positioning landmark is most superior?
   a. Nasion
   b. Gonion
   c. Glabella
   d. Acanthion

6. Where on the skull is the gonion located?
   a. Between the orbits
   A. On the anterior frontal bone
   b. On the posterior occipital bone
   c. On the lateroposterior part of the mandible

7. Where on the skull is the outer canthus located?
   a. Between the orbits
   b. At the mandibular angle
   c. Along each parietal eminence
   d. On the lateral border of each orbit

8. Which positioning landmark is located at the anterior portion of the mandible?
   a. Nasion
   b. Gonion
   c. Acanthion
   d. Mental point

9. Which suture articulates the frontal bone with both parietal bones?
   a. Sagittal
   b. Coronal
   c. Squamosal
   d. Lambdoidal

10. Which suture joins both parietal bones at the vertex of the skull?
    a. Sagittal
    b. Coronal
    c. Squamosal
    d. Lambdoidal

11. Which suture joins a parietal bone with both a sphenoid bone and a temporal bone?
    a. Sagittal
    b. Coronal
    c. Squamosal
    d. Lambdoidal

12. Which suture joins both parietal bones with the occipital bone?
    a. Sagittal
    b. Coronal
    c. Squamosal
    d. Lambdoidal

13. The bregma fontanelle is located at the junction of which two sutures?
    a. Coronal and sagittal
    b. Coronal and squamosal
    c. Lambdoidal and sagittal
    d. Lambdoidal and squamosal

14. The lambda fontanelle is located at the junction of which two sutures?
    a. Coronal and sagittal
    b. Coronal and squamosal
    c. Lambdoidal and sagittal
    d. Lambdoidal and squamosal

15. The bregma fontanelle is located at the junction of which cranial bones?
    a. Frontal and both parietals
    b. Occipital and both parietals
    c. Frontal and sphenoid
    d. Occipital and sphenoid

16. The lambda fontanelle is located at the junction of which cranial bones?
    a. Frontal and both parietals
    b. Occipital and both parietals
    c. Frontal and temporal
    d. Occipital and temporal

17. Which skull classification refers to a typical skull (in terms of width and length)?
    a. Mesocephalic
    b. Brachycephalic
    c. Dolichocephalic

18. Which skull classification refers to a long, narrow skull?
    a. Mesocephalic
    b. Brachycephalic
    c. Dolichocephalic

19. Which skull classification refers to a short, wide skull?
    a. Mesocephalic
    b. Brachycephalic
    c. Dolichocephalic

20. How many degrees are in the angle formed between the midsagittal plane and the petrous pyramids in the mesocephalic skull?
    a. 36 degrees
    b. 40 degrees
    c. 47 degrees
    d. 54 degrees

21. How many degrees are in the angle formed between the midsagittal plane and the petrous pyramids in the brachycephalic skull?
    a. 36 degrees
    b. 40 degrees
    c. 47 degrees
    d. 54 degrees

22. How many degrees are in the angle formed between the midsagittal plane and the petrous pyramids in the dolichocephalic skull?
    a. 36 degrees
    b. 40 degrees
    c. 47 degrees
    d. 54 degrees

23. On which cranial bone are the superciliary arches located?
    a. Frontal
    b. Parietal
    c. Ethmoid
    d. Occipital

24. On which cranial bone is the cribriform plate located?
    a. Frontal
    b. Ethmoid
    c. Temporal
    d. Sphenoid

25. On which cranial bone is the crista galli located?
    a. Ethmoid
    b. Occipital
    c. Temporal
    d. Sphenoid

26. Which cranial bone has a petrous pyramid?
    a. Parietal
    b. Ethmoid
    c. Temporal
    d. Sphenoid

27. On which cranial bone is the sella turcica located?
    a. Frontal
    b. Ethmoid
    c. Temporal
    d. Sphenoid

28. Which cranial bone has the mastoid process?
    a. Parietal
    b. Ethmoid
    c. Temporal
    d. Sphenoid

29. On which cranial bone is the perpendicular plate located?
    a. Parietal
    b. Ethmoid
    c. Temporal
    d. Sphenoid

30. Which cranial bone has both greater and lesser wings?
    a. Ethmoid
    b. Occipital
    c. Temporal
    d. Sphenoid

400

31. With which cranial bone does the first cervical vertebra articulate?
    a. Ethmoid
    b. Occipital
    c. Temporal
    d. Sphenoid

32. The pterygoid processes project inferiorly from
which cranial bone?
    a. Frontal
    b. Ethmoid
    c. Temporal
    d. Sphenoid

33. The foramen magnum is a part of which cranial
bone?
    a. Frontal
    b. Occipital
    c. Temporal
    d. Sphenoid

34. From which cranial bone does the zygomatic process
arise?
    a. Frontal
    b. Parietal
    c. Temporal
    d. Sphenoid

35. The EAM is a part of which cranial bone?
    a. Frontal
    b. Parietal
    c. Temporal
    d. Sphenoid

36. The temporal process projects posteriorly from
which facial bone?
    a. Vomer
    b. Maxilla
    c. Zygomatic
    d. Temporal

37. Which bones compose the bridge of the nose?
    a. Nasal
    b. Lacrimal
    c. Palatine
    d. Maxillae

38. With which bone does the mandible articulate?
    a. Hyoid
    b. Maxilla
    c. Zygoma
    d. Temporal

39. Where are the lacrimal bones located?
    a. Inside the nasal cavity
    b. On the lateral wall of each orbit
    c. On the medial wall of each orbit
    d. Inferior to the maxillary sinuses

40. Where is the vomer bone found?
    a. Posterior to the nasal bones
    b. On the floor of the nasal cavity
    c. On the lateral wall of the orbits
    d. In the posterior one fourth of the roof of the
       mouth

41. Which bone comprises most of the lateral wall of the
orbital cavities?
    a. Maxilla
    b. Lacrimal
    c. Palatine
    d. Zygomatic

42. Which term refers to the anterior process of the mandibular ramus?
    a. Cornu
    b. Condyle
    c. Coracoid
    d. Coronoid

43. Which term refers to the posterior process of the
mandibular ramus?
    a. Cornu
    b. Condyle
    c. Coracoid
    d. Coronoid

44. Which facial bones have alveolar processes?
    a. Vomer and mandible
    b. Vomer and zygomatic
    c. Maxillae and mandible
    d. Maxillae and zygomatic

45. Which bones form the posterior one fourth of the
roof of the mouth?
    a. Maxillae
    b. Palatine
    c. Zygomatic
    d. Inferior nasal conchae

46. Which positioning landmark is located on the maxillae?
    a. Gonion
    b. Nasion
    c. Acanthi
    d. Mental point

47. Which two positioning lines or planes should be
perpendicular to the IR for the PA projection of the
skull?
    a. OML and midsagittal plane
    b. OML and interpupillary line
    c. IOML and midsagittal plane
    d. IOML and interpupillary line

401

48. With reference to the patient, where should the IR be centered for the PA projection of the skull?
    a. Nasion
    b. Glabella
    c. Acanthion
    d. Mental point

49. With reference to the patient, where should the IR be centered for the lateral projection of the skull?
    a. Nasion
    b. EAM
    c. 2 inches (5 cm) above the EAM
    d. 2 inches (5 cm) below the EAM

50. With reference to the IR, how should the interpupillary line and the midsagittal plane be positioned for the lateral projection of the skull?
    a. Interpupillary line: parallel; midsagittal plane: parallel
    b. Interpupillary line: parallel; midsagittal plane: perpendicular
    c. Interpupillary line: perpendicular; midsagittal plane: parallel
    d. Interpupillary line: perpendicular; midsagittal plane: perpendicular

51. For the AP axial projection, Towne method, of the skull, how many degrees and in which direction should the central ray be directed when the OML is perpendicular to the IR?
    a. 30 degrees caudad
    b. 30 degrees cephalad
    c. 37 degrees caudad
    d. 37 degrees cephalad

52. For the AP axial projection, Towne method, of the skull, how many degrees and in which direction should the central ray be directed when the IOML is perpendicular to the IR?
    a. 30 degrees caudad
    b. 30 degrees cephalad
    c. 37 degrees caudad
    d. 37 degrees cephalad

53. Which positioning line should be parallel with the IR for the SMV projection of the skull?
    a. OML
    b. Glabellomeatal line
    c. Acanthiomeatal line
    d. IOML

54. Which projection of the skull can be correctly performed with the central ray angled 37 degrees?
    a. AP axial, Towne method
    b. PA axial, Haas method
    c. PA axial, Caldwell method
    d. SMV, Schüller method

55. Which projection of the skull can be correctly performed with the central ray angled 15 degree
    a. SMV
    b. AP axial, Towne method
    c. PA axial, Haas method
    d. PA axial, Caldwell method

56. Which projection of the skull produces a full basal image of the cranium?
    a. Lateral
    b. AP axial, Towne method
    c. PA with perpendicular central ray
    d. SMV, Schüller method

57. Which projection of the skull projects the petrous bones in the lower third of the orbits?
    a. PA axial, Haas method
    b. AP axial, Towne method
    c. PA axial, Caldwell method
    d. PA with perpendicular central ray

58. Which projection of the skull should be obtained when the frontal bone is of primary interest?
    a. PA axial, Haas method
    b. AP axial, Towne method
    c. PA axial, Caldwell method
    d. PA with perpendicular central ray

59. Which evaluation criterion pertains to the AP axial projection, Towne method, of the skull?
    a. The orbital roofs should be superimposed.
    b. The mental protuberance should superimpose the anterior frontal bone.
    c. Part of the sella turcica should be seen within the foramen magnum.
    d. The distance from the lateral border of the skull to the lateral margins of foramen magnum should be the same on both sides.

60. Which evaluation criterion pertains to the PA projection of the skull?
    a. The orbital roofs should be superimposed.
    b. The mental protuberance should superimpose the anterior frontal bone.
    c. Part of the sella turcica should be seen within the foramen magnum.
    d. The distance from the lateral border of the skull to the lateral border of the orbit should be the same on both sides.

61. Which evaluation criterion pertains to the lateral projection of the skull?
   a. The orbital roofs should be superimposed.
   b. The mental protuberance should superimpose the anterior frontal bone.
   c. Part of the sella turcica should be seen within the foramen magnum.
   d. The distance from the lateral border of the skull to the lateral border of the orbit should be the same on both sides.

62. Which evaluation criterion pertains to the SMV projection of the skull?
   a. The orbital roofs should be superimposed.
   b. The mental protuberance should superimpose the anterior frontal bone.
   c. Part of the sella turcica should be seen within the foramen magnum.
   d. The distance from the lateral border of the skull to the lateral border of the orbit should be the same on both sides.

63. For the PA axial projection, Haas method, of the skull, where should the central ray enter the patient's head?
   a. Nasion
   b. Acanthion
   c. 1½ inches (3.8 cm) above the external occipital protuberance
   d. 1½ inches (3.8 cm) below the external occipital protuberance

64. How many degrees and in which direction should the central ray be directed for the PA axial projection, Haas method, of the skull?
   a. 15 degrees caudad
   b. 15 degrees cephalad
   c. 25 degrees caudad
   d. 25 degrees cephalad

65. Which evaluation criterion pertains to the PA axial, Haas method, of the skull?
   a. The orbital roofs should be superimposed.
   b. The petrous ridges should be demonstrated in the lower third of the orbits.
   c. The dorsum sella and posterior clinoids should be projected within the foramen magnum.
   d. The mental protuberance should superimpose the anterior frontal bone.

66. With reference to the patient, where should the central ray be directed for the lateral projection of the facial bones?
   a. Zygomatic bone
   b. Nasal bones
   c. Outer canthus
   d. ¾ inch (1.9 cm) anterior and ¾ inch (1.9 cm) superior to the EAM

67. With reference to the IR, how should the central ray be directed for the parietoacanthial projection, Waters method?
   a. Perpendicular
   b. 15 degrees caudad
   c. 23 degrees caudad
   d. 37 degrees caudad

68. Where should the petrous ridges be seen in the image of the parietoacanthial projection of the facial bones?
   a. Superior to the orbits
   b. Lower third of the orbits
   c. Through the maxillary sinuses
   d. Below the maxillary sinuses

69. Which positioning line and angle indicate correct positioning of the head for the parietoacanthial projection, Waters method?
   a. OML; 37 degrees to the IR
   b. OML; perpendicular to the IR
   c. IOML; 37 degrees to the IR
   d. IOML; perpendicular to the IR

70. Which evaluation criterion pertains to the parietoacanthial projection, Waters method?
   a. The orbital roofs should be superimposed.
   b. The petrous ridges should be projected within the orbits.
   c. The zygomatic arches should be free from overlying structures.
   d. The petrous ridges should be projected immediately below the maxillary sinuses.

71. Which evaluation criterion pertains to the PA axial projection, Caldwell method?
   a. The orbital roofs should be superimposed.
   b. The zygomatic arches should be superimposed.
   c. The petrous pyramids should be projected within the orbits.
   d. The distance between the lateral border of the skull and orbit should be the same on both sides.

72. Which evaluation criterion pertains to the lateral projection of the facial bones?
   a. The orbital roofs should be superimposed.
   b. The petrous ridges should be projected within the orbits.
   c. The zygomatic arches should be free from overlying structures.
   d. The petrous ridges should be projected immediately below the maxillary sinuses.

73. Which evaluation criterion pertains to the SMV projection for bilateral zygomatic arches?
    a. The orbital roofs should be superimposed.
    b. The zygomatic arches should be superimposed.
    c. The petrous ridges should be projected within the orbits.
    d. The zygomatic arches should be free from overlying structures.

74. An AP axial projection (modified Towne method) of the bilateral zygomatic arches produces an image similar to the AP axial projection (Towne method) of the skull. How many degrees and in what direction should the central ray be directed for this projection to demonstrate zygomatic arches when the OML is perpendicular to the IR?
    a. 30 degrees caudad
    b. 37 degrees caudad
    c. 30 degrees cephalad
    d. 37 degrees cephalad

75. An AP axial projection (modified Towne method) of the bilateral zygomatic arches is performed similarly to the AP axial projection (Towne method) of the skull except that the projection for the zygomatic arches requires that which of the following be done?
    a. The central ray should be directed cephalically.
    b. The central ray should be directed to the glabella.
    c. The OML forms an angle of 37 degrees with the IR.
    d. The midsagittal plane forms an angle of 45 degrees with the IR.

76. With reference to the IR, how should the midsagittal plane be adjusted for the tangential projection demonstrating an individual zygomatic arch?
    a. Parallel with the IR
    b. 15 degrees from perpendicular
    c. 37 degrees to the IR
    d. 53 degrees to the IR

77. To demonstrate the mandibular body with the axiolateral oblique projection, how should the patient's head be positioned?
    a. Keep the head in a true lateral position.
    b. From true lateral, rotate the head 15 degrees toward the IR.
    c. From true lateral, rotate the head 30 degrees toward the IR.
    d. From true lateral, rotate the head 45 degrees toward the IR.

78. How many degrees and in which direction should the central ray be directed for the axiolateral projection of the mandible?
    a. 15 degrees caudad
    b. 15 degrees cephalad
    c. 25 degrees caudad
    d. 25 degrees cephalad

79. Which projection is performed with the patient's head positioned true lateral and the central ray directed 25 degrees cephalad?
    a. Axiolateral oblique projection of the TMJs
    b. Axiolateral projection of the mandible
    c. Parietoacanthial projection of the facial bones
    d. Tangential projection of the bilateral zygomatic arches

80. Which evaluation criterion pertains to the axiolateral oblique projection of the mandible?
    a. The mandibular rami should be superimposed.
    b. The opposite side of the mandible should not overlap the ramus.
    c. The mandibular condyles should be anterior to the petrous ridges.
    d. The mental protuberance should superimpose anterior frontal bone.

81. Which structure is of primary interest when the patient's head is rotated 15 degrees toward the IR from a true lateral position and the central ray is directed 15 degrees caudad, entering about 1½ inches (3.8 cm) superior to the upside EAM?
    a. Orbit
    b. Mandible
    c. Zygomatic arch
    d. TMJ

82. Which of the following structures can be well demonstrated with an axiolateral oblique projection?
    a. Facial bones
    b. Zygomatic arches
    c. Maxillary sinuses
    d. TMJs

83. How many degrees and in which direction should the central ray be directed for the axiolateral oblique projection for TMJs?
    a. 15 degrees caudad
    b. 15 degrees cephalad
    c. 25 degrees caudad
    d. 25 degrees cephalad

84. For the AP axial projection of the TMJs, where should the central ray be directed?
    a. Nasion
    b. Glabella
    c. Acanthion
    d. 3 inches (7.6 cm) above the nasion

85. With reference to the patient, where should the IR be centered for the axiolateral oblique projection of the TMJs?
    a. To the glabella
    b. ½ inch (1.2 cm) anterior to the EAM closest to IR
    c. 1 inch (2.5 cm) posterior to the EAM closest to IR
    d. 2 inches (5 cm) above the EAM closest to IR

404

86. Which structures should always be imaged with the patient in an upright position?
    a. Orbits
    b. Mastoids
    c. Zygomatic arches
    d. Paranasal sinuses

87. Which of the following is the only projection for paranasal sinuses that adequately demonstrates all four sinus groups?
    a. Lateral
    b. SMV
    c. PA axial, Caldwell method
    d. Parietoacanthial, Waters method

88. With reference to the outer canthus, where should the central ray be directed for the lateral projections of the sinus?
    a. Inferior
    b. Superior
    c. Anterior
    d. Posterior

89. Which sinus group is of primary importance in the lateral projection of the sinuses?
    a. Frontal
    b. Maxillary
    c. Ethmoidal
    d. Sphenoidal

90. Which sinus groups are best demonstrated with the PA axial projection, Caldwell method?
    a. Frontal and sphenoidal
    b. Frontal and anterior ethmoidal
    c. Maxillary and sphenoidal
    d. Maxillary and anterior ethmoidal

91. For the PA axial projection, Caldwell method, of the sinuses, which positioning line, in addition to the midsagittal plane, should be perpendicular to the IR?
    a. Orbitomeatal
    b. Interpupillary
    c. Glabellomeatal
    d. Infraorbitomeatal

92. Where should petrous ridges be seen in the image of the PA axial projection, Caldwell method, of the sinuses?
    a. Superior to the orbits
    b. Lower third of the orbits
    c. Through the maxillary sinuses
    d. Below the maxillary sinuses

93. Which positioning line should form an angle of 37 degrees with the IR for the parietoacanthial projection, Waters method?
    a. Orbitomeatal
    b. Glabellomeatal
    c. Acanthiomeatal
    d. Infraorbitomeatal

94. With reference to the IR, how should the central ray be directed for the parietoacanthial projection, Waters method?
    a. Perpendicular
    b. 15 degrees caudad
    c. 23 degrees caudad
    d. 37 degrees caudad

95. Which paranasal sinus group is best demonstrated with the parietoacanthial projection, Waters method?
    a. Frontal
    b. Maxillary
    c. Ethmoidal
    d. Sphenoidal

96. Where should the petrous ridges be seen in the image of the parietoacanthial projection, Waters method, of the paranasal sinuses?
    a. Superior to the orbits
    b. Lower third of the orbits
    c. Through the maxillary sinuses
    d. Below the maxillary sinuses

97. Where should the central ray exit the head for the parietoacanthial projection, Waters method?
    a. Nasion
    b. Glabella
    c. Acanthion
    d. Mental point

98. Which sinus group is not well demonstrated in the image produced by the parietoacanthial projection, Waters method?
    a. Frontal
    b. Maxillary
    c. Ethmoidal
    d. Sphenoidal

99. Which two paranasal sinus groups are better demonstrated than the other sinuses with the SMV projection?
    a. Frontal and maxillary
    b. Frontal and sphenoidal
    c. Ethmoidal and maxillary
    d. Ethmoidal and sphenoidal

100. Which projection of the sinuses demonstrates a symmetric image of the anterior portion of the base of the skull?
    a. Lateral
    b. SMV
    c. PA axial, Caldwell method
    d. Parietoacanthial, Waters method

101. In which projection of the sinuses is the IR centered to the nasion?
    a. Lateral
    b. SMV
    c. PA axial, Caldwell method
    d. Parietoacanthial, Waters method

102. In which projection of the sinuses is the mentomeatal line approximately perpendicular to the plane of the IR?
    a. Lateral
    b. SMV
    c. PA axial, Caldwell method
    d. Parietoacanthial, Waters method

103. In which projection of the sinuses must the OML form an angle of 15 degrees with the plane of the IR?
    a. Lateral
    b. SMV
    c. PA axial, Caldwell method
    d. Parietoacanthial, Waters method

104. Which evaluation criterion pertains to the lateral projection of the paranasal sinuses?
    a. All four sinus groups should be included.
    b. The petrous pyramids should lie in the lower third of the orbits.
    c. The mental protuberance should superimpose the anterior frontal bone.
    d. The petrous pyramids should lie immediately below the floor of the maxillary sinuses.

105. Which evaluation criterion pertains to the lateral projection of the paranasal sinuses?
    a. The orbital roofs should be superimposed.
    b. The petrous ridges should lie in the lower third of the orbits.
    c. The mandibular condyles should be anterior to the petrous ridges.
    d. The mental protuberance should superimpose the anterior frontal bone.

106. Which evaluation criterion pertains to the PA axial projection, Caldwell method, of the sinuses?
    a. All four sinus groups should be included.
    b. The frontal and ethmoidal sinuses should be seen.
    c. The mandibular condyles should be anterior to the petrous ridges.
    d. The petrous ridges should lie immediately below the floor of the maxillary sinuses.

107. Which evaluation criterion pertains to the PA axial projection, Caldwell method, for sinuses?
    a. Orbital roofs should be superimposed.
    b. Mandibular rami should be superimposed.
    c. Petrous ridges should lie in the lower third of the orbits.
    d. Petrous ridges should lie immediately below the floor of the maxillary sinuses.

108. Which evaluation criterion pertains to the parietoacanthial projection, Waters method, for paranasal sinuses?
    a. Mandibular rami should be superimposed.
    b. Petrous ridges should lie in the lower third of the orbits.
    c. Mental protuberance should superimpose anterior frontal bone.
    d. Petrous ridges should lie immediately below the floor of the maxillary sinuses.

109. Which evaluation criterion pertains to the SMV projection for paranasal sinuses?
    a. Mandibular rami should be superimposed.
    b. Frontal and ethmoidal sinuses should be clearly seen.
    c. Mental protuberance should superimpose anterior frontal bone.
    d. Petrous ridges should lie immediately below the floor of the maxillary sinuses.

110. Which evaluation criterion pertains to the SMV projection for sinuses?
    a. Petrous ridges should lie in the lower third of the orbits.
    b. Mandibular condyles should be anterior to the petrous ridges.
    c. Mandibular condyles should be posterior to the petrous ridges.
    d. Petrous ridges should lie immediately below the floor of the maxillary sinuses.

12 Trauma Radiography

The condition of some trauma patients sometimes requires a radiographer to alter procedures associated with routine radiographic examinations. All radiographers must be competent in performing trauma radiography. This exercise pertains to trauma radiography. Provide a short answer for each of the following questions.

1. Define *trauma*.

2. How does a level I trauma center differ from a level IV trauma center?

3. Within how many feet from the x-ray tube should appropriate shielding be provided to patients on nearby stretchers when performing mobile radiography?

4. Circle the symptoms of shock that can be readily observed by a radiographer.
   a. Cool, clammy skin
   b. Agitation or confusion
   c. Vomiting
   d. Excessive sweating
   e. Increased drowsiness
   f. Pale, bluish skin color

5. Concerning providing information to key personnel, what procedure should a radiographer perform if it is necessary to deviate from the routine projections?

6. What should be the first projection performed for a trauma patient with a cervical injury?
   a. Anteroposterior (AP) chest
   b. Lateral skull
   c. Lateral projection of cervical spine, dorsal decubitus position
   d. CT scan of the head with and without contrast

7. When is it necessary to perform the lateral projection for the cervicothoracic region?

8. What condition must be met before attempting to move the patient's arms for the lateral projection of the cervicothoracic region, dorsal decubitus position?

9. When performing the lateral projection for the cervico-thoracic region, dorsal decubitus position, on a patient who cannot move the shoulder closer to the x-ray tube,

   the central ray may be angled _____.

10. When performing the lateral projection of the cervicothoracic region, dorsal decubitus position, what is the purpose for using a long exposure time with the patient breathing normally?

11. When performing the AP axial projection on a patient who is not on a backboard or x-ray table, who should lift the patient's head and neck so that a radiographer can position the IR under the patient?

12. When performing the AP axial oblique projection for cervical vertebrae, why should a grid IR not be used?

13. When performing the AP axial oblique projection for cervical vertebrae on a supine trauma patient, how should the central ray be directed with a nongrid IR?

14. When performing the AP axial oblique projection for cervical vertebrae on a supine trauma patient, where should the central ray enter the patient?

15. When demonstrating lumbar vertebrae on a trauma patient who is supine on a backboard, what should be the first projection performed?

16. When performing the lateral projection for thoracic vertebrae on a trauma patient who is supine on a backboard, how should the central ray be directed?

17. When performing the AP projection of the abdomen on a trauma patient, what should be obtained before moving the patient to the radiographic table?

18. Circle the signs that require the radiographer to notify the emergency department physician immediately.
    a. Loss of consciousness
    b. Agitation without vomiting or other symptoms
    c. Extreme eversion of foot
    d. Bluish nail beds
    e. Increased abdominal distention

19. When performing the AP projection of the abdomen on a trauma patient on a gurney, why must the grid IR be perfectly horizontal and the central ray directed perpendicularly to the IR?

20. When performing the AP projection of the abdomen, left lateral decubitus position, why should the patient be placed in the left lateral recumbent position for at least 5 minutes before making the exposure?

21. What type of shock should radiographers be aware of when imaging patients with pelvic fractures?

22. What action should a radiographer initiate if a patient with head trauma has unequal pupils or experiences a decrease in the level of consciousness?

23. When performing the acanthioparietal projection, reverse Waters method, for facial bones on a supine trauma patient, how should the infraorbitomeatal line (IOML) be positioned with reference to the IR?

24. What is the general rule concerning demonstrating adjacent joints when imaging long bones on trauma patients?

25. What is the general rule concerning immobilization devices when imaging upper and lower limbs on trauma patients?

Define the following abbreviations:

26. CPR: _____

27. MVA: _____

28. GSW: _____

29. CVA: _____

30. ED: _____

31. OML: _____

32. IOML: _____

33. MML: _____

34. IVU: _____

35. EAM: _____

Answer the following questions by selecting the best choice.

1. Which of the following is an example of blunt trauma?
   a. Frostbite
   b. Gunshot wound
   c. Impalement injury
   d. Motor vehicle accident

2. Which procedure should be performed when taking images to localize a penetrating foreign object?
   a. Reduce kVp to produce less penetration.
   b. Mark entrance and exit wounds with a radiopaque marker.
   c. Provide a written description of the location of the entrance wound.
   d. Use twice the usual source-to-image distance to increase detail of structures.

3. Which procedure should a radiographer perform if a trauma patient begins to experience a seizure?
   a. Provide a drink of water.
   b. Roll the patient onto the side.
   c. Inform the attending physician.
   d. Cover the patient with a blanket.

4. Which of the following symptoms is associated with stroke injuries?
   a. Slurred speech
   b. Cool, clammy skin
   c. Excessive sweating
   d. Increased drowsiness

5. Which of the following statements is not an appropriate rule for trauma radiographers?
   a. Always make at least three images for each area of injury.
   b. Never leave a trauma patient unattended during imaging procedures.
   c. Never remove any immobilization device without physician's orders.
   d. Always ask the attending physician before giving a trauma patient anything to eat or drink.

6. Which of the following projections should be the first one performed for a multiple-trauma patient?
   a. AP lumbar spine
   b. Lateral lumbar spine, dorsal decubitus position
   c. AP cervical spine
   d. Lateral cervical spine, dorsal decubitus position

7. When performing the AP axial oblique projection for cervical vertebrae on a supine trauma patient, how should the central ray be directed if only one angle is used?
   a. 15 degrees cephalad
   b. 45 degrees cephalad
   c. 15 degrees lateromedially
   d. 45 degrees lateromedially

8. When performing the AP projection of the abdomen on a trauma patient, what should be obtained before moving the patient to the radiographic table?
   a. Vital signs
   b. Written consent from the patient
   c. Permission from the attending physician
   d. Lateral cervical spine projection in dorsal decubitus position

9. Which of the following procedures should the radiographer perform if a trauma patient has bleeding wounds?
   a. Protect the IR with plastic.
   b. Enclose the IR inside a pillowcase.
   c. Provide fluids to the patient by mouth or intravenously.
   d. Have emergency department personnel assist with the procedure.

10. Why should the left lateral decubitus position be used for demonstrating free air within the abdominal cavity?
    a. Free air will collect under the left hemidiaphragm.
    b. Fluid levels will collect under the right hemidiaphragm.
    c. The density of the liver provides good contrast for free air.
    d. The density of the stomach provides good contrast for free air.

11. How should a radiographer determine if an AP projection of the abdomen, left lateral decubitus position, is being requested for demonstrating free air or fluid levels?
    a. Ask the patient.
    b. Ask the attending physician.
    c. Examine for penetrating wounds.
    d. Examine for distended or firm abdomen.

12. When performing the AP projection of the abdomen, left lateral decubitus position, which of the following procedures should be performed when fluid levels are of primary interest?
    a. Ensure the entire left side is demonstrated.
    b. Ensure the entire right side is demonstrated.
    c. Center the IR 4 inches above the iliac crests to include the diaphragm.
    d. Have the patient drink one full glass of water before making the image.

13. Which projection of the abdomen should be performed to demonstrate air or fluid levels when a trauma patient is unable to be positioned either upright or in the lateral recumbent position?
    a. AP
    b. Left AP oblique
    c. Right AP oblique
    d. Lateral, dorsal decubitus position

14. When performing the AP projection for the pelvis in a trauma patient, which of the following procedures should not be performed?
    a. Use a grid IR directly under the patient.
    b. Rotate the femurs 15 degrees medially.
    c. Transfer the patient to a radiographic table.
    d. Center the IR to a level of 2 inches inferior to the anterior superior iliac spine (ASIS).

15. Which action should a radiographer perform if a semiconscious patient with head trauma begins vomiting during radiographic procedures?
    a. Obtain vital signs.
    b. Give the patient a plastic bag.
    c. Move the patient to a sitting position.
    d. Logroll the patient to the lateral recumbent position.

16. Which of the following procedures should a radiographer perform if a trauma patient with a head injury displays unequal pupils?
    a. Give the patient a drink of water.
    b. Remove restrictive immobilization devices.
    c. Immediately inform the attending physician.
    d. Logroll the patient into a lateral recumbent position.

17. Which of the following projections of the cranium would best demonstrate a suspected fracture of the posterior cranium?
    a. AP
    b. PA
    c. AP axial, Towne method
    d. Lateral, dorsal decubitus position

18. Which positioning line of the head should be nearly perpendicular to the IR when performing the acanthioparietal projection, reverse Waters method, for facial bones on a supine trauma patient?
    a. Mentomeatal
    b. Orbitomeatal
    c. Glabellomeatal
    d. Infraorbitomeatal

19. How should the central ray be directed when performing the acanthioparietal projection, reverse Waters method, for facial bones on a supine trauma patient?
    a. 37 degrees cephalad
    b. Perpendicular to the IR
    c. Parallel with the mentomeatal line
    d. Parallel with the IOML

20. Which of the following general rules should be followed when imaging upper and lower extremities on trauma patients?
    a. Always obtain two images, 90 degrees apart.
    b. Always position for true AP and lateral projections.
    c. When demonstrating long bones, always remove immobilization devices.
    d. When demonstrating long bones, always transfer the patient to the radiographic table.

21. Which procedure is performed on patients with suspected bilateral hip fractures?
    a. Cleaves
    b. Danelius-Miller
    c. Clements-Nakayama
    d. Lauenstein

22. How should the central ray be directed when performing the axiolateral projection, Danelius-Miller for trauma hip?
    a. 15 degrees posteriorly and aligned perpendicular to the femoral neck and grid IR
    b. Horizontal and perpendicular to femoral neck
    c. Perpendicular midway between the ASIS and the pubic symphysis for the Lauenstein method
    d. Cephalic angle of 20 to 25 degrees and 1 inch (2.5 cm) inferior through the hip joint

23. How should the central ray be directed when performing the modified axiolateral projection, Clements-Nakayama, for trauma hip?
    a. 15 degrees posteriorly and aligned perpendicular to the femoral neck and grid IR
    b. Horizontal and perpendicular to femoral neck
    c. Perpendicular midway between the ASIS and the pubic symphysis for the Lauenstein method
    d. Cephalic angle of 20 to 25 degrees and 1 inch (2.5 cm) inferior through the hip joint

24. How should the central ray be directed when performing the lateral projection, dorsal decubitus position for the abdomen?
    a. Perpendicular entering the patient at MSP at the level of the iliac crests
    b. Perpendicular entering the patient at MSP at the level 2 inches (5 cm) above the iliac crests
    c. Horizontal and perpendicular entering MSP at a level 2 inches (5 cm) above the iliac crests
    d. Horizontal and perpendicular entering MCP at a level 2 inches (5 cm) above the iliac crests

25. How should the central ray be directed when performing the AP axial projection, reverse Caldwell method for the cranium?
    a. Perpendicular to MSP at the nasion
    b. Angled 15 degrees cephalad entering MSP at the nasion
    c. Angled 30 degrees caudad to the OML or 37 degrees to the IOML passing through the EAM
    d. Angled cephalad until parallel with the MML entering the acanthion

412

13 Contrast Arthrography

Contrast arthrography is a procedure that greatly enhances the visibility of joint structures compared with plain-image radiography. Other imaging modalities have reduced the need for radiographic contrast arthrography. This exercise pertains to contrast arthrography. Fill in missing words, provide a short answer, or choose true or false (explaining any statement you believe to be false) for each item.

1. Define *arthrography*.

2. List the imaging modalities that have significantly reduced the number of arthrograms performed in radiography departments.

3. List four soft tissue structures of joints that are often demonstrated with arthrographic examinations.

4. Identify the type of contrast media used for each of the following examinations.

   a. Opaque arthrography: _____

   _____

   b. Pneumoarthrography: _____

   _____

   c. Double-contrast arthrography: _____

   _____

5. The joint that is demonstrated by contrast arthrography more often than any other joint is the _____

   _____.

6. True or false. Contrast arthrography is usually performed with a local anesthetic.

7. True or false. The radiographer injects the contrast medium under carefully maintained aseptic conditions.

8. Who should manipulate the joint to ensure good distribution of the contrast medium?

9. For arthrography of the knee, what is the purpose of a stress device?

10. For arthrography of the knee, what is the purpose of "opening up" the side of the joint space being examined?

11. For the vertical ray method of knee arthrography, what five conventional projections are made to complement fluoroscopy?

12. Hip arthrography is most often performed on children to evaluate congenital _____ _____.

13. Give two reasons why hip arthrography is frequently performed on adults.

14. List the conventional projections that comprise a shoulder arthrogram.

15. In addition to conventional radiography, what imaging modality is frequently used to demonstrate the shoulder after a double-contrast arthrogram?

16. Arthrography of the shoulder is performed to evaluate which conditions?

17. When performing shoulder arthrography, why is a spinal needle recommended?

18. What is the recommended patient position when performing knee arthrography using the horizontal central ray method to demonstrate the medial and lateral meniscus?

19. True or false. Essentially any joint can be evaluated by arthrography.

20. True or false. The American College of Radiology (ACR) ranks radiographic contrast arthrography from very low or not at all as an appropriate diagnostic tool.

Answer the following questions by selecting the best choice.

1. Which examination demonstrates joint structures after the introduction of only a water-soluble, iodinated contrast medium?
   a. Pneumoarthrography
   b. Opaque arthrography
   c. Double-contrast arthrography

2. Which examination combines radiopaque and radiolucent contrast media in a joint to demonstrate soft tissue structures?
   a. Pneumoarthrography
   b. Opaque arthrography
   c. Single-contrast arthrography
   d. Double-contrast arthrography

3. Which examination room should be used for contrast arthrography?
   a. Surgical
   b. Sonographic
   c. Urologic-radiographic
   d. Fluoroscopic-radiographic

4. Which arthrogram would most likely include subtraction technique images with conventional radiography?
   a. Shoulder arthrography for rotator cuff tear
   b. Wrist arthrography for carpal tunnel syndrome
   c. Hip arthrography for congenital hip dislocation
   d. Hip arthrography to detect a loose hip prosthesis

5. Which articulation is examined by contrast arthrography more often than any other joint?
   a. Hip
   b. Knee
   c. Wrist
   d. Shoulder

6. What is the most common reason for performing hip arthrography on children?
   a. Child abuse
   b. Automobile accidents
   c. Long bone measurement
   d. Congenital hip dislocation

7. What is one of the two most common reasons for performing hip arthrography on adults?
   a. Automobile accidents
   b. Long bone measurement
   c. Congenital hip dislocation
   d. Detection of a loose hip prosthesis

8. For a single-contrast arthrogram, approximately how many milliliters of positive contrast medium is injected into the shoulder?
   a. 6 to 8 mL
   b. 10 to 12 mL
   c. 14 to 16 mL

9. Which structures are demonstrated with contrast arthrography?
   a. Bursae
   b. Tendons
   c. Ventricles
   d. Intervertebral disks

10. What are the two methods for performing contrast arthrography of a knee?
    a. Immediate and delayed
    b. Invasive and noninvasive
    c. Vertical ray and horizontal ray
    d. Perpendicular ray and angled ray

11. Contrast arthrography is recommended for all of the following EXCEPT:
    a. after knee arthroplasty as a routine follow-up or for complications.
    b. aspiration in suspected septic or inflammatory arthropathies of the shoulder.
    c. superficial skin infections.
    d. to rule out the hip as the referred pain source after other negative imaging.

12. Which arthrography is performed primarily for the evaluation of partial or complete tears in the rotator cuff?
    a. Knee
    b. Hip
    c. Shoulder
    d. Elbow

13. Which arthrography is performed primarily for the evaluation of meniscal tears?
    a. Knee
    b. Hip
    c. Shoulder
    d. Elbow

14. Which arthrography is performed primarily to evaluate lateral femoral head displacement and after closed reduction to ensure that there is no folding or impingement of soft tissues?
    a. Knee
    b. Hip
    c. Shoulder
    d. Elbow

15. Which of the following can be evaluated by arthrography?
    a. Wrist
    b. Ankle
    c. Elbow
    d. Any joint

ANATOMY OF THE CENTRAL NERVOUS SYSTEM

Section 1: Exercise 1

This exercise pertains to the anatomic structures of the central nervous system (CNS). Identify structures, fill in missing words, or provide a short answer for each item.

1. Identify each lettered structure shown in Fig. 14.1.

   A. _____

   B. _____

   C. _____

   D. _____

   E. _____

   F. _____

   G. _____

   H. _____

2. Identify each lettered structure shown in Fig. 14.2.

   A. _____

   B. _____

   C. _____

   D. _____

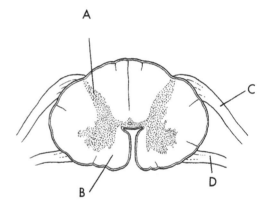

Fig. 14.2 Transverse section of the spinal cord.

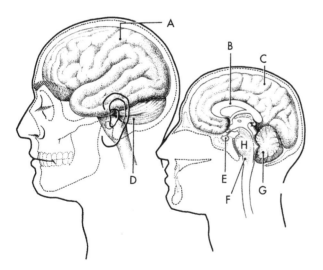

Fig. 14.1 Lateral surface and midsection of the brain.

3. Identify each lettered structure shown in Fig. 14.3.

A. _____

B. _____

C. _____

D. _____

4. Identify each lettered structure shown in Fig. 14.4.

A. _____

B. _____

C. _____

D. _____

E. _____

F. _____

G. _____

H. _____

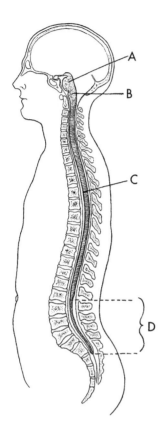

Fig. 14.3 Sagittal section showing the spinal cord.

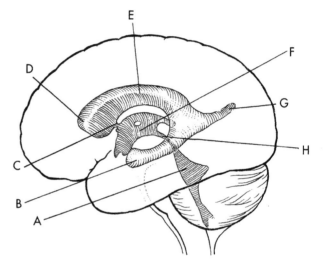

Fig. 14.4 Lateral aspect of the cerebral ventricles in relation to the surface of the brain.

5. Identify each lettered structure shown in Fig. 14.5.

A. _____

B. _____

C. _____

6. Identify each lettered structure shown in Fig. 14.6.

A. _____

B. _____

C. _____

D. _____

E. _____

F. _____

G. _____

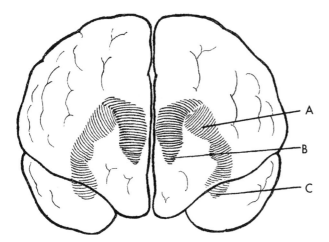

Fig. 14.5 Anterior aspect of the lateral cerebral ventricles in relation to the surface of the brain.

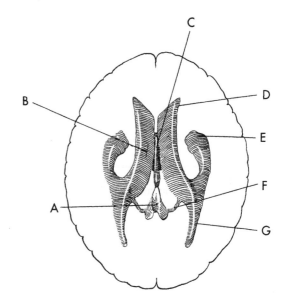

Fig. 14.6 Superior aspect of the cerebral ventricles in relation to the surface of the brain.

7. Name the two main parts of the CNS.

8. Name the three parts of the brain.

9. Name the four parts of the brainstem.

10. Name the three parts of the hindbrain.

11. The largest part of the brain is the _____ _____.

12. Another name for the cerebrum is the _____ _____.

13. The stemlike portion of the brain that connects the cerebrum to the hindbrain is the _____ _____.

14. The deep cleft that separates the cerebrum into right and left hemispheres is the _____.

15. The master endocrine gland of the body is located in the brain and is the _____.

16. The largest part of the hindbrain is the _____ _____.

17. The portion of the hindbrain that connects the pons to the spinal cord is the _____.

18. The protective membranes that enclose the brain and spinal cord are the _____.

19. The membrane that closely adheres to the brain and spinal cord is the _____.

20. The outermost membrane that forms the tough fibrous covering for the brain and spinal cord is the _____.

21. The two uppermost ventricles are called the right and left _____ ventricles.

22. The lateral ventricles are located in the portion of the brain called the _____.

23. Each lateral ventricle communicates with the third ventricle by way of the _____ foramen.

24. Another name for the interventricular foramen is the foramen of _____.

25. What are the two names for the passage between the third and fourth ventricles?

IMAGING OF THE CENTRAL NERVOUS SYSTEM

Section 2: Exercise 1

This exercise pertains to radiographic examinations that demonstrate CNS structures. Fill in missing words, provide a short answer, or choose true or false (explaining any statement you believe to be false) for each item.

1. Define *myelography*.

2. Identify three common sites for the injection of contrast medium during myelography.

3. What abnormality is demonstrated using myelography?

4. What type or group of contrast media is preferred for myelography? Explain why.

5. When the exposure room is prepared for myelography, why should the image intensifier be locked in place?

6. What should be done to reduce patient apprehension?

7. What are the two body positions most frequently used when contrast medium is injected for myelography?

8. During myelography, what procedure is used to control the movement of the contrast medium after its injection?

9. During myelography, why should the patient hyperextend the neck?

10. When using plain radiography, what image is recommended to be performed first on a trauma patient with possible CNS involvement?

11. Myelography continues to be the preferred examination method for assessing disk disease in patients with contraindications to what other imaging modality?

12. List some common pathologic conditions that result from traumatic injury that may compress the spinal cord?

13. True or false. The patient should be well hydrated for a myelogram procedure.

14. True or false. Premedication of the patient for myelography is common.

15. The Centers for Disease Control and Prevention (CDC) require _____ _____ be worn when placing a catheter or injecting material into the _____ _____ or _____ _____.

16. True or false. To reduce the chance of infection, multidose vials of contrast media are recommended.

17. True or false. Improvements in nonionic contrast agents have resulted in fewer side effects.

18. The patient should be informed that the _____ of the examining table will change repeatedly and acutely.

19. The patient should be told why the head must be maintained in a fully _____ position when the table is tilted to the _____ position.

20. Most facilities require an _____ _____ form to be completed and signed by the patient and physician.

21. What scout image is often requested before beginning a myelogram procedure?

22. Approximately how many milliliters of nonionic contrast medium is slowly injected into the subarachnoid space?

23. Most myelograms are performed on an outpatient basis, with patients recovering for approximately how many hours after the procedure?

24. When performing the conus projection to show the conus medullaris, the patient is placed in the _____ position with the central ray centered to _____.

25. Most physicians recommend that the patient's head and shoulders be elevated how many degrees during recovery?

Section 2: Exercise 2

This exercise pertains to interventional radiology procedures of the vertebral column. Fill in missing words, provide a short answer, or choose true or false (explaining any statement you believe to be false) for each item.

1. Define *percutaneous vertebroplasty.*

2. How does percutaneous kyphoplasty differ from *vertebroplasty?*

3. Describe the function of a percutaneous mesh container.

4. Vertebroplasty, kyphoplasty, and mesh-container-plasty are interventional radiology procedures used to treat what type of fractures?

5. What is the most common complication that occurs in patients treated for compression fractures before the cement hardens?

6. Why is diskography performed?

7. True or false. Some authors suggest diskography may increase the chance of later disk disruption.

8. Interventional pain management physicians perform a variety of injections using _____ and _____ to reduce inflammation and improve symptoms.

9. True or false. Interventional pain management procedures can be performed at all levels of the spine.

10. What are the two body positions most frequently used during interventional pain management procedures?

Answer the following questions by selecting the best choice.

1. Which two structures make up the CNS?
   a. Brain and cerebellum
   b. Brain and spinal cord
   c. Cerebrum and cerebellum
   d. Cerebrum and spinal cord

2. Which part of the brain is also referred to as the forebrain?
   a. Pons
   b. Cerebrum
   c. Cerebellum
   d. Diencephalon

3. Which three parts of the CNS make up the hindbrain?
   a. Cerebrum, cerebellum, and spinal cord
   b. Cerebrum, pons, and medulla oblongata
   c. Pons, cerebellum, and medulla oblongata
   d. Pons, spinal cord, and medulla oblongata

4. Which cerebral structure is the largest part of the brain?
   a. Pons
   b. Cerebrum
   c. Cerebellum
   d. Medulla oblongata

5. Which structure is divided into right and left hemispheres by the longitudinal fissure?
   a. Pons
   b. Cerebrum
   c. Cerebellum
   d. Medulla oblongata

6. What other term refers to the hypophysis cerebri?
   a. Pituitary gland
   b. Medulla spinalis
   c. Corpus callosum
   d. Conus medullaris

7. Which membrane forms the tough, fibrous outer covering for the meninges?
   a. Pia mater
   b. Arachnoid
   c. Dura mater

8. Which structure connects the lateral ventricles to the third ventricle?
   a. Cerebral aqueduct
   b. Foramen of Luschka
   c. Foramen of Magendie
   d. Interventricular foramen

9. In which part of the brain is the fourth ventricle found?
   a. Midbrain
   b. Forebrain
   c. Hindbrain

10. Which projection should be the first image for a trauma patient with possible CNS involvement?
    a. Anteroposterior (AP) axial
    b. AP oblique
    c. Upright lateral
    d. Cross-table lateral

11. Which examination is performed to demonstrate the contour of the subarachnoid space?
    a. Diskography
    b. Myelography
    c. Ventriculography
    d. Vertebroplasty

12. For which examination is the contrast medium injected directly into the fibrous cartilage between two vertebral bodies?
    a. Diskography
    b. Myelography
    c. Ventriculography
    d. Angiography

13. Which interventional procedure uses a balloon catheter to expand a collapsed vertebra before injecting cement?
    a. Diskography
    b. Myelography
    c. Kyphoplasty
    d. Vertebroplasty

14. During myelography, which procedure should be performed to prevent contrast medium from entering the cerebral ventricles?
    a. Tilt the head of the table down.
    b. Instruct the patient to hyperflex the neck.
    c. Place the patient in the lateral recumbent position.
    d. Have the patient hyperextend the neck.

15. What is the purpose of tilting the table during myelography?
    a. To attach the footboard
    b. To facilitate patient comfort
    c. To control the flow of contrast medium
    d. To remove cerebrospinal fluid from the patient

16. Bone cement is injected into the vertebral body for all of the following procedures EXCEPT:
    a. vertebroplasty.
    b. diskography.
    c. mesh-container-plasty.
    d. kyphoplasty.

17. Myelography is performed by introducing a nonionic, water-soluble contrast medium into the subarachnoid space by spinal puncture, most commonly at what interspace level? (More than one answer may apply.)
    a. T12-L1
    b. L2-3
    c. L3-4
    d. L5-S1

18. All of the following interventional radiology procedures are used to treat spinal osteoporotic compression fractures EXCEPT:
    a. vertebroplasty.
    b. kyphoplasty.
    c. diskography.
    d. mesh-container-plasty.

19. Which of the following imaging types is commonly performed after diskography to look for clefts or tears?
    a. Magnetic resonance imaging (MRI)
    b. Ultrasound (US)
    c. Plain radiographs
    d. Computed tomography (CT)

20. All of the following may be used to provide imaging for needle placement during interventional pain management EXCEPT for:
    a. CT.
    b. MRI.
    c. ultrasound.
    d. fluoroscopy.

15 Digestive System: Salivary Glands, Alimentary Canal, and Biliary System

CHAPTER 15: SECTION 1

ANATOMY OF THE ALIMENTARY CANAL

Section 1: Exercise 1

This exercise pertains to the digestive system. Identify structures for each question and provide short answers.

1. Identify each lettered structure shown in Fig. 15.1.

    A. _____

    B. _____

    C. _____

    D. _____

    E. _____

    F. _____

    G. _____

2. Identify each lettered structure shown in Fig. 15.2.

    A. _____

    B. _____

    C. _____

    D. _____

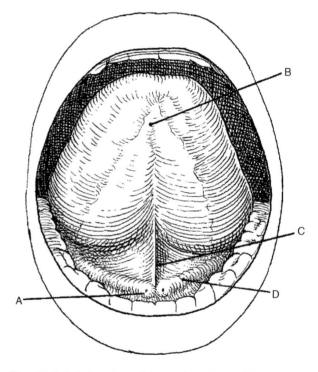

Fig. 15.2 Anterior view of the undersurface of the tongue and the floor of the mouth.

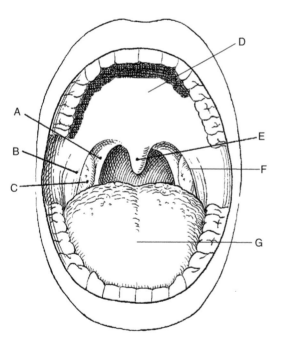

Fig. 15.1 Anterior aspect of the oral cavity.

426

Chapter **15** Digestive System: Salivary Glands, Alimentary Canal, and Biliary System

3. Identify each lettered structure shown in Fig. 15.3.

A. _____

B. _____

C. _____

D. _____

E. _____

F. _____

4. Identify each lettered structure shown in Fig. 15.4.

A. _____

B. _____

C. _____

D. _____

E. _____

F. _____

G. _____

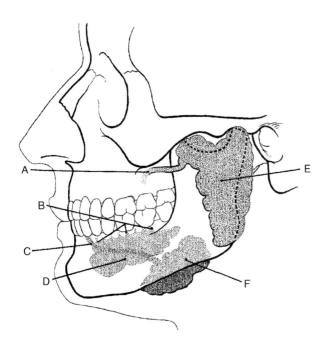

Fig. 15.3 The salivary glands from the left lateral aspect.

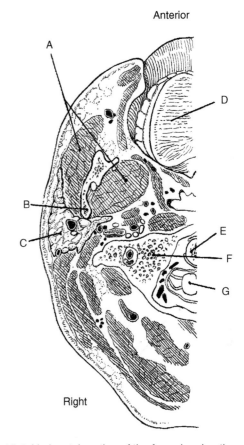

Fig. 15.4 Horizontal section of the face showing the relation of the parotid gland to the mandibular ramus.

Chapter **15 Digestive System: Salivary Glands, Alimentary Canal, and Biliary System**

5. Identify each lettered structure shown in Fig. 15.5.

   A. _____

   B. _____

   C. _____

   D. _____

   E. _____

   F. _____

6. What is the first division of the digestive system?

7. Define *mastication*.

8. Which structures function in mastication?

9. What is the purpose of saliva?

10. Name the three pairs of salivary glands.

Anterior

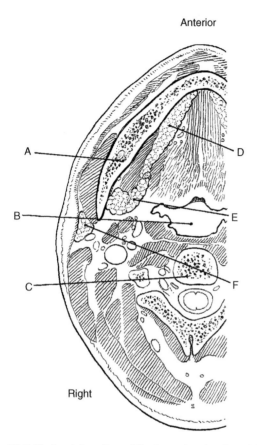

Right

Fig. 15.5 Horizontal section of the face showing the relation of the submandibular and sublingual glands to surrounding structures.

Chapter **15** **Digestive System: Salivary Glands, Alimentary Canal, and Biliary System**

11. Identify each lettered structure shown in Fig. 15.6.

A. _____

B. _____

C. _____

D. _____

E. _____

F. _____

G. _____

H. _____

I. _____

J. _____

K. _____

L. _____

M. _____

N. _____

O. _____

12. Identify each lettered structure shown in Fig. 15.7.

A. _____

B. _____

C. _____

D. _____

E. _____

F. _____

G. _____

H. _____

I. _____

J. _____

K. _____

L. _____

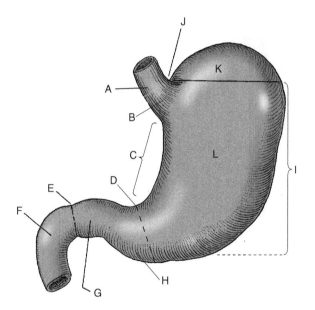

Fig. 15.7 Anterior surface of the stomach.

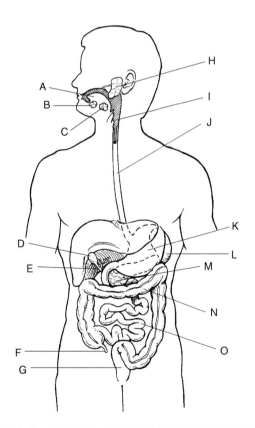

Fig. 15.6 The alimentary canal and its accessory organs.

Chapter **15 Digestive System: Salivary Glands, Alimentary Canal, and Biliary System**

13. Identify each lettered structure shown in Fig. 15.8.

A. _____

B. _____

C. _____

D. _____

E. _____

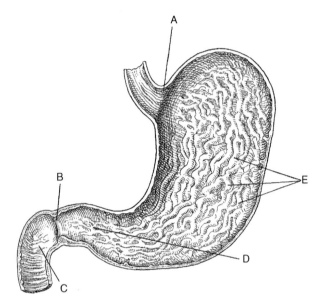

Fig. 15.8 Section of the stomach showing rugae.

14. Identify each lettered structure shown in Fig. 15.9.

A. _____

B. _____

C. _____

D. _____

E. _____

F. _____

G. _____

H. _____

I. _____

J. _____

K. _____

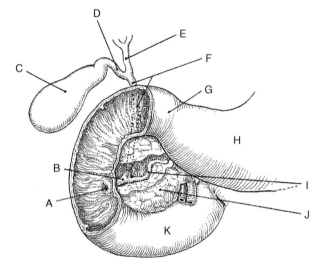

Fig. 15.9 The duodenal loop in relation to the biliary and pancreatic ducts.

15. Identify each lettered structure shown in Fig. 15.10.

A. _____

B. _____

C. _____

D. _____

E. _____

F. _____

G. _____

H. _____

I. _____

J. _____

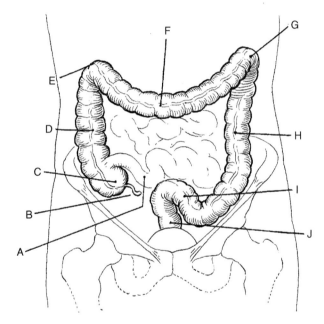

Fig. 15.10 Anterior aspect of the large bowel.

16. Identify each lettered structure shown in Fig. 15.11.

A. _____

B. _____

C. _____

D. _____

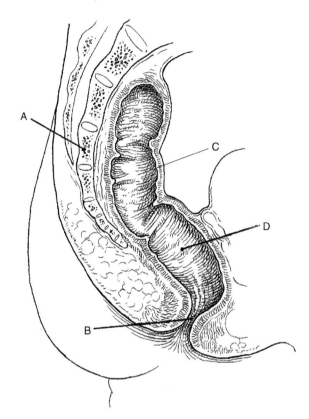

Fig. 15.11 Sagittal section showing the anal canal and rectum.

Chapter **15 Digestive System: Salivary Glands, Alimentary Canal, and Biliary System**

17. Identify each lettered structure shown in Fig. 15.12.

A. _____

B. _____

C. _____

D. _____

E. _____

F. _____

G. _____

H. _____

I. _____

J. _____

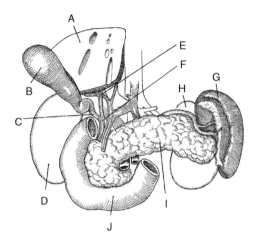

Fig. 15.12 Visceral (inferoposterior) surface of the gallbladder and bile ducts.

Section 1: Exercise 2

Use the following clues to complete the crossword puzzle. All answers refer to the alimentary canal.

Across

1. Stores bile
5. Gastric folds
8. Attached to cecum
10. Terminates alimentary canal
11. Widest part of alimentary canal
15. Contraction waves
18. Proximal part of small bowel
19. Left colic flexure
22. Between cecum and right colic flexure
23. Average body build
24. Precedes anal canal

Down

2. Digestive juice
3. Musculomembranous tube
4. Upper part of stomach
6. Lower than sthenic
7. Proximal part of large intestine
9. Precedes esophagus
12. Large body build
13. Middle part of small bowel
14. Very slender body build
16. Intestinal bend
17. Between left colic flexure and sigmoid
20. Produces bile
21. Distal part of small bowel

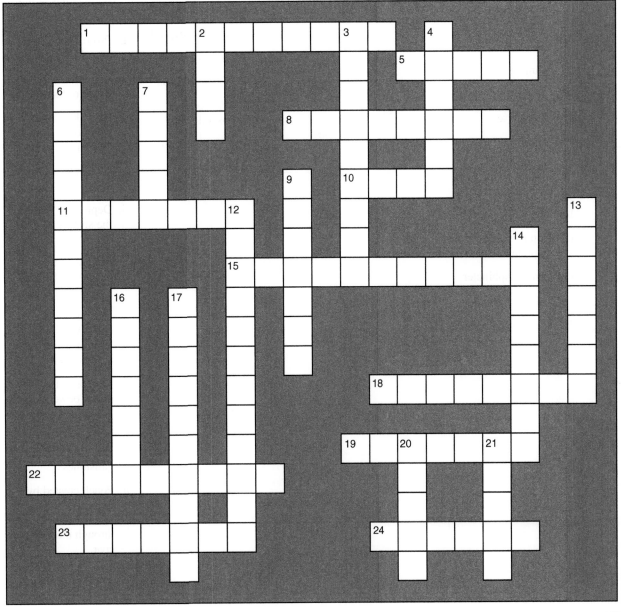

Chapter **15** **Digestive System: Salivary Glands, Alimentary Canal, and Biliary System**

Section 1: Exercise 3

Match the structures or portions of organs found in the alimentary canal from the list in Column A with the major organs to which they most closely relate as listed in Column B.

Column A

_____ 1. Bulb

_____ 2. Body

_____ 3. Rugae

_____ 4. Ileum

_____ 5. Cecum

_____ 6. Rectum

_____ 7. Fundus

_____ 8. Pylorus

_____ 9. Sigmoid

_____ 10. Jejunum

_____ 11. Duodenum

_____ 12. Transverse

_____ 13. Ascending

_____ 14. Descending

_____ 15. Lesser curvature

_____ 16. Greater curvature

_____ 17. Hepatopancreatic ampulla

_____ 18. Cardiac sphincter

_____ 19. Left colic flexure

_____ 20. Right colic flexure

Column B

a. Stomach

b. Small intestine

c. Large intestine

Section 1: Exercise 4

Match the pathology terms in Column A with the appropriate definition in Column B.

Column A

_____ 1. Ulcer

_____ 2. Polyp

_____ 3. Gastroesophageal reflux

_____ 4. Colitis

_____ 5. Gastritis

_____ 6. Volvulus

_____ 7. Diverticulum

_____ 8. Diverticulosis

_____ 9. Intussusception

_____ 10. Inguinal hernia

_____ 11. Cholelithiasis

_____ 12. Pancreatic pseudocyst

_____ 13. Biliary stenosis

_____ 14. Pancreatitis

Column B

a. Collection of fluid, debris, pancreatic enzymes, and blood; complication of acute pancreatitis

b. Inflammation of the colon

c. Twisting of a bowel loop on itself

d. Acute or chronic inflammation of the pancreas

e. Protrusion of the bowel into the groin

f. Inflammation of the lining of the stomach

g. Growth or mass protruding from a mucous membrane

h. Narrowing of the bile ducts

i. Depressed lesion of the surface of the alimentary canal

j. Backward flow of the stomach contents into the esophagus

k. Diverticula in the colon without inflammation or symptoms

l. Prolapse of a portion of the bowel into the lumen of an adjacent part

m. Presence of gallstones

n. Pouch created by the herniation of the mucous membrane through the muscular coat

434

Chapter **15** **Digestive System: Salivary Glands, Alimentary Canal, and Biliary System**

Copyright © 2019, Elsevier Inc. All Rights Reserved.

Section 1: Exercise 5

This exercise pertains to the alimentary canal and its related organs. Fill in missing words or provide a short answer for each question.

1. The musculomembranous passage that extends from the pharynx to the stomach is the _____ _____.

2. The expanded part of the distal end of the esophagus is the _____.

3. The opening into the stomach through which food and liquids pass is the _____ _____.

4. The organ in which gastric digestion begins is the _____.

5. The gastric folds of the stomach are the _____ _____.

6. The border of the stomach with the lesser curvature is the _____ border.

7. The lesser curvature extends from the esophagogastric junction to the _____ _____.

8. The left and inferior borders of the stomach are _____ .

9. The stomach is located _____ and more _____ in the hypersthenic body habitus.

10. The stomach is located lower and closer to midline in the _____ body habitus.

11. Name the four parts of the stomach.

12. The part of the stomach immediately surrounding the esophageal opening is the _____ _____.

13. The most superior part of the stomach is the _____ _____.

14. The most inferior part of the stomach is the _____ portion.

15. The opening between the stomach and the small intestine is the _____.

16. The three parts of the small intestine are the _____, _____, and _____.

17. The proximal part of the small intestine is the _____ _____.

18. The radiographically significant first segment of the proximal part of the small intestine is the _____ _____.

19. The small intestine terminates at the _____ _____.

20. The common bile and the pancreatic ducts empty into the _____.

21. The middle part of the small intestine is the _____ _____.

22. The distal part of the small intestine is the _____ _____.

23. The shortest part of the small intestine is the _____; the longest part is the _____.

24. The passage from the small intestine to the large intestine is the _____.

25. The proximal part of the large intestine is the _____ _____.

26. The vermiform appendix attaches to the large intestine at the _____.

435

27. Located between the ascending colon and the transverse colon is the _____ flexure.

28. The part of the colon that extends from the cecum to the right colic flexure is the _____ colon.

29. The part of the colon that extends between the two flexures is the _____ colon.

30. Located between the transverse colon and the descending colon is the _____ flexure.

31. The part of the colon that extends inferiorly from the left colic flexure is the _____ colon.

32. The sigmoid colon is located between the two parts of the large intestine known as the _____ and the _____.

33. The sigmoid colon terminates in the _____ _____.

34. The part of the large intestine that extends between the rectum and the anus is the _____.

35. The external opening at the terminal end of the anal canal is the _____.

36. The largest organ in the abdominal cavity is the _____.

37. The right and left hepatic ducts join to form the _____.

38. The cystic duct enables bile from the liver to be stored in the _____.

39. The gallbladder is usually located on the inferior side of the right lobe of the _____ _____.

40. The common hepatic duct unites with the cystic duct to form the _____ _____.

41. In 20% of subjects, before entering the duodenum, the common bile duct joins with the _____ _____.

42. The muscular contraction of the gallbladder is activated by a hormone called _____.

43. The gland that produces insulin is the _____.

44. True or false. In a hypersthenic patient, the gallbladder is situated high and well away from the midsagittal plane.

45. True or false. The gallbladder is located posterior to the liver in the retroperitoneal space.

46. True or false. The pancreas cannot be demonstrated using plain radiography.

47. True or false. The spleen is an organ of the lymphatic system.

48. True or false. The pancreas and the liver secrete specialized digestive juices into the small intestine.

POSITIONING OF THE ALIMENTARY CANAL

Section 2: Exercise 1: Sialography

1. Define *sialography*.

2. What type of contrast medium is used for sialography?

3. Why can only one salivary gland at a time be examined by the sialographic method?

4. List two reasons why preliminary radiographs are made before the introduction of the contrast medium.

5. Name the two projections that demonstrate the salivary glands and ducts.

6. Which salivary glands are demonstrated with the lateral projection?
   a. Parotid and sublingual
   b. Parotid and submandibular
   c. Sublingual and submandibular

7. How is the central ray directed for the tangential projection of a sialographic procedure?

8. True or false. The patient may be positioned prone or supine for the tangential projection.

9. True or false. The mandibular ramus should be parallel with the plane of the image receptor (IR) for the tangential projection.

10. True or false. Parotid glands on both sides of the face should be demonstrated with the same tangential exposure.

11. Examine Fig. 15.13 and answer the questions that follow.
    a. Which projection does this image represent?
    b. Which salivary gland is demonstrated?
    c. What is the special breathing technique that can be performed by the patient to improve the radiographic demonstration of the gland with this type of projection?

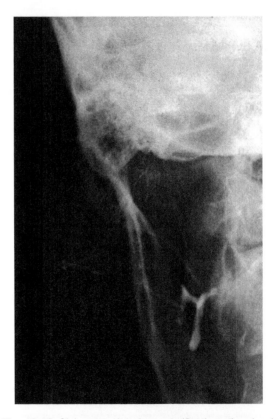

Fig. 15.13 Sialogram showing opacification of a gland.

Chapter **15 Digestive System: Salivary Glands, Alimentary Canal, and Biliary System**

12. Examine Fig. 15.14 and answer the questions that follow.
    a. Which projection does this image represent?
    b. Which salivary gland is demonstrated?
    c. To which duct does the arrow point?

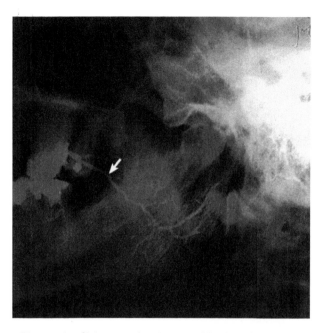

Fig. 15.14 Sialogram showing opacification of a gland.

13. Examine Fig. 15.15 and answer the questions that follow.
    a. Which projection does this image represent?
    b. Which salivary gland is demonstrated?
    c. To which duct does the arrow point?

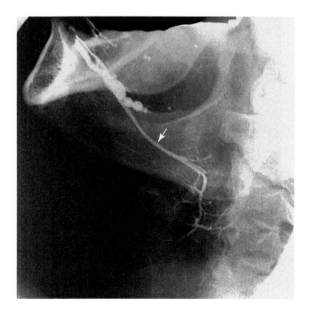

Fig. 15.15 Sialogram showing opacification of a gland.

14. List the various conditions that are detected when performing sialography.

15. When performing the sialographic procedure, what is an example of a secretory stimulant that can be given to a patient to open the duct for easier passage of a catheter and for evacuation of contrast medium?

Section 2: Exercise 2: Positioning for the Esophagus

The esophagus can be radiographically examined after a contrast medium has been introduced. This exercise pertains to procedures used to obtain the required images of the esophagus. Fill in missing words, provide a short answer, or choose true or false (explaining any statement you believe to be false) for each item.

1. List the projections that comprise the typical esophageal study.

2. What two types of contrast media are used for double-contrast esophageal studies?

3. Why is the PA oblique projection, left anterior oblique (LAO) position, not included in the typical esophageal study?

4. When demonstrating the entire esophagus, to what level of the patient should the IR be centered?

5. What two oblique positions can be used to demonstrate the entire esophagus effectively?

6. Why is the recumbent right anterior oblique (RAO) position preferred over the upright position?

7. For anteroposterior (AP) or posteroanterior (PA) projections, how is it determined that the selection of exposure factors was acceptable?

8. In relation to the surrounding structures, where should the esophagus appear in images with the patient in the RAO position?

9. In images of a contrast-filled esophagus with the patient in the RAO position, how does the esophagus appear in relation to the surrounding structures when rotation of the patient was insufficient?

10. In the lateral projection, what structures are used to determine whether the patient was rotated? How should these structures appear?

11. For images with the patient in the RAO position, the patient should be rotated approximately

_____ to _____ degrees.

12. The esophagus should be clearly seen from the lower

neck to the _____.

13. True or false. Single-contrast and double-contrast studies can be used to demonstrate the esophagus.

14. True or false. A barium sulfate mixture is the preferred contrast medium for esophagrams.

15. True or false. A high-density barium (210% to 250% weight/volume) is recommended for double-contrast esophageal and gastric examinations.

Section 2: Exercise 3: Gastrointestinal Series

A commonly performed study employing contrast media is the gastrointestinal (GI) series. This exercise pertains to GI studies. Identify structures, fill in missing words, provide a short answer, select from a list, or choose true or false (explaining any statement you believe to be false) for each item.

Items 1 to 16 pertain to upper gastrointestinal (UGI) examination procedures.

1. What acronym refers to the upper gastrointestinal series?

2. As part of patient preparation, why should the patient maintain a soft, low-residue diet for 2 days?

3. How can the UGI study be affected if the patient smokes cigarettes shortly before the examination?

4. What type of radiopaque contrast medium is usually used in routine UGI studies?

5. List the two general GI studies routinely used to examine the stomach.

6. What weight per volume concentration for the barium sulfate suspension is recommended for single-contrast examinations?

7. List two advantages of performing the double-contrast examination.

8. What are the two types of contrast media used in double-contrast procedures?

9. True or false. The barium sulfate suspension used for double-contrast examinations should have a higher weight-per-volume ratio than the barium sulfate suspension used for single-contrast examinations.

10. Why should patients undergoing double-contrast examinations turn from side to side or roll over a few times during the procedure?

11. During double-contrast examinations, what instructions should be given to the patient after the patient swallows the carbon dioxide crystals or tablets to ensure a double-contrast effect?

12. What is the purpose of using glucagon during the double-contrast examination?

13. What is a biphasic GI examination?

14. Which method of examination (single-contrast or double-contrast) is performed first as part of a biphasic examination?

15. True or false. During a normal UGI examination, the contrast medium normally begins to pass into the duodenum almost immediately.

16. True or false. Nervous tension of the patient may accelerate transit of the contrast material.

441

Items 17 to 25 pertain to the *PA projection.* Examine Fig. 15.16 and answer the following questions.

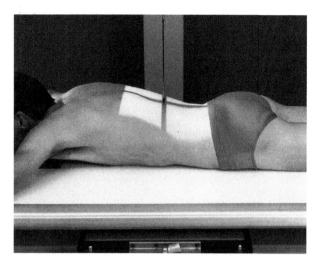

Fig. 15.16 PA stomach and duodenum.

17. True or false. The PA projection with the patient in the prone position demonstrates the contour of the barium-filled stomach and duodenal bulb.

18. True or false. The PA projection with the patient in the upright position shows the size, shape, and relative position of the barium-filled stomach.

19. True or false. A compression band may be placed across the patient's abdomen to immobilize the patient and reduce involuntary movement of the viscera.

20. How should the prone position of the patient be adjusted to prevent the full weight of the abdomen from causing the stomach and duodenum to press against the vertebral column?

21. How should the patient's position be adjusted to center the stomach over the midline of the table?

22. When performing the PA projection on a prone patient, to what level of the patient should the IR be centered?

23. How should the centering of the IR be adjusted if the patient is repositioned from the prone position to the upright position?

24. With which body habitus does the greatest visceral movement occur between the prone position and the upright position?

25. What breathing instructions should be given to the patient when making the exposure?

Items 26-30 pertain to the *PA oblique projection, RAO position*. Examine Fig. 15.17 and answer the following questions.

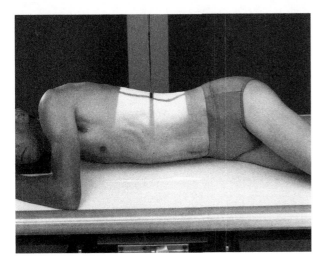

Fig. 15.17 PA oblique stomach and duodenum, RAO position.

26. Describe how the patient should be adjusted from the prone position to the RAO position.

27. How and to where should the central ray be directed?

28. How many degrees should the patient be rotated from the prone position?
    a. 10 to 15
    b. 20 to 35
    c. 40 to 70

29. Which type of body habitus requires the most rotation?
    a. Sthenic
    b. Hyposthenic
    c. Hypersthenic

30. True or false. For the average patient, the PA oblique projection, RAO position, produces the best image of the pyloric canal and the duodenal bulb filled with barium.

Items 31 to 35 pertain to the *AP oblique projection, left posterior oblique (LPO) position*. Examine Fig. 15.18 and answer the following questions.

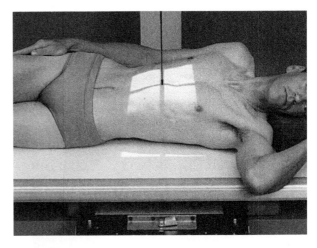

Fig. 15.18 AP oblique stomach and duodenum, LPO position.

31. The AP oblique projection, LPO position, requires the patient's _____ side be elevated away from the table _____ degrees.

32. To what level of the patient should the IR be centered?

33. Where exactly should the central ray enter the patient?

34. The AP oblique projection, LPO position, demonstrates the _____ portion of the stomach filled with barium.

35. Identify each lettered structure shown in Fig. 15.19.

A. _____

B. _____

C. _____

D. _____

E. _____

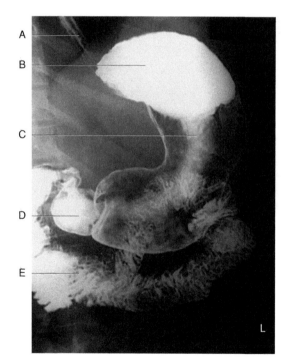

Fig. 15.19 AP oblique stomach and duodenum, LPO position.

Items 36 to 43 pertain to the *right lateral projection*. Examine Fig. 15.20 and answer the following questions.

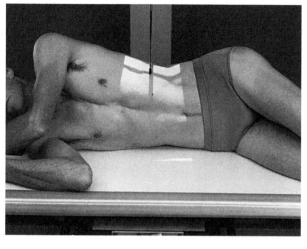

Fig. 15.20 Right lateral stomach and duodenum.

36. Which radiographic body position should be used to demonstrate best the duodenal loop and the duodenojejunal junction filled with contrast medium?
   a. Upright RAO position
   b. Recumbent LPO position
   c. Upright left lateral position
   d. Recumbent right lateral position

37. At which vertebral level should the central ray enter the patient if the patient is in the recumbent position?
   a. T10-T11
   b. L1-L2
   c. L5-S1

38. Approximately how many inches above the lower rib margin should the IR be centered to the recumbent patient?
   a. 1 to 2
   b. 3 to 4
   c. 5 to 6

39. At which vertebral level should the central ray enter the patient if the patient is moved from the recumbent position to the upright lateral position?
   a. T12
   b. L1
   c. L3
   d. L5

40. When examining images of the right lateral projection, which osteologic structures should be examined to determine whether the patient was rotated?
    a. Ribs
    b. Vertebrae
    c. Pelvic bones

41. Describe how and to where the central ray should be directed to the IR and the patient.

42. Examine Fig. 15.21 and indicate whether the following gastric structures are mostly barium-filled or mostly gas-filled:

    a. Stomach fundus: _____

    b. Duodenal bulb: _____

    c. Duodenum: _____

    d. Pyloric portion: _____

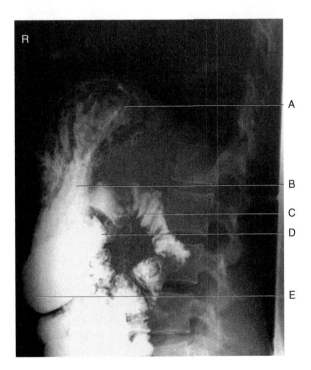

Fig. 15.21 Right lateral stomach.

43. Identify each lettered structure shown in Fig. 15.21.
    A. _____
    B. _____
    C. _____
    D. _____
    E. _____

Items 44 to 49 pertain to the *AP projection*. Examine Fig. 15.22 and answer the following questions.

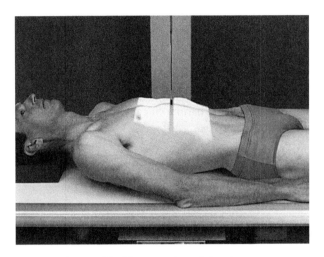

Fig. 15.22 AP stomach and duodenum.

44. Which body position should be used?
    a. Prone
    b. Supine
    c. Upright

45. Which procedure should be performed to help demonstrate a diaphragmatic herniation (hiatal hernia)?
    a. Tilt the table to the Fowler angulation.
    b. Place the patient in the upright position.
    c. Tilt the table to the Trendelenburg angulation.
    d. Place the patient in the right lateral recumbent position.

46. Describe where to center the stomach when a 14-inch × 17-inch (35-cm × 43-cm) exposure field (or CR plate) is used.

47. Describe where to center the stomach when a 10-inch × 12-inch (24-cm × 30-cm) exposure field (or CR plate) is used.

48. How should each of the following structures be demonstrated—barium-filled or gas-filled (double-contrast)?

    a. Body: _____

    b. Fundus: _____

    c. Pylorus: _____

    d. Duodenal bulb: _____

49. Identify each lettered structure shown in Fig. 15.23.

    A. _____

    B. _____

    C. _____

    D. _____

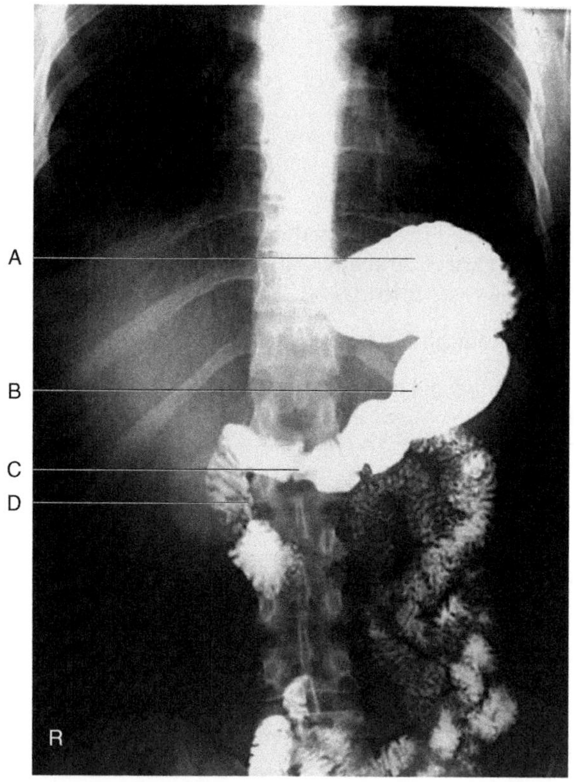

Fig. 15.23 AP stomach and duodenum.

Section 2: Exercise 4: Small Intestine Examination

The small intestine can be radiographically examined by more than one method, often after the stomach is examined. This exercise pertains to the small intestine examination, often referred to as the small bowel series. Provide a short answer or select the answer from a list for each item.

1. List the three methods by which a barium sulfate mixture can be administered for a small bowel series.

2. Which small bowel series method is most commonly used?
   a. Oral
   b. Enteroclysis
   c. Complete reflux

3. Select the four instructions from the following list that are usually given to patients preparing for the oral method of performing a small bowel series.
   a. Have a cleansing enema.
   b. Do not eat breakfast on the morning of the examination.
   c. Do not eat an evening meal the night before the examination.
   d. Swallow laxatives the morning of the examination.
   e. Drink three to four glasses of water the morning of the examination.
   f. Consume nothing by mouth after the evening meal the night before the examination.
   g. Eat a restricted diet (soft, low-residue foods) for 2 days before the examination.

4. Why is a time marker displayed on each image made during the oral method small bowel series?
   a. To show the time of day the exposure was made
   b. To indicate the interval between the exposure of the image and the previous one
   c. To indicate the interval between the exposure of the image and the ingestion of the barium

5. How should the patient be placed for timed images when compression of the abdominal contents is desired?
   a. Prone
   b. Supine
   c. Lateral recumbent

6. Approximately how long after the patient swallows the barium sulfate mixture should the first image be made?
   a. 5 minutes
   b. 15 minutes
   c. 30 minutes

7. Approximately how long after the exposure of the first image should subsequent images be exposed?
   a. 5 to 10 minutes
   b. 15 to 30 minutes
   c. 35 to 45 minutes

8. How might the oral method of small bowel examination be affected by giving the patient a cup of cold water after the administration of the contrast medium?
   a. Peristalsis is accelerated.
   b. Peristalsis is slowed down.
   c. The stomach becomes distended.

9. Which small bowel series method often requires the administration of glucagon or diazepam (Valium) to relax the intestine and reduce patient discomfort during the initial filling of the small intestine?
   a. Oral
   b. Enteroclysis
   c. Complete reflux

10. How should the patient be positioned when the small intestine is to be filled by the complete reflux method?
    a. Prone
    b. Supine
    c. Lateral recumbent

11. Which small bowel series method injects contrast medium through an intestinal tube?
    a. Oral
    b. Enteroclysis
    c. Complete reflux

12. Where in the small intestine should the tube be inserted for the enteroclysis method of performing a small bowel series?
    a. Ileum
    b. Jejunum
    c. Duodenum

13. Which method of performing a small bowel series does not use a cleansing enema as part of patient preparation?
    a. Oral
    b. Enteroclysis
    c. Complete reflux

Items 14 to 20 pertain to the *AP or PA projection*. Examine Fig. 15.24 and answer the following questions.

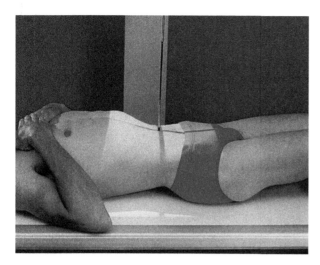

Fig. 15.24 AP small intestine.

14. For the AP projection demonstrating the small intestine, which plane of the body should be centered to the grid?
    a. Horizontal
    b. Midsagittal
    c. Midcoronal

15. For the AP projection demonstrating the small intestine of a sthenic patient within 30 minutes after the administration of contrast medium, to which level of the patient should the IR be centered?
    a. T12
    b. L2
    c. L5

16. For delayed AP projections demonstrating the small intestine of a sthenic patient, to which level of the patient should the IR be centered?
    a. T12
    b. L2
    c. Iliac crests

17. For the AP projection, when should the exposure be made?
    a. At the end of expiration
    b. At the end of inspiration

18. How should the central ray be directed?
    a. Perpendicularly
    b. Angled caudally
    c. Angled cephalically

19. When examining images of a small bowel series, which structure usually indicates adequate demonstration of the entire small intestine?
    a. Cecum
    b. Jejunum
    c. Duodenum

20. From the following list, circle the seven evaluation criteria that indicate small bowel series images were properly performed.
    a. The patient should not be rotated.
    b. A time marker should be included.
    c. No ribs should be seen below the diaphragm.
    d. The exposure factors should demonstrate the anatomy.
    e. The stomach should be included on the initial image.
    f. The vertebral column should be in the middle of the image.
    g. The entire small intestine should be included on each image.
    h. The entire alimentary canal should be included on each image.
    i. The examination is usually completed when barium is visualized in the cecum.
    j. The examination is usually completed when barium is visualized in the jejunum.
    k. The postevacuation image is accomplished after the administration of a cleansing enema.

448

Section 2: Exercise 5: Large Intestine Examination

The large intestine is frequently examined radiographically after the introduction of a suitable contrast medium. This type of examination is called a barium enema (BE). This exercise pertains to the procedures and images used for the two BE methods. Identify structures, fill in missing words, provide a short answer, match columns, select from a list, or choose true or false (explaining any statement you believe to be false) for each item.

1. What are the two basic methods of performing a BE?
   a. Oral and double-contrast
   b. Oral and enteroclysis (intubation)
   c. Single-contrast and double-contrast
   d. Single-contrast and enteroclysis (intubation)

2. What is the most common type of contrast medium used for a BE?

3. Why should a high-density barium product be used as the contrast medium for double-contrast studies?

4. What two radiolucent contrast media can be used during the double-contrast study?

5. When might an orally administered, water-soluble, iodinated contrast medium be used in place of a barium sulfate mixture?

6. What should be included in the instructions generally given to a patient in preparation for a BE?

7. What is considered the most important aspect of patient preparation for the BE?

8. When a patient has a suspected colon perforation or leak, what type of contrast media is used when performing a BE?

9. How could the patient be affected if the barium solution is too warm?

449

10. List three instructions that can be given to the patient to help the patient retain the barium during the examination.

11. What is the maximum height above the level of the anus that a BE bag may be placed on an IV stand?

12. Approximately how far into the rectum should an enema tip be inserted?

13. What wording refers to the last image usually performed as part of a BE examination?

Items 14 to 16 pertain to the *PA projection*. Examine Fig. 15.25 and answer the following questions.

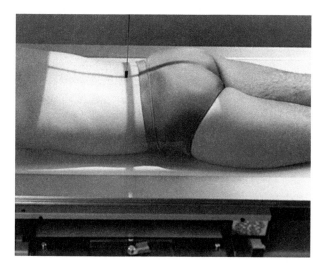

Fig. 15.25 PA large intestine.

14. How should the patient be placed for the PA projection?
    a. Prone
    b. Supine
    c. Upright
    d. Lateral recumbent

15. To which level of the patient should the IR be centered?
    a. T12
    b. L2
    c. Iliac crests
    d. Symphysis pubis

16. How should the central ray be directed for the PA projection?
    a. Perpendicularly
    b. Angled caudally
    c. Angled cephalically

450

17. Identify each lettered structure shown in Fig. 15.26.

A. _____ (flexure)

B. _____ (flexure)

C. _____

D. _____

E. _____

F. _____

G. _____

H. _____

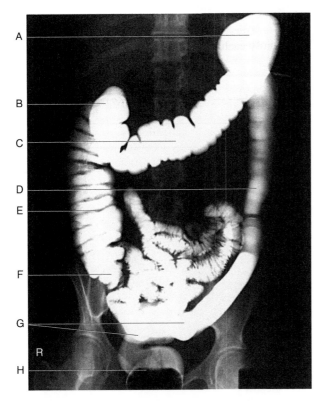

Fig. 15.26 PA large intestine.

Items 18 to 23 pertain to the *PA axial projection*. Examine Fig. 15.27 and answer the following questions.

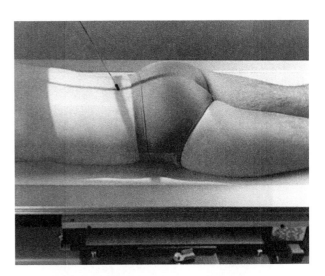

Fig. 15.27 PA axial large intestine.

18. For the PA axial projection, which plane of the body should be centered to the midline of the table?
    a. Transverse
    b. Midsagittal
    c. Midcoronal

19. To which level of the patient should the central ray be directed for the PA axial projection?
    a. L2
    b. Symphysis pubis
    c. Anterior superior iliac spine (ASIS)

20. How should the central ray be directed for the PA axial projection?
    a. Perpendicularly
    b. Angled caudally
    c. Angled cephalically

21. Which area of the large intestine is best demonstrated with the PA axial projection?
    a. Ileocecal
    b. Superior
    c. Rectosigmoid

22. True or false. Both colic flexures should be seen with the PA axial projection.

23. Identify each lettered structure shown in Fig. 15.28.

A. _____ (flexure)

B. _____

C. _____

D. _____

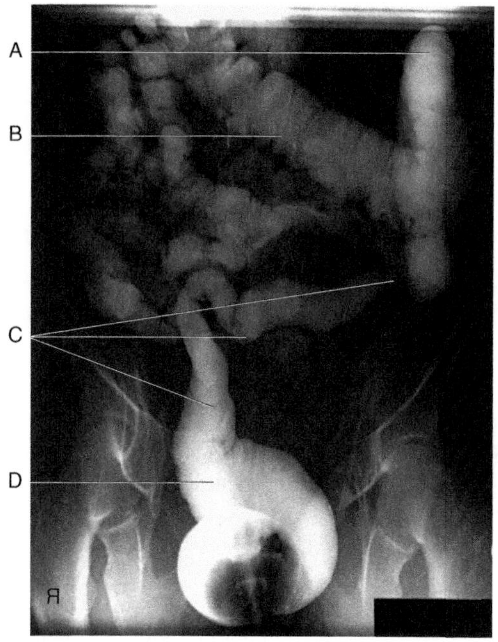

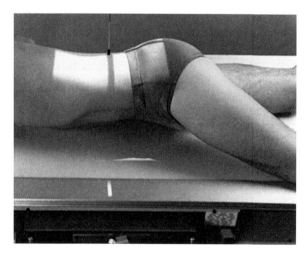

Fig. 15.28 PA axial large intestine.

Items 24 to 28 pertain to the *PA oblique projection, RAO position*. Examine Fig. 15.29 and answer the following questions.

Fig. 15.29 PA oblique large intestine, RAO position.

24. True or false. For the PA oblique projection, RAO position, the patient should be rotated 35 to 45 degrees from the prone position.

25. True or false. For the PA oblique projection, RAO position, the central ray should be directed 35 to 45 degrees caudally.

26. True or false. Both colic flexures should be seen in the RAO position image.

27. True or false. The PA oblique projection, RAO position, is performed primarily to demonstrate the right colic flexure.

28. Identify each lettered structure shown in Fig. 15.30.

A. _____ (flexure)

B. _____ (flexure)

C. _____

D. _____

E. _____

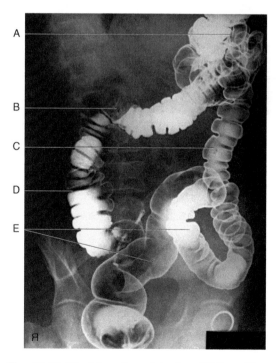

Fig. 15.30 PA oblique large intestine, RAO position.

Items 29 to 31 pertain to the *PA oblique projection, LAO position*. Examine Fig. 15.31 as you answer the following questions.

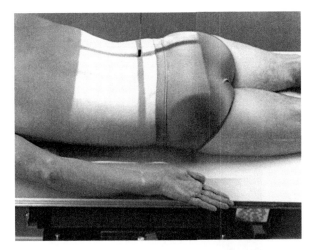

Fig. 15.31 PA oblique large intestine, LAO position.

29. To which level of the patient should the IR be centered for the PA oblique projection, LAO position?
    a. T12
    b. L2
    c. Iliac crests
    d. Symphysis pubis

30. Which two structures of the large intestine are demonstrated primarily with the PA oblique projection, LAO position?
    a. Left colic flexure and ascending colon
    b. Left colic flexure and descending colon
    c. Right colic flexure and ascending colon
    d. Right colic flexure and descending colon

31. Identify each lettered structure shown in Fig. 15.32.
    A. _____ (flexure)
    B. _____ (flexure)
    C. _____
    D. _____
    E. _____
    F. _____
    G. _____

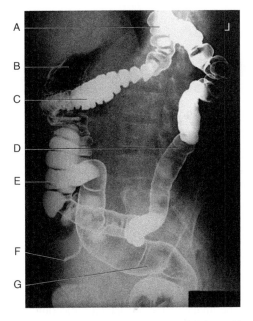

Fig. 15.32 PA oblique large intestine, LAO position.

Chapter **15** **Digestive System: Salivary Glands, Alimentary Canal, and Biliary System**

Items 32 to 36 pertain to the *lateral projection*. Examine Fig. 15.33 and answer the following questions.

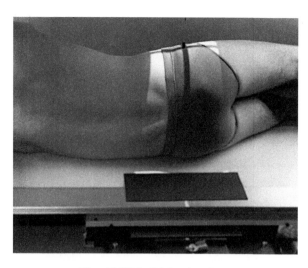

Fig. 15.33 Left lateral rectum.

32. For the lateral projection, to what level of the patient should an IR that is 10 × 12 inches (24 × 30 cm) be centered?

33. In the image of the left lateral projection, how is it determined that the patient was not rotated?

34. Which portions of the large intestine are of prime interest with the lateral projection?
    a. Sigmoid and rectum
    b. Cecum and ascending colon
    c. Lift colic flexure and descending colon
    d. Right colic flexure and ascending colon

35. For the lateral projection, which plane of the body should be centered to the midline of the table?
    a. Transverse
    b. Midsagittal
    c. Midcoronal

36. Identify each lettered structure shown in Fig. 15.34.

    A. _____

    B. _____

    C. _____

    D. _____

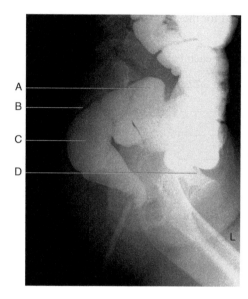

Fig. 15.34 Left lateral rectum.

Items 37 to 41 pertain to the *AP projection*. Examine Fig. 15.35 and answer the following questions.

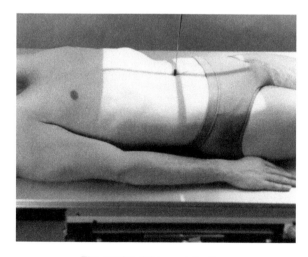

Fig. 15.35 AP large intestine.

37. Which plane of the body should be centered to the grid for the AP projection?

38. To what level of the patient should the IR be centered?

_____

39. True or false. The patient should suspend respiration for the exposure.

40. True or false. The entire colon should be demonstrated for the AP projection.

41. Identify each lettered structure shown in Fig. 15.36.

A. _____ (flexure)

B. _____

C. _____ (flexure)

D. _____

E. _____

F. _____

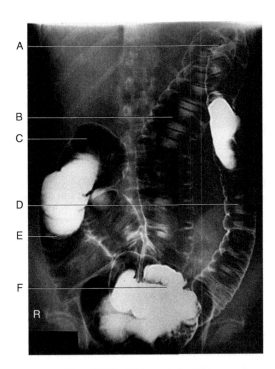

Fig. 15.36 AP large intestine.

Items 42 to 46 pertain to the *AP axial projection*. Examine Fig. 15.37 and answer the following questions.

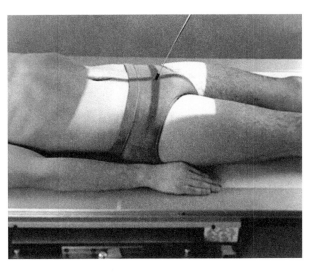

Fig. 15.37 AP axial large intestine.

42. Which projection produces an image similar to the AP axial projection?
   a. AP projection
   b. PA axial projection
   c. PA oblique projection, LAO position
   d. PA oblique projection, RAO position

43. In which direction and how many degrees should the central ray be directed?
   a. Caudally 10 to 20 degrees
   b. Caudally 30 to 40 degrees
   c. Cephalically 10 to 20 degrees
   d. Cephalically 30 to 40 degrees

Chapter **15 Digestive System: Salivary Glands, Alimentary Canal, and Biliary System**

44. For the AP axial projection, where on the patient's anterior surface should the central ray enter when a 14-inch × 17-inch (35-cm × 43-cm) IR is used?

45. To produce a coned-down image of the AP axial projection on an IR that is 10 × 12 inches (24 × 30 cm), where on the patient should the central ray enter?

46. Identify each lettered structure shown in Fig. 15.38.

A. _____

B. _____

C. _____

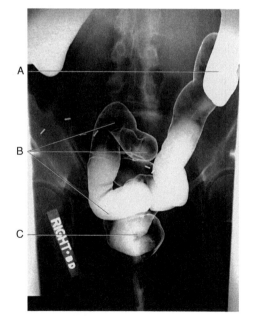

Fig. 15.38 AP axial large intestine.

Items 47 to 51 pertain to the *AP oblique projection, LPO position*. Examine Fig. 15.39 and answer the following questions.

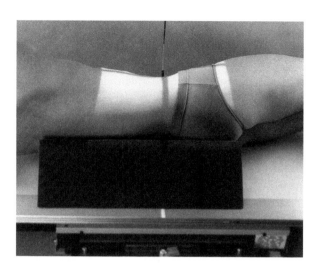

Fig. 15.39 AP oblique large intestine, LPO position.

47. The AP oblique projection, LPO position, produces an image similar to the _____ projection (_____ position).

48. For the AP oblique projection, LPO position, the patient should be rotated _____ to _____ degrees.

49. For the AP oblique projection, LPO position, which side of the patient (right or left) should be elevated away from the x-ray table?

50. Which flexure (right colic or left colic) should be well demonstrated with the AP oblique projection, LPO position?

51. Identify each lettered structure shown in Fig. 15.40.

A. _____ (flexure)

B. _____ (flexure)

C. _____

D. _____

E. _____

F. _____

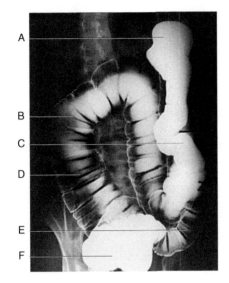

Fig. 15.40 AP oblique large intestine, LPO position.

Items 52 to 55 pertain to the *AP oblique projection, right posterior oblique (RPO) position.* Examine Fig. 15.41 and answer the following questions.

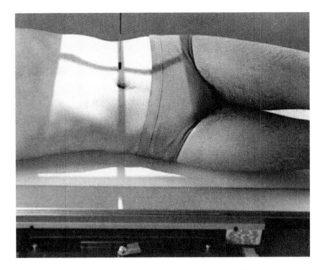

Fig. 15.41 AP oblique large intestine, RPO position.

52. What other oblique position produces an image similar to the AP oblique projection, RPO position?

53. Which flexure (right colic or left colic) should be well demonstrated with the AP oblique projection, RPO position?

Chapter **15 Digestive System: Salivary Glands, Alimentary Canal, and Biliary System**

54. How many degrees should the patient be rotated from the supine position for the AP oblique projection, RPO position?

55. Identify each lettered structure shown in Fig. 15.42.

A. _____ (flexure)

B. _____

C. _____ (flexure)

D. _____

E. _____

F. _____

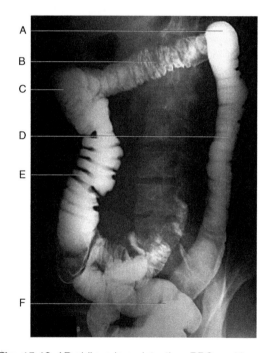

Fig. 15.42 AP oblique large intestine, RPO position.

Items 56 to 60 pertain to *AP or PA projections, right and left lateral decubitus positions*. Examine Figs. 15.43 and 15.44 and answer the following questions.

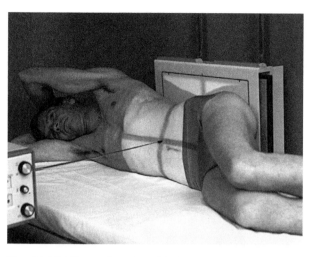

Fig. 15.43 AP large intestine, right lateral decubitus position.

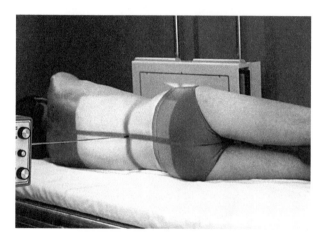

Fig. 15.44 PA large intestine, left lateral decubitus position.

56. Which BE projection requires that the patient be placed in the right lateral recumbent position and that a horizontal central ray be directed to the midline of the patient at the level of the iliac crests?
a. Right lateral
b. AP oblique, RPO position
c. PA oblique, RAO position
d. AP, right lateral decubitus position

57. For lateral decubitus positions, what should be accomplished to ensure that the dependent side of the patient is demonstrated?

59. Name the lateral decubitus position that best demonstrates each of the following intestinal structures.

    a. Left colic flexure: _____

    b. Right colic flexure: _____

58. How much of the colon should be demonstrated in the image of a lateral decubitus position?

_____

60. Figs. 15.45 and 15.46 are lateral decubitus images. Examine the images and answer the questions that follow.

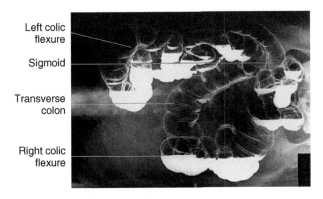

Fig. **15.45** Image of the large intestine, lateral decubitus position.

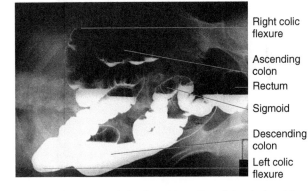

Fig. **15.46** Image of the large intestine, lateral decubitus position.

    a. Which image shows the left lateral decubitus position?

    _____.

    b. Which image shows the right lateral decubitus position?

    _____.

    c. Which image best demonstrates the left colic flexure?

    _____.

    d. Which image best demonstrates the right colic flexure?

    _____.

    e. Which image requires that the patient be placed in the left lateral recumbent position?

    _____.

    f. Which image requires that the patient be placed in the right lateral recumbent position?

    _____.

Questions 61 and 62 pertain to BE images performed with the patient in the upright position.

61. For upright frontal, oblique, and lateral projections, how is the centering of the IR adjusted from that used for the recumbent positions? Why is this compensation necessary?

62. Examine Fig. 15.47 and answer the questions that follow.

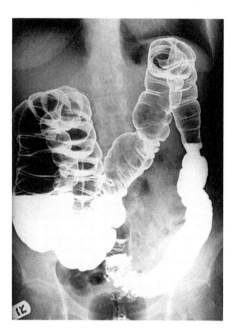

Fig. 15.47 AP large intestine.

a. What body position was used to make this image?

b. What image characteristics led you to that conclusion?

63. Figs. 15.48 to 15.55 represent different projections used to obtain BE images. Examine the images, then match the figures in Column A with the positions/projections in Column B.

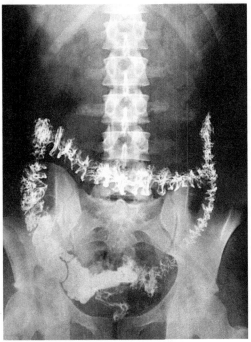

Fig. 15.48 BE image.

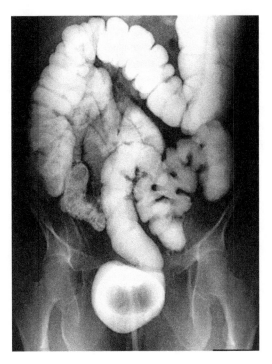

Fig. 15.49 BE image.

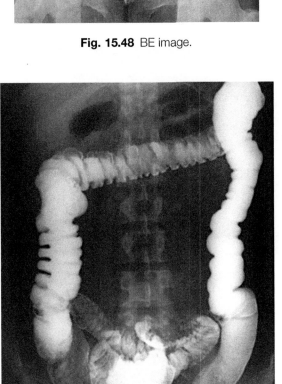

Fig. 15.50 BE image.

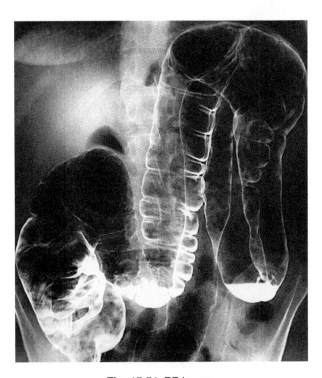

Fig. 15.51 BE image.

Chapter **15** **Digestive System: Salivary Glands, Alimentary Canal, and Biliary System**

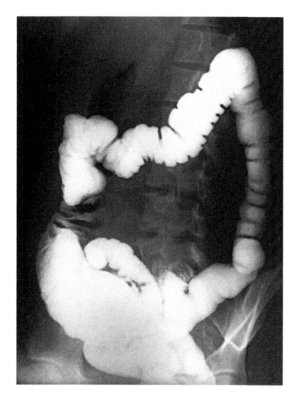

Fig. 15.52 BE image.

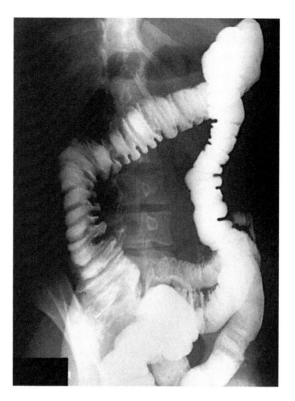

Fig. 15.53 BE image.

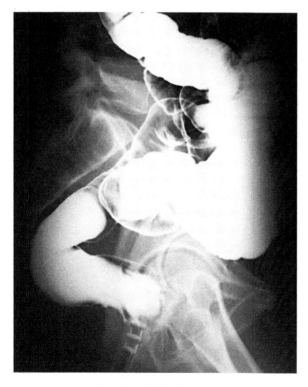

Fig. 15.54 BE image.

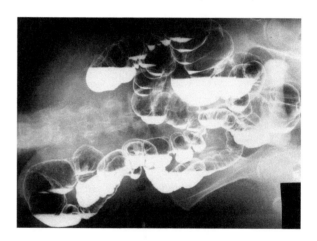

Fig. 15.55 BE image.

Column A		Column B
_____	1. Fig. 15.48	a. LAO position
_____	2. Fig. 15.49	b. LPO position
_____	3. Fig. 15.50	c. AP axial projection
_____	4. Fig. 15.51	d. PA, upright position
_____	5. Fig. 15.52	e. AP, recumbent position
_____	6. Fig. 15.53	f. Left lateral position
_____	7. Fig. 15.54	g. Postevacuation
_____	8. Fig. 15.55	h. Lateral decubitus position

CHAPTER 15: SELF-TEST: ANATOMY AND POSITIONING OF THE DIGESTIVE SYSTEM: SALIVARY GLANDS, ALIMENTARY CANAL, AND BILIARY SYSTEM

Answer the following questions by selecting the best choice.

1. What is the first division of the digestive system?
   a. Mouth
   b. Stomach
   c. Small intestine
   d. Salivary glands

2. Which salivary gland is the largest?
   a. Parotid
   b. Sublingual
   c. Submandibular

3. Which salivary glands are the smallest?
   a. Parotid
   b. Sublingual
   c. Submandibular

4. Which salivary glands are located along the lateral aspect of the mandibular ramus?
   a. Parotid
   b. Sublingual
   c. Submandibular

5. Which salivary duct opens into the oral vestibule opposite the second upper molar?
   a. Parotid
   b. Sublingual
   c. Submandibular

6. Which two imaging modalities have greatly reduced the frequency of sialography?
   a. Computed tomography and ultrasonography
   b. Computed tomography and magnetic resonance imaging
   c. Conventional tomography and ultrasonography
   d. Conventional tomography and magnetic resonance imaging

7. For sialography, into which structure is the contrast medium injected?
   a. Vein
   b. Artery
   c. Muscle
   d. Salivary duct

8. Which sialographic projection directs the central ray along the mandibular ramus?
   a. Lateral projection
   b. Tangential projection
   c. Verticosubmental projection
   d. Submentovertical projection

9. Which sialographic projection demonstrates a parotid gland superimposed over a mandibular ramus?
   a. Lateral projection
   b. Tangential projection
   c. Verticosubmental projection
   d. AP axial projection

10. Which two sialographic projections best demonstrate the parotid gland?
   a. Axiolateral and lateral projections
   b. Axiolateral and verticosubmental projections
   c. Tangential and lateral projections
   d. Tangential and verticosubmental projections

11. Which gland is demonstrated with tangential projections?
   a. Parotid
   b. Sublingual
   c. Submandibular

12. Which sialographic projection demonstrates parotid and submandibular glands?
   a. Lateral projection
   b. Tangential projection
   c. AP axial projection

13. Which salivary gland can be demonstrated with a lateral projection when the patient's head is adjusted so that the midsagittal plane is rotated approximately 15 degrees toward the IR from true lateral and the central ray is directed to a point 1 inch (2.5 cm) above the mandibular ramus?
   a. Parotid
   b. Sublingual
   c. Submandibular

14. Which salivary gland can be demonstrated with a lateral projection when the patient's head is positioned true lateral and a perpendicular central ray is directed to the inferior margin of the mandibular angle?
   a. Parotid
   b. Sublingual
   c. Submandibular

15. For the lateral projection demonstrating the submandibular gland, what is the purpose of pressing the tongue to the floor of the mouth?
   a. To hold the intraoral film in place
   b. To displace the submandibular gland below the mandible
   c. To prevent the tongue from superimposing the submandibular gland

16. In which body habitus type is the stomach almost horizontal and high in the abdomen?
    a. Sthenic
    b. Asthenic
    c. Hyposthenic
    d. Hypersthenic

17. Which curvature is located on the right (medial) border of the stomach?
    a. Lesser
    b. Greater
    c. Inferior
    d. Superior

18. Which area is the most superior part of the stomach?
    a. Head
    b. Body
    c. Fundus
    d. Pylorus

19. Which area is the most inferior part of the stomach?
    a. Body
    b. Cardia
    c. Fundus
    d. Pylorus

20. The distal esophagus empties its contents into which of the following?
    a. Duodenum
    b. Pyloric canal
    c. Duodenal bulb
    d. Cardiac antrum

21. Which opening is located between the stomach and small intestine?
    a. Cardiac orifice
    b. Pyloric orifice
    c. Ileocecal orifice
    d. Hepatopancreatic ampulla

22. Which opening is at the distal end of the small intestine?
    a. Anus
    b. Cardiac orifice
    c. Pyloric orifice
    d. Ileocecal orifice

23. Which structure is the proximal part of the small intestine?
    a. Ileum
    b. Pylorus
    c. Jejunum
    d. Duodenum

24. Which structure is the distal part of the small intestine?
    a. Ileum
    b. Cecum
    c. Jejunum
    d. Duodenum

25. In which abdominal region does the large intestine originate?
    a. Left iliac
    b. Right iliac
    c. Left lumbar
    d. Right lumbar

26. Which structure is the proximal part of the large intestine?
    a. Ileum
    b. Cecum
    c. Rectum
    d. Sigmoid

27. Which part of the large intestine is located between the ascending and descending parts of the colon?
    a. Cecum
    b. Rectum
    c. Sigmoid
    d. Transverse colon

28. Which structure is located between the ascending colon and the transverse colon?
    a. Sigmoid
    b. Left colic flexure
    c. Right colic flexure
    d. Descending colon

29. Where in the large intestine is the left colic flexure located?
    a. Between the cecum and the ascending colon
    b. Between the ascending colon and the transverse colon
    c. Between the transverse colon and the descending colon
    d. Between the descending colon and the sigmoid

30. Which structure is the pouchlike part of the large intestine situated below the junction of the ileum and the colon?
    a. Cecum
    b. Rectum
    c. Sigmoid
    d. Vermiform appendix

31. Where in the large intestine is the sigmoid located?
    a. Between the cecum and the transverse colon
    b. Between the ascending colon and the transverse colon
    c. Between the descending colon and the rectum
    d. Between the transverse colon and the descending colon

32. Approximately how long does it usually take the first part of a barium meal to reach the ileocecal valve?
    a. 30 minutes to 1 hour
    b. 2 to 3 hours
    c. 4 to 5 hours
    d. 24 hours

33. Approximately how long does it usually take a barium meal to reach the rectum?
    a. 2 to 3 hours
    b. 4 to 5 hours
    c. 6 to 8 hours
    d. 24 hours

34. Which two imaging modalities are most commonly used to examine the alimentary canal after the introduction of a barium product?
    a. Fluoroscopy and sonography
    b. Fluoroscopy and radiography
    c. Computed tomography and sonography
    d. Computed tomography and radiography

35. Which type of contrast medium is most commonly used for examining the upper GI tract?
    a. An oily, viscous compound
    b. A barium sulfate suspension
    c. A nonionic injectable compound
    d. A water-soluble, iodinated solution

36. To demonstrate swallowing function best, in which position should the patient be placed to begin the fluoroscopic phase of single-contrast examinations of the esophagus?
    a. Upright
    b. Left lateral decubitus
    c. Recumbent LAO
    d. Recumbent RPO

37. Which two recumbent oblique positions can be used to demonstrate best an unobstructed image of a barium-filled esophagus between the vertebrae and the heart?
    a. LAO and LPO
    b. LAO and RPO
    c. RAO and LPO
    d. RAO and RPO

38. Which of the following is a major advantage of double-contrast UGI examination over single-contrast UGI examination?
    a. The patient can tolerate the procedure better.
    b. Radiation exposure to the patient is reduced.
    c. Small lesions on the mucosal lining are better demonstrated.
    d. The examination can be performed with the patient upright instead of recumbent.

39. Which description refers to the biphasic GI examination?
    a. Single-contrast study of the entire alimentary canal
    b. Single-contrast study of the upper GI tract
    c. Double-contrast study of the upper GI tract
    d. Combination single-contrast and double-contrast study of the upper GI tract

40. Which body habitus produces the greatest visceral movement when a patient is moved from the prone position to the upright position?
    a. Sthenic
    b. Asthenic
    c. Hyposthenic
    d. Hypersthenic

41. For the PA projection as part of the UGI examination, why should the lower lung fields be included on a 14-inch × 17-inch (35-cm × 43-cm) radiation field?
    a. To demonstrate pneumothorax
    b. To demonstrate a possible hiatal hernia
    c. To demonstrate fluid levels in the thorax
    d. To demonstrate the gas bubble in the fundus of the stomach

42. For the double-contrast UGI examination, which projection produces the best image of a gas-filled duodenal bulb and pyloric canal?
    a. AP oblique projection, upright LPO position
    b. AP oblique projection, recumbent LPO position
    c. PA oblique projection, upright RAO position
    d. PA oblique projection, recumbent RAO position

43. For the single-contrast UGI examination with the patient recumbent, which projection produces the best image of a barium-filled pyloric canal and duodenal bulb in patients whose habitus approximates the sthenic type?
    a. AP projection
    b. Left lateral projection
    c. AP oblique projection, LPO position
    d. PA oblique projection, RAO position

44. For the UGI examination with the patient recumbent, which projection best stimulates gastric peristalsis to demonstrate the pyloric canal and duodenal bulb better?
    a. AP projection
    b. Left lateral projection
    c. AP oblique projection, LPO position
    d. PA oblique projection, RAO position

45. Which breathing procedure should the patient perform when UGI images are exposed?
    a. Slow, deep breathing
    b. Quick, panting breaths
    c. Suspended expiration
    d. Suspended inspiration

46. For the double-contrast UGI examination with the patient recumbent, which projection produces the best image of a gas-filled fundus?
    a. Left lateral projection
    b. AP projection, left lateral decubitus position
    c. AP oblique projection, LPO position
    d. PA oblique projection, RAO position

47. For the UGI examination with the patient recumbent, which projection best demonstrates the right retro-gastric space?
    a. Right lateral projection
    b. AP projection, right lateral decubitus position
    c. AP oblique projection, LPO position
    d. PA oblique projection, RAO position

48. For the AP projection with the patient supine (as part of the UGI examination), which procedure should be performed to demonstrate best a diaphragmatic herniation (hiatal hernia)?
    a. Angle the central ray 30 to 35 degrees caudally.
    b. Tilt the table and patient into a full Trendelenburg position.
    c. Instruct the patient to suspend respiration after full inspiration.
    d. Place radiolucent cushions under the thorax to elevate the shoulders.

49. To which level of the patient should the central ray be directed for the PA oblique projection, RAO position, as part of the UGI examination?
    a. T9-T10
    b. T11-T12
    c. L1-L2
    d. L3-L4

50. Which examination of the alimentary canal requires that a series of images be taken at specific time intervals after the ingestion of the contrast medium?
    a. UGI series
    b. BE
    c. Esophagography
    d. Small bowel series

51. For a small bowel series of a patient with hypomotility of the small intestine, which procedure should be performed to accelerate peristalsis?
    a. Roll the patient 360 degrees.
    b. Instruct the patient to drink a glass of ice water.
    c. Instruct the patient to perform the Valsalva maneuver.
    d. Tilt the table and patient into a full Trendelenburg position.

52. Which structure, when visualized on an image as part of a small bowel series, usually indicates the completion of the examination?
    a. Ileum
    b. Cecum
    c. Jejunum
    d. Duodenum

53. What is the proper sequence for filling the large intestine with barium when performing a BE?
    a. Rectum, sigmoid, ascending colon, transverse colon, and descending colon
    b. Rectum, sigmoid, descending colon, transverse colon, and ascending colon
    c. Sigmoid, rectum, ascending colon, transverse colon, and descending colon
    d. Sigmoid, rectum, descending colon, transverse colon, and ascending colon

54. Which instructions should be given to the patient if cramping is experienced during filling of the large intestine for a BE?
    a. Perform the Valsalva maneuver.
    b. Contract the anus tightly.
    c. Concentrate on deep oral breathing.
    d. Take shallow, rapid breaths or pant.

55. Before the enema tip is inserted during a BE, why should a small amount of barium sulfate mixture be allowed to run into a waste basin?
    a. To lubricate the enema tip
    b. To remove air from the tube
    c. To determine if the mixture is too warm or too cold
    d. To ensure that the consistency of the mixture is adequate

56. Which procedure should be accomplished when inserting the enema tip for a BE?
    a. Lubricate the tip with petroleum jelly.
    b. Place the patient in the Trendelenburg position.
    c. Inflate the air-filled retention tip before insertion.
    d. Ensure that the tip is inserted no more than 3½ to 4 inches (8.9 to 10 cm).

57. For the PA projection during a BE, what is the advantage of placing the x-ray table and patient in a slight Trendelenburg position?
    a. To demonstrate the ileocecal valve
    b. To enable more air to be injected into the colon
    c. To help separate overlapping loops of the distal bowel
    d. To move the transverse colon higher in the abdomen

58. Which structures of the large intestine are of primary interest with AP axial or PA axial projections during a BE?
    a. Sigmoid and rectum
    b. Cecum and ileocecal valve
    c. Left and right colic flexures
    d. Ascending and descending colons

59. How many degrees and in which direction should the central ray be directed for the PA axial projection during a BE?
    a. 20 to 25 degrees caudal
    b. 20 to 25 degrees cephalic
    c. 30 to 40 degrees caudal
    d. 30 to 40 degrees cephalic

60. Which structure of the large intestine is of primary interest for the PA oblique projection, RAO position, during BE examinations?
    a. Anal canal
    b. Left colic flexure
    c. Right colic flexure
    d. Descending colon

61. Which two oblique projections can be performed to demonstrate best the left colic flexure during a BE?
    a. PA oblique projection, LAO position; AP oblique projection, LPO position
    b. PA oblique projection, LAO position; AP oblique projection, RPO position
    c. PA oblique projection, RAO position; AP oblique projection, LPO position
    d. PA oblique projection, RAO position; AP oblique projection, RPO position

62. Which structure of the large intestine is best demonstrated if the patient is rotated 45 degrees from a supine position to move the right side of the abdomen away from the x-ray table during a BE?
    a. Ileum
    b. Cecum
    c. Left colic flexure
    d. Right colic flexure

63. For the right lateral decubitus position as part of a BE, which procedure should be done to ensure that the ascending colon is demonstrated in the image?
    a. Center the IR to the iliac crests.
    b. Elevate the patient on a radiolucent support.
    c. Tilt the table and patient into a full Trendelenburg position.
    d. Make the exposure after the patient suspends respiration.

64. Which BE projection requires that a 10-inch × 12-inch (24-cm × 30-cm) lengthwise exposure field or CR plate be centered to the level of the ASIS?
    a. AP projection
    b. Lateral projection
    c. AP projection, left lateral decubitus position
    d. AP oblique projection, LPO position

65. Which BE projection does not require colic flexures to be included in the image?
    a. AP projection
    b. Lateral projection
    c. AP projection, lateral decubitus position
    d. PA oblique projection, RAO position

Chapter **15** **Digestive System: Salivary Glands, Alimentary Canal, and Biliary System**

16 Urinary System and Venipuncture

ANATOMY OF THE URINARY SYSTEM

Section 1: Exercise 1

This exercise pertains to urinary structures. Identify structures for each question.

1. Identify each lettered structure shown in Fig. 16.1.

    A. _____

    B. _____

    C. _____

    D. _____

    E. _____

    F. _____

2. Identify each lettered structure shown in Fig. 16.2.

    A. _____

    B. _____

    C. _____

    D. _____

    E. _____

    F. _____

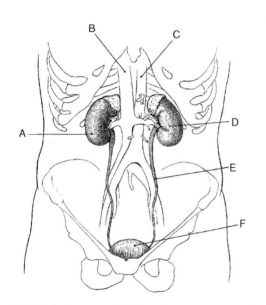

Fig. 16.1 Anterior aspect of the urinary system in relation to the surrounding structures.

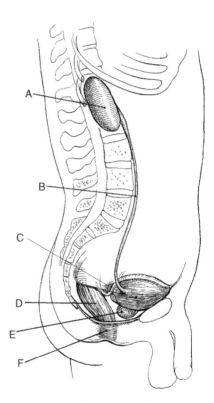

Fig. 16.2 Lateral aspect of the male urinary system in relation to the surrounding structures.

3. Identify each lettered part of the kidney shown in Fig. 16.3.

A. _____

B. _____

C. _____

D. _____

E. _____

F. _____

G. _____

H. _____

I. _____

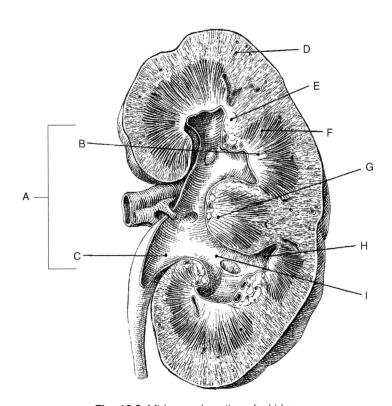

Fig. 16.3 Midcoronal section of a kidney.

4. Identify each lettered structure shown in Fig. 16.4.

A. _____

B. _____

C. _____

D. _____

E. _____

F. _____

G. _____

H. _____

I. _____

J. _____

K. _____

5. Identify each lettered structure shown in Fig. 16.5.

A. _____

B. _____

C. _____

D. _____

E. _____

F. _____

G. _____

H. _____

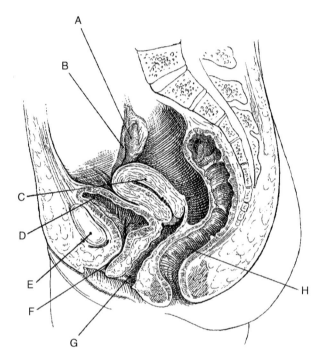

Fig. 16.5 Midsagittal section through the female pelvis.

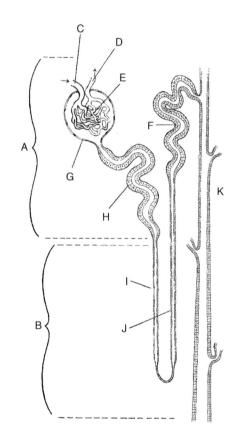

Fig. 16.4 Diagram of a nephron and collecting duct.

6. Identify each lettered structure shown in Fig. 16.6.

A. _____

B. _____

C. _____

D. _____

E. _____

F. _____

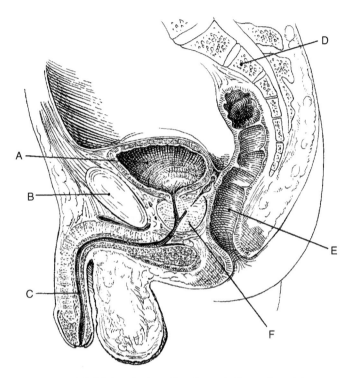

Fig. 16.6 Midsagittal section through the male pelvis.

Section 1: Exercise 2

Use the following clues to complete the crossword puzzle. All answers refer to the urinary system.

Across

3. Outer renal tissue
4. This arteriole leaves the capsule
6. Filtrate derivative
7. Another term for suprarenal
8. Urine vessel from glomerular capsule
10. Cup-shaped urine receivers
12. Cone-shaped renal segments
15. Cluster of blood vessels
16. Urinary reservoir
17. Functional renal unit
18. Musculomembranous excretory duct
19. Medial opening of a kidney

Down

1. This arteriole enters the capsule
2. Inner renal tissue
3. Membranous cup; Bowman _____
5. Central renal cavity
6. External excretory tube
9. Male gland
11. Gland that is found on a kidney
13. Glomerular fluid
14. Primary organ of urinary system

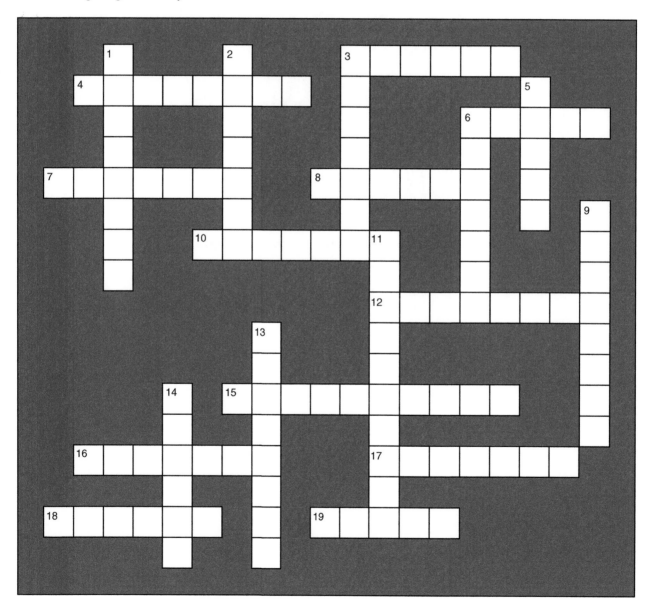

Chapter **16** **Urinary System and Venipuncture**

Section 1: Exercise 3

Match the pathology terms in Column A with the appropriate definition in Column B. Not all choices from Column B should be selected.

Column A

_____ 1. Wilms tumor

_____ 2. Fistula

_____ 3. Cystitis

_____ 4. Stenosis

_____ 5. Calculus

_____ 6. Renal cell carcinoma

_____ 7. Ureterocele

_____ 8. Pyelonephritis

_____ 9. Hydronephrosis

_____ 10. Polycystic kidney

_____ 11. Renal obstruction

_____ 12. Renal hypertension

_____ 13. Glomerulonephritis

_____ 14. Congenital anomaly

_____ 15. Vesicoureteral reflux

Column B

a. Inflammation of the bladder

b. Enlargement of the prostate

c. Abnormality present since birth

d. Narrowing or contraction of a passage

e. Increased blood pressure to the kidneys

f. Inflammation of the kidney and renal pelvis

g. Most common childhood abdominal malignant neoplasm

h. Distention of the renal pelvis and calyces with urine

i. Backward flow of urine from the bladder into the ureters

j. Ballooning of the lower end of the ureter into the bladder

k. Abnormal concretion of mineral salts, often called a stone

l. Malignant new growth located in the kidney

m. Inflammation of the capillary loops in the glomeruli of the kidneys

n. Massive enlargement of the kidney with the formation of many cysts

o. Condition preventing the normal flow of urine through the urinary system

p. Abnormal connection between two internal organs or between an organ and the body surface

Section 1: Exercise 4

This exercise pertains to the anatomy of the urinary system. Fill in missing words for each question.

1. The kidneys and ureters are part of the _____ system.

2. The organ that removes waste products from the blood is the _____.

3. The gland that sits on the superior pole of each kidney is the _____ gland.

4. Blood vessels, nerves, and the ureter enter a kidney through an opening known as the _____.

5. The hilum is located on the _____ border of the kidney.

6. In the average (sthenic) person, the superior pole of the kidney is located at the _____ vertebral level.

7. The microscopic functional unit of the kidney is the _____.

8. Nephron units are found in the layer of renal tissue known as the _____.

9. The proximal portion of a nephron consisting of a double-walled membranous cup is the _____ capsule.

10. A cluster of blood capillaries surrounded by a Bowman capsule is a _____.

11. A glomerulus branches off the _____ artery.

12. The blood vessel entering a glomerular capsule is the _____ arteriole; the blood vessel leaving a glomerular capsule is the _____ arteriole.

13. The fluid that passes from the glomerulus to the glomerular capsule is _____.

14. Urine from collecting ducts drains into minor _____.

15. Minor calyces drain urine into major _____.

16. Major calyces unite to form the expanded, funnel-shaped renal _____.

17. The long tubes that transport urine from the kidneys are the _____.

18. Ureters transport urine from the kidneys to the _____.

19. The musculomembranous tube that conveys urine from the urinary bladder to outside the body is the _____.

20. The gland that surrounds the proximal part of the male urethra is the _____.

Section 1: Exercise 5: Abbreviations

This exercise provides practice in the use of the common abbreviations related to urinary system radiography and the imaging profession. Write out the expanded form beside each abbreviation.

1. VCUG: _____

2. IVU: _____

3. ACR: _____

4. BPH: _____

5. UVJ: _____

6. GFR: _____

Section 1: Exercise 6: Venipuncture and IV Contrast Media Administration

This exercise pertains to venipuncture and intravenous (IV) contrast media administration. Items require you to write a short answer or select from a list.

1. Which condition should be prevented if strict aseptic techniques are used when administering IV medications?
   a. The patient lapsing into shock
   b. Introducing infection into the patient
   c. Injecting an excessive amount of medication

2. How does the use of an IV filter affect a bolus injection?
   a. The rate of injection will be reduced.
   b. The introduction of foreign matter will increase.
   c. The time required to inject the medication will be reduced.

3. What are the three parts of a syringe?
   a. Tip, barrel, and bevel
   b. Tip, barrel, and plunger
   c. Hub, cannula, and bevel
   d. Hub, cannula, and plunger

4. What are the three parts of a hypodermic needle?
   a. Tip, barrel, and bevel
   b. Tip, barrel, and plunger
   c. Hub, cannula, and bevel
   d. Hub, cannula, and plunger

5. To what does the term *needle gauge* refer?
   a. The angle of the bevel
   b. The length of the needle
   c. The diameter of the needle

6. What injection apparatus is preferred for most IV administrations?
   a. Butterfly set
   b. Over-the-needle cannula
   c. Seldinger-technique needle

7. Which procedure should be performed to maintain a closed system with a multiple-dose vial of medication?
   a. Discard the vial after the second use.
   b. Inject into the bottle an amount of air equal to the amount of fluid to be withdrawn.
   c. Inject into the bottle an amount of sterile saline solution equal to the amount of fluid to be withdrawn.

8. When assessing vessels for venipuncture, why should a vessel not be used if a pulse is detected?
   a. A pulse indicates the vessel is an artery.
   b. A pulse indicates the patient is hypertensive.
   c. A pulse indicates the patient has low blood pressure.
   d. A pulse indicates the patient has a fistula in that vessel.

9. Circle the four sites that are most often used for establishing IV access.
   a. Anterior hand
   b. Posterior hand
   c. Femoral artery
   d. Anterior forearm
   e. Posterior forearm
   f. Ulnar aspect of the wrist
   g. Radial aspect of the wrist
   h. Anterior aspect of the elbow

10. Describe how the skin should be prepared before inserting a needle into a vein.

11. How far above the site of a venipuncture should the tourniquet be placed?

12. How should the IV needle be inserted (bevel up or bevel down)?

13. When inserting an IV needle into the patient, what angle should exist between the needle and the patient's skin surface?

475

14. What is the significance of a backflow of blood into the syringe during a venipuncture procedure?

15. What procedure should a radiographer perform if the needle has punctured both walls of the vein?

16. What is infiltration?
    a. The procedure for using an IV filter in tubing
    b. The introduction of a hypodermic needle into a vein
    c. The process of injecting fluid into tissues instead of a vein

17. Which other term refers to infiltration?
    a. Extraction
    b. Extirpation
    c. Extravasation

18. Which procedure should a radiographer perform after a needle has been removed from a vein?
    a. Apply a tourniquet 3 to 4 inches (7.6 to 10 cm) above the puncture site.
    b. Using a 2-inch × 2-inch (5-cm × 5-cm) pad of gauze, apply pressure directly to the injection site.
    c. Clean the area using a circular motion covering an area that is approximately 2 inches (5 cm) in diameter.

19. Circle the four symptoms that may indicate the occurrence of infiltration.
    a. Pain
    b. Burning
    c. Redness
    d. Swelling
    e. Dyspnea
    f. Sneezing
    g. Rapid pulse
    h. Hypotension

20. Circle the five golden rules of medication administration.
    a. The right time
    b. The right route
    c. The right patient
    d. The right syringe
    e. The right amount
    f. The right medication
    g. The right technologist
    h. The right body position

21. Number the following ten steps in the correct order that a technologist would perform venipuncture:

    _____ Anchor the needle with tape and a dressing.

    _____ Release the tourniquet.

    _____ Using the dominant hand, the technologist places the needle bevel up at a 45-degree angle to the skin's surface.

    _____ The technologist puts on gloves and cleans the area.

    _____ The technologist holds the patient's limb with the nondominant hand, using that thumb to stabilize and anchor the selected vein.

    _____ After the vein is punctured and blood return is noted, the cannula is advanced.

    _____ A local anesthetic is administered according to facility policy (optional).

    _____ The technologist uses a quick, sharp darting motion to enter the skin with the needle.

    _____ A tourniquet is placed 6 to 8 inches (15 to 20 cm) above the intended site of puncture.

    _____ If a backflow of blood does not occur, verify venous access before injecting the medication.

POSITIONING OF THE URINARY SYSTEM

Section 2: Exercise 1: Excretory Urography

Radiography of the urinary system comprises numerous specialized procedures. The most common radiographic examination of the urinary system is the excretory urogram. This exercise pertains to excretory urography. Identify structures, fill in missing words, select from a list, provide a short answer, or choose true or false (explain any item you believe to be false) for each question.

Questions 1 to 22 pertain to general information concerning excretory urography.

1. The radiographic investigation of the renal drainage system is accomplished by various procedures classified under the general term _____.

2. Which two terms refer to the excretory urogram examination?
   a. Cystourethrography and retrograde urography
   b. Cystourethrography and IV pyelography
   c. IV urography and retrograde urography
   d. IV urography and IV pyelography

3. Circle four terms that identify the typical contrast media currently used in excretory urography.
   a. Ionic
   b. Nonionic
   c. Water-soluble iodinated
   d. Noniodinated
   e. Injectable
   f. Noninjectable

4. Circle the mild adverse reactions to iodinated contrast medium administration.
   a. Hives
   b. Death
   c. Nausea
   d. Dyspnea
   e. Vomiting
   f. Warm feeling
   g. Cardiac arrest
   h. Renal shutdown
   i. Respiratory arrest
   j. Flushed appearance
   k. Edema of the respiratory mucous membranes

5. How soon after the injection of a contrast medium are symptoms of a reaction most likely to occur?

6. Circle the four typical recommendations for a patient preparing for an intravenous urography (IVU) examination.
   a. Laxative
   b. Cleansing enema
   c. Light evening meal
   d. Liquid diet for 3 to 4 days
   e. Low-residue diet for 1 or 2 days
   f. Drinking 32 ounces of water to fill the bladder
   g. Nothing by mouth (NPO) after midnight on the day of the examination

7. What is the purpose of giving a child 12 oz of carbonated beverage just before the start of an IVU?

8. What patient preparation is required for retrograde urography? Why?

9. What is the purpose of applying compression over the distal ends of the ureters?

477

10. Where on the abdomen should compression pads be located to compress the ureters?

11. When ureteral compression is used, why should the pressure be slowly released when the compression device is no longer needed?

12. Why is ureteral compression currently not often used in excretory urography?

13. Why might an upright anteroposterior (AP) projection of the abdomen be made before the injection of the contrast medium?

14. What identification data should be included on every postinjection image?

15. Why is it desirable to have the patient remove his or her underwear?

16. Why should the patient be instructed to empty his or her bladder just before IVU begins?
    a. To locate the ureteral openings
    b. To measure the capacity of the bladder
    c. To prevent dilution of the opacified urine

17. What is the normal creatinine range?

18. What is a normal glomerular filtration rate (GFR)? At what level is the GFR considered abnormal?

19. Circle the five reasons that AP projections with the patient recumbent are performed as the scout image.
    a. To demonstrate the bladder
    b. To identify the location of the kidneys
    c. To demonstrate the presence of calculi
    d. To demonstrate the contour of the kidneys
    e. To check the radiographic exposure factors
    f. To demonstrate the mobility of the kidneys
    g. To examine for radiopaque artifacts on the positioning table
    h. To determine how well the patient's gastrointestinal tract was cleaned

20. Approximately how long after a bolus injection of the contrast medium should the exposure be made to best demonstrate a nephrogram?
    a. 30 seconds
    b. 3 minutes
    c. 5 minutes

21. How long after the completion of the contrast medium injection does the contrast agent usually begin to appear in the renal pelvis?
    a. 30 seconds to 1 minute
    b. 2 to 8 minutes
    c. 10 to 14 minutes
    d. 15 to 20 minutes

22. How long after the injection of the contrast medium does the greatest concentration usually appear within the kidneys?
    a. 30 seconds to 1 minute
    b. 2 to 8 minutes
    c. 15 to 20 minutes
    d. 30 to 45 minutes

23. A postvoiding image is usually the last image taken to demonstrate which structure(s)?
    a. Ureters
    b. Bladder
    c. Kidneys

Items 24 to 32 pertain to the AP projection. Examine Fig. 16.7 and answer the following questions.

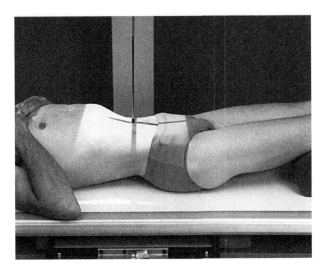

Fig. 16.7 Supine urogram, AP projection.

24. True or false. Preliminary (scout) images are most often obtained with the patient supine.

25. True or false. Postinjection images are most often obtained with the patient upright.

26. What is the most likely purpose for obtaining an AP projection image with the patient standing?
    a. To elongate the ureters
    b. To demonstrate ureteral reflux
    c. To demonstrate air-fluid levels
    d. To demonstrate the mobility of the kidneys

27. What adjustment in the position of the supine patient can be made to help demonstrate the distal ends of the ureters?
    a. Place supports under the patient's knees.
    b. Place a support under the patient's lumbar region.
    c. Tilt the table and patient 15 to 20 degrees toward the Trendelenburg position.
    d. Position a compression band around the patient's abdomen.

28. What should be done to reduce the lordotic curvature when performing the AP projection with the patient recumbent?
    a. Place supports under the patient's knees.
    b. Tilt the table and patient 10 to 15 degrees toward the Trendelenburg position.
    c. Position a compression band around the patient's abdomen.

29. Which procedure should be performed if the bladder is not seen in the AP projection to demonstrate the entire urinary system?
    a. Center the IR to the level of L3.
    b. Direct the central ray 10 to 15 degrees cephalically.
    c. Make a separate AP projection image of the bladder.
    d. Tilt the table and patient 10 to 15 degrees toward the Trendelenburg position.

30. Why is it desirable to include the area below the pubic symphysis for older male patients?
    a. To demonstrate distal ureters
    b. To demonstrate ureteral reflux
    c. To demonstrate the prostate region
    d. To demonstrate urinary bladder calculi

31. If a device is used for ureteral compression, to which level of the patient should it be centered?
    a. L1-L3
    b. At the level of the ASIS
    c. 2 inches (5 cm) above the iliac crests
    d. 1 inch (2.5 cm) above the superior border of the pubic symphysis

32. Identify each lettered structure shown in Fig. 16.8.

A. _____

B. _____

C. _____

D. _____

E. _____

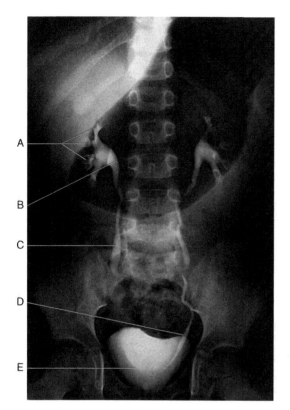

Fig. 16.8 AP projection of the urinary system.

Questions 33 to 38 pertain to *AP oblique projections.* Examine Fig. 16.9 and answer the following questions.

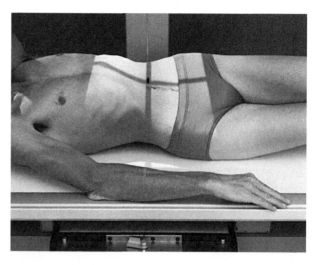

Fig. 16.9 Urogram, AP oblique projection (RPO position).

33. Into which position should the patient be placed when beginning to position for either type of AP oblique projection?
    a. Prone
    b. Supine
    c. Lateral recumbent

34. When performing the AP oblique projection, right posterior oblique (RPO) position, which kidney will be parallel with the plane of the IR?
    a. Left
    b. Right

35. Approximately how many degrees should the patient be rotated from the supine position to an oblique position to demonstrate renal and urinary structures?
    a. 10 degrees
    b. 20 degrees
    c. 30 degrees
    d. 40 degrees

36. Which structure should be centered to the grid for the AP oblique projection, left posterior oblique (LPO) position?
    a. Left kidney
    b. Right kidney
    c. Vertebral column

37. To which level of the patient should the IR be centered?
   a. L3
   b. Iliac crests
   c. Anterior superior iliac crests
   d. Pubic symphysis

38. Where should the central ray enter the patient?
   a. 2 inches (5 cm) lateral to the midline on the elevated side
   b. 2 inches (5 cm) lateral to the midline on the dependent side
   c. Centered to the midline 2 inches (5 cm) below the iliac crests

Items 39 to 43 pertain to the *lateral projection (lateral recumbent position)*. Examine Fig. 16.10 and answer the following questions.

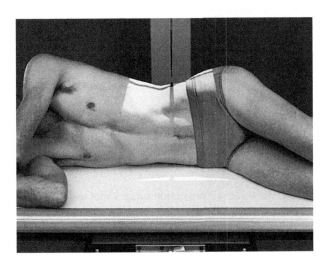

Fig. 16.10 Urogram, lateral projection.

39. Which plane of the body should be centered to the grid?

40. Describe how the patient's arms and hands should be placed.

41. Which areas of the patient should be examined to ensure that the patient is not rotated?

42. The exposure should be made at the end of _____ _____ (inspiration or expiration).

43. The exposure technique should clearly show the contrast medium in the _____, _____, and _____.

Items 44 to 50 pertain to *the lateral projection (dorsal decubitus position)*. Examine Fig. 16.11 and answer the following questions.

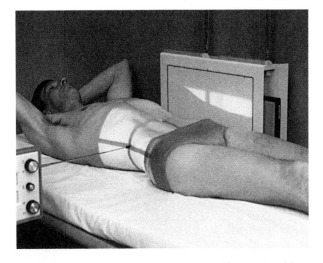

Fig. 16.11 Urogram, lateral projection (dorsal decubitus position).

44. The dorsal decubitus position requires that the patient be _____ (prone or supine).

45. The long axis of the IR should be centered to the _____ plane.

Chapter **16 Urinary System and Venipuncture**

46. Which area of the patient should be closest to the grid?
    a. Side
    b. Anterior
    c. Posterior

47. To which level of the patient should the IR be centered?
    a. L3
    b. Iliac crests
    c. Anterior superior iliac spines
    d. Pubic symphysis

48. True or false. Only male patients should have gonadal shielding for this type of projection.

49. True or false. The exposure should be made at the end of inspiration.

50. True or false. The central ray should be directed horizontal and perpendicular to the center of the IR.

Section 2: Exercise 2: Retrograde Urography

Retrograde urography is a radiographic procedure that demonstrates certain urinary structures. This exercise pertains to retrograde urography. Provide a short answer, select from a list, or choose true or false (explaining any statement you believe to be false) for each item.

Examine Fig. 16.12 and answer the following questions about retrograde urography.

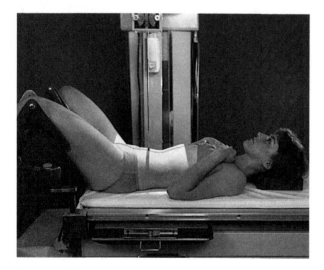

Fig. 16.12 Patient positioned on the table for retrograde urography.

1. True or false. Retrograde urography differs from excretory urography in that the contrast medium is injected directly into the kidney by means of a percutaneous injection through the skin.

2. True or false. Retrograde urography is performed on a regular x-ray table.

3. At the beginning of the retrograde urographic examination, the patient should be placed in the modified

    _____ position.
    a. prone
    b. upright
    c. lithotomy
    d. lateral recumbent

4. True or false. Retrograde urography is indicated for evaluation of the collecting system in patients who have renal insufficiency or who are allergic to iodinated contrast media.

5. Who should inject the contrast medium?
    a. The urologist
    b. The radiologist
    c. The radiographer

6. Describe how a kidney function test can be performed during retrograde urography.

7. List the three AP projection images that usually comprise a retrograde urographic examination.

8. Why might the head of the x-ray table be lowered 10 to 15 degrees during the retrograde pyelography procedure?

9. Which retrograde urographic image sometimes requires that the head of the table be elevated 35 to 40 degrees?
    a. Pyelogram
    b. Ureterogram
    c. Preliminary image showing catheter insertion

482

10. After necessary AP projections are made, which oblique positions are often used for oblique projections?
   a. RPO and LPO
   b. RPO and LAO
   c. RAO and LPO
   d. RAO and LAO

11. True or false. Because the contrast medium is not introduced into the circulatory system, the incidence of reactions is reduced.

Section 2: Exercise 3: Retrograde Cystography

Projections obtained during retrograde cystography often include an AP projection, both AP oblique projections (RPO and LPO positions), and a lateral projection. This exercise pertains to those projections. Fill in missing words or provide a short answer for each item.

1. Describe how the contrast medium is introduced into the patient for retrograde cystography.

Questions 2 to 11 pertain to AP *axial or posteroanterior (PA) axial projections.* Examine Fig. 16.13 and answer the following questions.

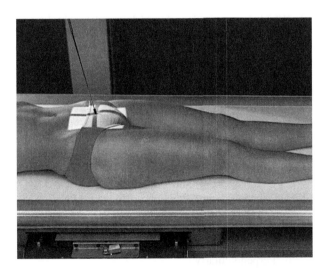

Fig. 16.13 AP axial bladder.

2. At what level should the exposure field or CR plate be centered?

3. Which structures are sometimes better demonstrated with the head of the table lowered 15 to 20 degrees?
   a. Prostate gland and urethra
   b. Lower (distal) ends of the ureters
   c. Upper (proximal) ends of the ureters

4. Why should patients in the supine position extend the lower limbs?
   a. To demonstrate ureteral reflux
   b. To retard the excretion of opacified urine from the bladder
   c. To enable the lumbar lordotic curve to arch the pelvis enough to tilt the pubic bones inferiorly

5. Which breathing instructions should be given to the patient?
   a. Breathe slowly.
   b. Suspend breathing after expiration.
   c. Suspend breathing after inspiration.

6. To demonstrate the bladder during cystography, how many degrees and in which direction should the central ray be directed for the AP axial projection?
   a. 5 degrees caudal
   b. 5 degrees cephalic
   c. 10 to 15 degrees caudal
   d. 10 to 15 degrees cephalic

7. To which level of the patient should the central ray enter for the AP axial projection?
   a. The iliac crests
   b. 2 inches (5 cm) above the upper border of the pubic symphysis
   c. 2 inches (5 cm) below the upper border of the pubic symphysis

8. How should the patient be positioned for the best demonstration of the prostate?
   a. Prone
   b. Supine
   c. Upright
   d. Lateral recumbent

9. How should the central ray be directed for the best demonstration of the prostate?
   a. Caudally
   b. Cephalically
   c. Perpendicularly

10. If minor reflux is present at the bladder, what other structures will most likely be demonstrated?
   a. Both kidneys
   b. Distal ureters
   c. Prostate gland

11. How should the pubic bones be demonstrated in the image of the AP axial projection?
   a. They should superimpose both the bladder neck and the proximal urethra.
   b. They should be projected above both the bladder neck and the proximal urethra.
   c. They should be projected below both the bladder neck and the proximal urethra.

Items 12 to 16 pertain to *AP oblique projections*. Examine Fig. 16.14 and answer the following questions.

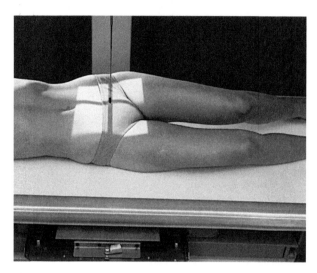

Fig. 16.14 Retrograde cystogram, AP oblique projection (RPO position).

12. In which position should the patient be placed?
   a. Semiprone
   b. Semisupine
   c. Lateral recumbent

13. How should the patient's uppermost thigh be positioned to prevent it from superimposing the bladder in AP oblique projections?
   a. Crossed over the other thigh
   b. Flexed and placed at right angles to the abdomen
   c. Extended and abducted enough to prevent its superimposition on the bladder area

14. How many degrees should the patient be rotated for AP oblique projections?
   a. 10 to 15
   b. 20 to 30
   c. 40 to 60

15. Circle the two ways that the central ray can be directed for AP oblique projections.
   a. Perpendicularly
   b. 10 degrees caudally
   c. 10 degrees cephalically
   d. 20 degrees caudally
   e. 20 degrees cephalically

16. With reference to the pubic bones, where should the bladder neck be seen in the AP oblique projection image, RPO position?
   a. Above
   b. Below
   c. To the left side
   d. To the right side

Questions 17 to 20 pertain to the *lateral projection*. Examine Fig. 16.15 and answer the following questions.

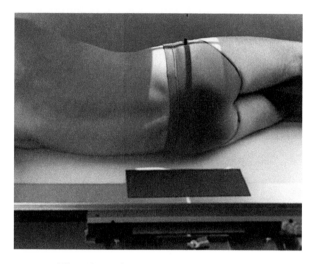

Fig. 16.15 Cystogram, lateral projection.

17. Which body position should be used for the lateral projection for cystography?
   a. Upright lateral
   b. Lateral recumbent
   c. Ventral decubitus (prone)
   d. Dorsal decubitus (supine)

18. Where should the IR be centered for the lateral projection?
   a. At the level of the iliac crests
   b. At the level of the pubic symphysis
   c. 2 inches (5 cm) above the iliac crests
   d. 2 inches (5 cm) above the pubic symphysis

19. How should the central ray be directed?
   a. Horizontally
   b. Perpendicularly
   c. Angled caudally
   d. Angled cephalically

20. Which imaged structures can determine whether the patient was rotated from the lateral position?
   a. Lumbar vertebrae
   b. Crests of the ilia
   c. Hips and femora

484

Section 2: Exercise 4: Male Cystourethrography

This exercise pertains to male cystourethrography. Provide a short answer, select from a list, or choose true or false (explaining any statement you believe to be false) for each item.

Examine Fig. 16.16 and answer the following questions.

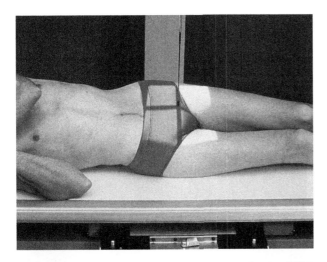

Fig. 16.16 Cystourethrogram, AP oblique projection (RPO position).

1. Define *cystourethrography*.

2. Describe how the contrast medium is introduced into the urinary structures of interest.

3. After the contrast medium is introduced into the patient, in which two positions can the patient be placed to demonstrate urinary structures?
   a. RAO and LAO
   b. RAO and LPO
   c. RPO and LAO
   d. RPO and LPO

4. How many degrees should the patient be rotated for the desired oblique projection?
   a. 15 to 20 degrees
   b. 25 to 30 degrees
   c. 35 to 40 degrees

5. To which level of the patient should the IR be centered?
   a. Crests of the ilia
   b. Anterior superior iliac spines
   c. 2 inches (5 cm) above the superior border of the pubic symphysis
   d. Superior border of the pubic symphysis

6. True or false. To ensure adequate coverage, the IR should be placed lengthwise.

7. True or false. To ensure that the entire urethra is filled, the exposure should be made while the physician is injecting the contrast medium.

8. True or false. After the bladder is filled with contrast medium, the voiding image can be exposed with the patient in a posterior oblique or an upright position.

9. True or false. The radiation field should be large enough to include the entire urinary system on all images.

10. Identify each lettered structure shown in Fig. 16.17.
    A. _____
    B. _____
    C. _____
    D. _____

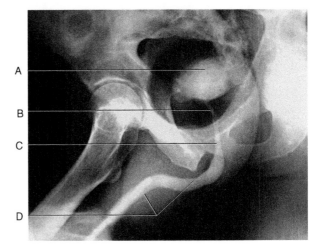

Fig. 16.17 Cystourethrogram, AP oblique projection (RPO position).

Chapter **16 Urinary System and Venipuncture**

Section 2: Exercise 5: Identifying Urinary System Images

Identify each of the following images by selecting the best choice from the list provided for each image.

1. Fig. 16.18:
   a. Excretory urogram, AP projection
   b. Retrograde urogram, AP projection
   c. Excretory cystogram, AP projection
   d. Preliminary (scout) image, AP projection

2. Fig. 16.19:
   a. Excretory urogram, AP projection
   b. Retrograde urogram, AP projection
   c. Excretory cystogram, AP projection
   d. Preliminary (scout) image, AP projection

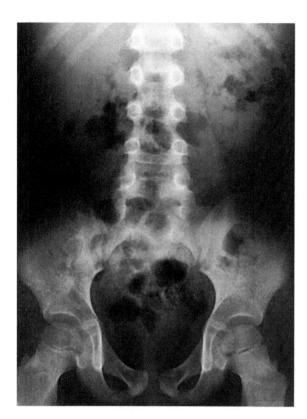

Fig. 16.18 Urinary examination image.

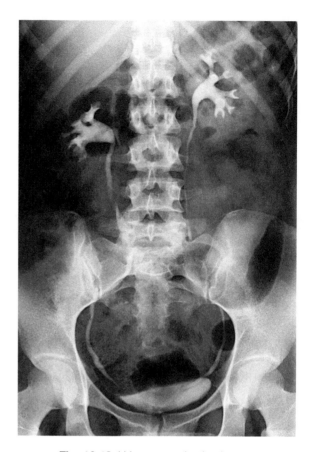

Fig. 16.19 Urinary examination image.

3. Fig. 16.20:
   a. Excretory urogram, AP projection
   b. Retrograde urogram, AP projection
   c. Excretory cystogram, AP projection
   d. Preliminary (scout) image, AP projection

4. Fig. 16.21:
   a. Excretory urogram, AP oblique projection, LPO position
   b. Excretory urogram, AP oblique projection, RPO position
   c. Retrograde cystogram, AP oblique projection, LPO position
   d. Retrograde cystogram, AP oblique projection, RPO position

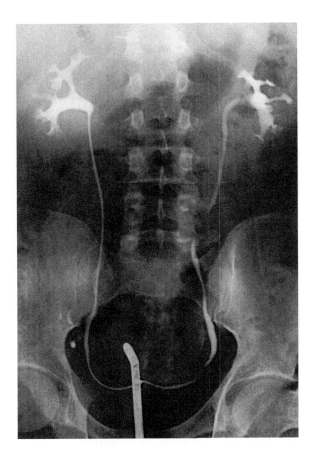

Fig. 16.20 Urinary examination image.

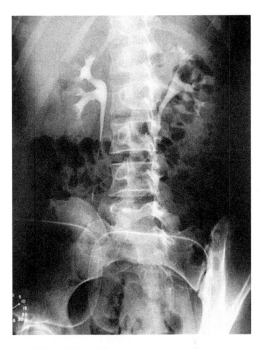

Fig. 16.21 Urinary examination image.

Chapter **16 Urinary System and Venipuncture**

5. Fig. 16.22:
   a. Urogram, lateral projection
   b. Urogram, left lateral decubitus
   c. Excretory urogram, AP oblique projection, RPO position
   d. Excretory urogram, AP oblique projection, LPO position

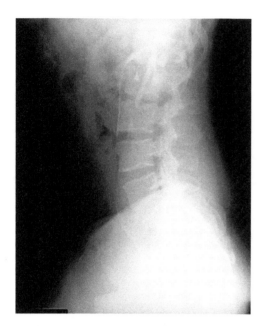

Fig. 16.22 Urinary examination image

6. Fig. 16.23:
   a. Prevoiding filled bladder, AP projection
   b. Postvoiding emptied bladder, AP projection
   c. Retrograde cystogram, AP oblique projection, RPO position
   d. Injection cystourethrogram, AP oblique projection, RPO position

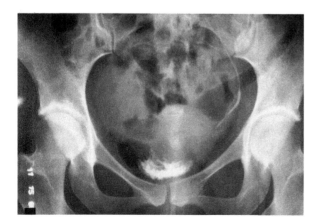

Fig. 16.23 Urinary examination image.

7. Fig. 16.24:
   a. Prevoiding filled bladder, AP projection
   b. Postvoiding emptied bladder, AP projection
   c. Retrograde cystogram, AP oblique projection, RPO position
   d. Injection cystourethrogram, AP oblique projection, RPO position

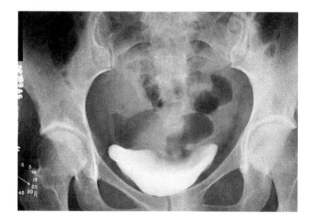

Fig. 16.24 Urinary examination image.

8. Fig. 16.25:
   a. Excretory cystogram, AP projection
   b. Retrograde cystogram, AP projection
   c. Postvoiding emptied bladder, AP projection
   d. Retrograde cystogram, AP oblique projection, RPO position

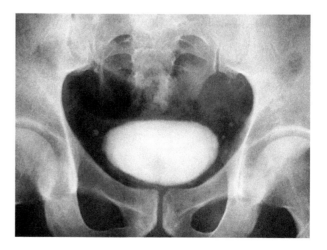

Fig. 16.25 Urinary examination image.

9. Fig. 16.26:
    a. Excretory cystogram, AP projection
    b. Retrograde cystogram, AP projection
    c. Postvoiding emptied bladder, AP projection
    d. Retrograde cystogram, AP oblique projection, RPO position

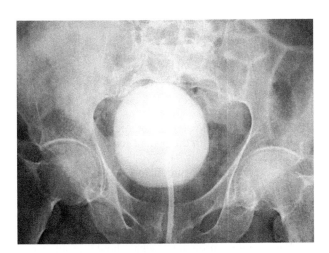

Fig. 16.26 Urinary examination image.

10. Fig. 16.27:
    a. Excretory cystogram, AP projection
    b. Retrograde cystogram, AP projection
    c. Postvoiding emptied bladder, AP projection
    d. Retrograde cystogram, AP oblique projection, RPO position

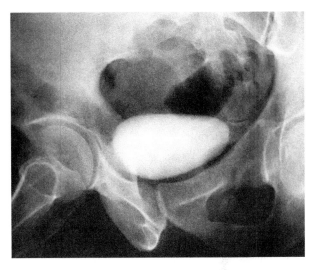

Fig. 16.27 Urinary examination image.

CHAPTER 16: SELF-TEST: URINARY SYSTEM AND VENIPUNCTURE

Answer the following questions by selecting the best choice.

1. Which renal structure filters the blood?
   a. Glomerulus
   b. Major calyx
   c. Efferent arteriole
   d. Afferent arteriole

2. Which urinary excretory duct conveys urine from the bladder to outside the body?
   a. Ureter
   b. Urethra
   c. Efferent arteriole
   d. Afferent arteriole

3. Which body organ filters blood and produces urine as a by-product of waste material?
   a. Liver
   b. Spleen
   c. Kidney
   d. Pancreas

4. At which vertebral level is the superior border of the kidneys usually found?
   a. T10
   b. T12
   c. L2
   d. L4

5. What is the name of the opening on the medial border of a kidney?
   a. Pole
   b. Base
   c. Apex
   d. Hilum

6. Which of the following is an excretory examination used to demonstrate the upper urinary tract?
   a. Cystourethrography
   b. Retrograde urography
   c. Intravenous urography
   d. Retrograde cystography

7. Which examination has the ability to produce a radiographic image demonstrating renal cortical tissue well saturated with contrast medium?
   a. Cystourethrography
   b. Retrograde urography
   c. Intravenous urography
   d. Retrograde cystography

8. Which projection best demonstrates the mobility of the kidneys?
   a. AP projection with the patient supine
   b. AP projection with the patient upright
   c. Lateral projection with the patient lateral recumbent
   d. Lateral projection with the patient in dorsal decubitus position

9. In IVU, what is the purpose of applying compression pads over the distal ends of both ureters?
   a. To demonstrate ureteral reflux
   b. To demonstrate the mobility of the kidneys
   c. To retard the flow of opacified urine into the bladder
   d. To retard the flow of opacified urine from the bladder

10. Which of the following is not a reason for obtaining a scout image with the patient recumbent for excretory urography?
    a. To evaluate exposure factors
    b. To demonstrate urinary calculi
    c. To determine the location of the kidneys
    d. To demonstrate the mobility of the kidneys

11. For excretory urography, what should an adult patient do just before getting on the examination table?
    a. Empty the bladder
    b. Remove all jewelry
    c. Drink 12 oz of cold water
    d. Drink 12 oz of a carbonated beverage

12. What is the purpose of obtaining an AP projection image of the kidneys 30 seconds after the bolus injection of a contrast medium in excretory urography?
    a. To demonstrate ureteral reflux
    b. To demonstrate opacified renal cortex
    c. To demonstrate opacified renal arteries
    d. To demonstrate the mobility of the kidneys

13. What is the purpose of tilting the patient and table 15 to 20 degrees toward the Trendelenburg position for the AP projection during excretory urography?
    a. To demonstrate distal ureters
    b. To demonstrate opacified renal cortex
    c. To demonstrate the base of the bladder
    d. To demonstrate the mobility of the kidneys

14. How many degrees should the patient be rotated for AP oblique projection, posterior oblique position, during excretory urography?
    a. 15
    b. 30
    c. 45
    d. 60

15. For intravenous urography of a child, what should the patient be given when the scout image shows an excessive amount of intestinal gas overlying the kidneys?
    a. A laxative
    b. A cleansing enema
    c. 12 oz of ice water
    d. 12 oz of a carbonated beverage

16. Which examination requires that the patient be placed on a special urographic-radiographic examination table?
    a. Cystourethrography
    b. Retrograde urography
    c. Intravenous urography
    d. Retrograde cystography

17. Which renal structures are not demonstrated during retrograde urographic examinations?
    a. Ureters
    b. Nephrons
    c. Minor calyces
    d. Major calyces

18. In addition to the AP projection, which projection would most likely be included in the images for retrograde urography?
    a. PA projection
    b. PA oblique projection
    c. AP oblique projection
    d. AP projection, lateral decubitus position

19. What is the purpose of tilting the table 10 to 15 degrees toward the Trendelenburg position for retrograde urography?
    a. To demonstrate the ureters
    b. To demonstrate the mobility of the kidneys
    c. To produce a nephrogram effect in the kidneys
    d. To prevent contrast medium from escaping the kidneys

20. What is the purpose of raising the head of the table 35 to 40 degrees for retrograde urography?
    a. To demonstrate the ureters
    b. To position the patient for catheterization
    c. To produce a nephrogram effect in the kidneys
    d. To prevent contrast medium from escaping the kidneys

21. Which condition would most likely be demonstrated during voiding cystography?
    a. Renal cyst
    b. Renal calculi
    c. Ureteral reflux
    d. Hydronephrosis

22. For the AP axial projection of the bladder, how many degrees and in which direction should the central ray be directed?
    a. 15 degrees caudal
    b. 15 degrees cephalic
    c. 25 degrees caudal
    d. 25 degrees cephalic

23. For retrograde cystography, which projection should be performed to demonstrate the anterior and posterior walls of the bladder?
    a. Upright AP projection
    b. Recumbent AP projection
    c. Recumbent lateral projection
    d. AP projection, lateral decubitus position

24. For cystourethrography with an adult male patient, to which level of the patient should the IR be centered?
    a. T12 vertebra
    b. L3 vertebra
    c. L5 vertebra
    d. Pubic symphysis

25. For cystourethrography with an adult male patient, which of the following should be used to obtain an image while the patient is urinating?
    a. Recumbent PA projection
    b. Dorsal decubitus position
    c. Lateral decubitus position
    d. Recumbent AP oblique projection

26. A technologist may administer all of the following medications for radiographic procedures EXCEPT:
    a. contrast media.
    b. pain management.
    c. sedation.
    d. diabetic.

27. What is the normal range for glomerular filtration rate (GFR)?
    a. 0.05 to 1.2 mg/dL
    b. 10 to 20 mg/dL
    c. 110 to 115 mL/min
    d. 90 to 120 mL/min

28. What is the normal average range for blood urea nitrogen (BUN) level?
    a. 0.05 to 1.2 mg/dL
    b. 5 to 10 mg/dL
    c. 7 to 20 mg/dL
    d. 120 to 125 mL/min

29. What is the normal average range for creatinine level?
    a. 0.5 to 1.2 mg/dL
    b. 1.5 to 2.0 mg/dL
    c. 10 to 20 mg/dL
    d. 120 to 125 mL/min

30. All of the following are prime factors to consider in selecting a vein EXCEPT:
    a. condition of the vein.
    b. purpose of the infusion.
    c. a good pulse.
    d. duration of therapy.

31. All of the following veins are most often used in establishing IV access EXCEPT:
    a. basilic or cephalic veins on the back of the hand.
    b. saphenous vein on the dorsal foot.
    c. basilic vein on the medial, anterior forearm and elbow.
    d. cephalic vein on the lateral, anterior forearm and elbow.

32. Which vein site is overused and can become scarred or sclerotic?
    a. Anterior surface of the elbow
    b. Back of the hand
    c. Superficial foot
    d. Dorsal wrist

33. During venipuncture, the technologist places the needle bevel _____ at a _____ degree angle to the skin's surface.
    a. Up, 15
    b. Down, 15
    c. Up, 45
    d. Down, 45

34. Which of the following are moderate reactions to contrast media?
    a. Respiratory distress
    b. Sensation of warmth
    c. Metallic taste, or sneezing
    d. Nausea, vomiting, or itching

35. What is the most common cause of extravasation?
    a. Tourniquet placement
    b. Needle displacement
    c. Local anesthetic
    d. Indirect, two-step puncture technique

17 Reproductive System

ANATOMY OF THE REPRODUCTIVE SYSTEM

Section 1: Exercise 1

This exercise pertains to the anatomy of the female reproductive system. Identify structures, fill in missing words, provide a short answer, or match columns for each item.

1. Identify each lettered structure shown in Fig. 17.1.

A. _____

B. _____

C. _____

D. _____

E. _____

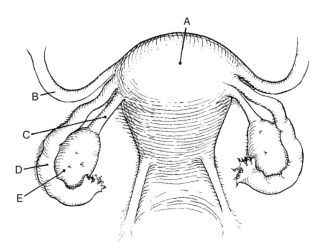

Fig. 17.1 Superoposterior view of the uterus, ovaries, and uterine tubes.

2. Identify each lettered structure shown in Fig. 17.2.

A. _____

B. _____

C. _____

D. _____

E. _____

F. _____

G. _____

H. _____

I. _____

J. _____

K. _____

L. _____

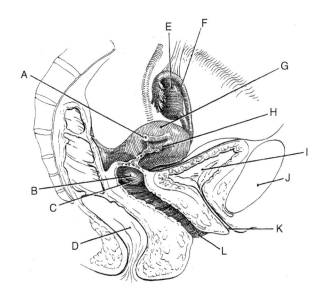

Fig. 17.2 Sagittal section showing the relationship of the internal genitalia to the surrounding structures.

493

3. The female gonads are called the _____.

4. Female reproductive cells are called _____.

5. The structure that conveys an ovum from a gonad to the uterus is the _____ tube.

6. The number of uterine tubes in the typical woman is _____.

7. The pear-shaped muscular organ of the female reproductive system is the _____.

8. Name the four main parts of the uterus.

9. What part of the uterus is referred to as the neck?

10. Match the uterine structures in Column A with the definitions in Column B.

Column A

_____ 1. Body

_____ 2. Fundus

_____ 3. Cervix

_____ 4. Isthmus

_____ 5. Endometrium

Column B

a. Superiormost portion

b. Cylindrical vaginal end

c. Mucosal lining of the uterine cavity

d. Constricted area adjacent to the vaginal end

e. Where ligaments attach the uterus within the pelvis

Section 1: Exercise 2

This exercise pertains to the anatomy of the male reproductive system. Identify structures or fill in missing words for each item.

1. Identify each lettered structure shown in Fig. 17.3.

A. _____

B. _____

C. _____

D. _____

E. _____

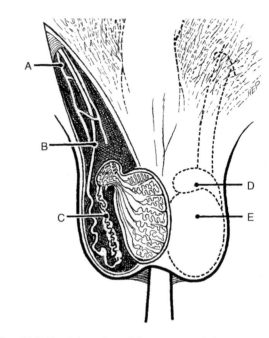

Fig. 17.3 Frontal section of the testes and ductus deferens.

2. Identify each lettered structure shown in Fig. 17.4.

A. _____

B. _____

C. _____

D. _____

E. _____

F. _____

G. _____

3. Identify each lettered structure shown in Fig. 17.5.

A. _____

B. _____

C. _____

D. _____

E. _____

F. _____

G. _____

H. _____

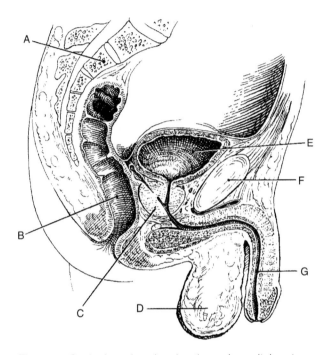

Fig. 17.4 Sagittal section showing the male genital system.

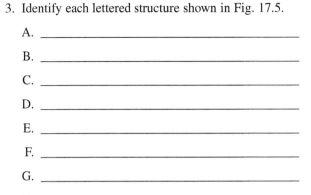

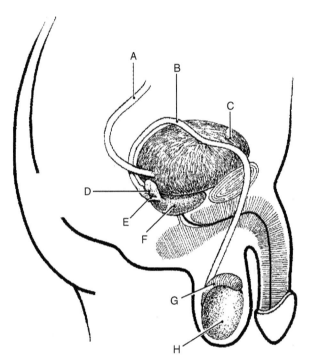

Fig. 17.5 Sagittal section through the male pelvis.

4. The male gonads are called the _____.

5. Male reproductive cells are called _____.

6. The oblong structure attached to each testicle is the _____.

7. The excretory channel that allows male germ cells to pass from a gonad to the urethra is the _____.

8. The union of the ductus deferens and the seminal vesicle duct forms the _____ duct.

9. The accessory genital organ that is composed of muscular and glandular tissues is the _____.

10. The ducts from the prostate open into the proximal portion of the _____.

Section 1: Exercise 3

Match the pathology terms in Column A with the appropriate definition in Column B.

Column A

_____ 1. Uterine fibroid

_____ 2. Dermoid cyst

_____ 3. Tumor

_____ 4. Fistula

_____ 5. Testicular torsion

_____ 6. Seminoma

_____ 7. Epididymitis

_____ 8. Uterine tube obstruction

_____ 9. Endometrial polyp

_____ 10. Adhesion

_____ 11. Prostate cancer

_____ 12. Cryptorchidism

Column B

a. Condition of undescended testis

b. Inflammation of the epididymis

c. Abnormal connection between two internal organs or between an organ and the body surface

d. Second most common malignancy in men

e. Smooth muscle tumor of the uterus

f. Union of two surfaces that are normally separate

g. Growth or mass protruding from endometrium

h. Most common type of testicular tumor

i. Condition preventing normal flow through uterine tube

j. Twisting of the testis at its base, causing acute ischemia

k. Tumor of the ovary filled with sebaceous material and hair

l. New tissue growth where cell proliferation is uncontrolled

RADIOGRAPHY OF THE REPRODUCTIVE SYSTEM

Section 2: Exercise 1: Radiography of the Female Reproductive System

Although other imaging modalities have reduced the demand for radiographic examinations of the female reproductive system, some facilities still radiographically demonstrate female reproductive structures. This exercise pertains to radiographic visualization of the female reproductive system. Match columns of relevant information or select the correct answer from a list for each item.

1. Match each radiographic examination from Column A with the type of patient from Column B who is most likely to undergo that type of examination.

Column A

_____ 1. Fetography

_____ 2. Vaginography

_____ 3. Placentography

_____ 4. Pelvic pneumography

_____ 5. Hysterosalpingography

Column B

a. Pregnant patient

b. Nongravid patient

2. Match the descriptions in Column A with the corresponding type of examination in Column B. Some descriptions may have more than one examination associated with them. Examinations will be used more than once.

Column A

_____ 1. Helps determine placenta previa

_____ 2. Requires a gaseous contrast agent

_____ 3. Requires the use of a contrast agent

_____ 4. Requires a radiopaque contrast agent

_____ 5. Investigates the patency of uterine tubes

_____ 6. Largely replaced by diagnostic ultrasound

_____ 7. Performed to demonstrate a fetus in utero

_____ 8. Introduces a contrast agent into the vaginal canal

_____ 9. Introduces a contrast agent through a uterine cannula

_____ 10. Introduces a contrast agent directly into the peritoneal cavity

_____ 11. Should be performed about 10 days after the onset of menstruation

_____ 12. Performed to determine the size, shape, and position of the uterus and uterine tubes

_____ 13. Performed to investigate congenital malformations and pathologic conditions such as vesicovaginal and enterovaginal fistulae

Column B

a. Fetography

b. Vaginography

c. Placentography

d. Pelvic pneumography

e. Hysterosalpingography

497

Figs. 17.6 through 17.9 are representative examinations of the female reproductive system.
Examine the images, then select the best answer from the list provided for each image.

3. Fig. 17.6:
   a. Pelvimetry
   b. Vaginography
   c. Pelvic pneumography
   d. Hysterosalpingography

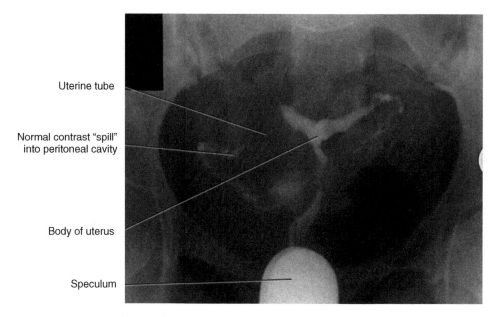

Fig. 17.6 Image of the female reproductive system.

4. Fig. 17.7:
   a. Fetography
   b. Vaginography
   c. Pelvic pneumography
   d. Hysterosalpingography

5. Fig. 17.8:
   a. Pelvimetry
   b. Vaginography
   c. Pelvic pneumography
   d. Hysterosalpingography

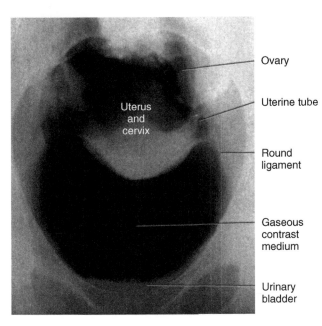

Fig. 17.7 Image of the female reproductive system.

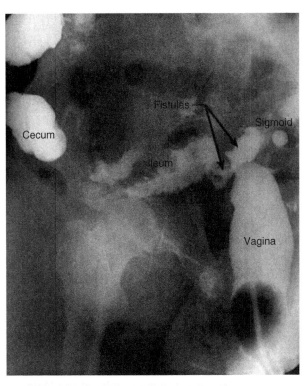

Fig. 17.8 Image of the female reproductive system.

6. Fig. 17.9:
   a. Pelvimetry
   b. Fetography
   c. Placentography
   d. Hysterosalpingography

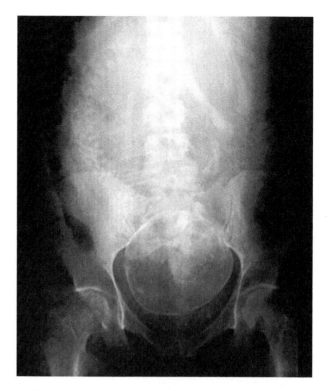

Fig. 17.9 Image of the female reproductive system.

Section 2: Exercise 2: Radiography of the Male Reproductive System

Although the demand for radiographic visualization of the male reproductive system has greatly decreased in recent years because of advances with diagnostic ultrasound, some facilities still radiographically demonstrate male reproductive structures. This exercise pertains to radiographic visualization of the male reproductive system. Provide a short answer for each question.

1. What type of contrast medium is used for radiographic examination of the seminal ducts?

2. List some genitourinary abnormalities in which imaging examinations of the seminal ducts are performed to investigate genitourinary abnormalities.

3. What accessory organ of the male reproductive system can be radiographically examined?

5. Today, the prostate is primarily imaged via

_____.

4. Define *prostatography*.

CHAPTER 17: SELF-TEST: REPRODUCTIVE SYSTEM

Answer the following questions by selecting the best choice.

1. Which structures are parts of the female reproductive system?
   a. Ovaries, uterus, and fallopian tubes
   b. Ovaries, testes, and ductus deferens
   c. Epididymis, uterus, and fallopian tubes
   d. Epididymis, testes, and ductus deferens

2. Which part of the uterus is most superior?
   a. Body
   b. Cervix
   c. Fundus
   d. Isthmus

3. Which structure conveys female reproductive cells from a gonad to the uterus?
   a. Urethra
   b. Uterine tube
   c. Ductus deferens
   d. Ejaculatory duct

4. Which structure produces female reproductive cells?
   a. Ovary
   b. Uterus
   c. Testicle
   d. Epididymis

5. Which structure produces spermatozoa?
   a. Ovary
   b. Testicle
   c. Prostate
   d. Epididymis

6. Which structure conveys male reproductive cells from a gonad to the urethra?
   a. Uterine tube
   b. Fallopian tube
   c. Ductus deferens
   d. Ejaculatory duct

7. Which structure is attached to each male gonad?
   a. Urethra
   b. Prostate
   c. Epididymis
   d. Ejaculatory duct

8. Which examination can be performed on a pregnant patient?
   a. Fetography
   b. Prostatography
   c. Pelvic pneumography
   d. Hysterosalpingography

9. Which examination can be performed on a non-gravid patient?
   a. Fetography
   b. Pelvimetry
   c. Placentography
   d. Hysterosalpingography

10. Which examination introduces contrast medium through a uterine cannula?
    a. Fetography
    b. Pelvimetry
    c. Vaginography
    d. Hysterosalpingography

11. Which examination is performed to verify the patency of uterine tubes?
    a. Fetography
    b. Pelvimetry
    c. Placentography
    d. Hysterosalpingography

12. Which examination demonstrates the architecture of the maternal pelvis to compare with the size of the fetal head?
    a. Fetography
    b. Pelvimetry
    c. Placentography
    d. Hysterosalpingography

13. Which type of contrast medium is preferred for hysterosalpingography?
    a. Oily viscous
    b. Water-soluble
    c. Barium sulfate

14. When should a hysterosalpingographic examination be performed?
    a. After the first trimester
    b. During the first trimester
    c. 10 days after the onset of menstruation
    d. 10 days before the onset of menstruation

15. Which of the following conditions can be investigated by radiographic imaging of the male reproductive system?
    1. Inflammation
    2. Tumors
    3. Sterility

    a. 1 and 2 only
    b. 1 and 3 only
    c. 2 and 3 only
    d. 1, 2, and 3

16. Which term describes the investigation of the prostate by radiographic, cystographic, or vesiculographic procedures?
    a. Fetography
    b. Pelvimetry
    c. Prostatography
    d. Hysterosalpingography

17. Radiation for any purpose is avoided during pregnancy, especially during what trimester of gestation?
    a. First trimester
    b. Second trimester
    c. Third trimester

18. All of the following radiologic examinations of the female pelvic organs are performed via intraperitoneal gas insufflation EXCEPT:
    a. pneumography.
    b. gynecography.
    c. fetography.
    d. pangynecography.

19. Hysterosalpingography is performed approximately how many months after insertion of the permanent type of intrauterine device?
    a. One month
    b. Two months
    c. Three months
    d. Four months

20. When performing hysterosalpingography, where is the IR centered?
    a. 1 inch (2.5 cm) distally to the pubic symphysis
    b. 1 inch (2.5 cm) proximally to the pubic symphysis
    c. 2 inches (5 cm) distally to the pubic symphysis
    d. 2 inches (5 cm) proximally to the pubic symphysis

503

18 Mammography

ANATOMY AND PHYSIOLOGY OF THE BREAST

Section 1: Exercise 1

This exercise pertains to the anatomy of the breast. Identify structures for each figure.

1. Identify each lettered structure shown in Fig. 18.1.

   A. _____

   B. _____

   C. _____

   D. _____

2. Identify each lettered structure shown in Fig. 18.2.

   A. _____

   B. _____

   C. _____

   D. _____

   E. _____

   F. _____

   G. _____

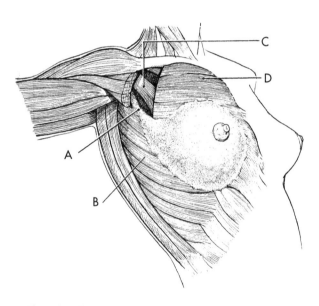

Fig. 18.1 Relationship of the breast to the chest wall.

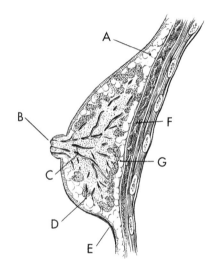

Fig. 18.2 Sagittal section through the breast illustrating structural anatomy.

Section 1: Exercise 2

1. Another term for the female breast is the _____ gland.

2. The female breast functions as an accessory gland to the reproductive system by producing and secreting _____.

3. The axillary prolongation of the breast is also called the axillary _____.

4. The posterior surface of the breast overlying the muscles is the _____.

5. The female breast tapers anteriorly from the base, ending in the _____.

6. The circular area of pigmented skin that surrounds the nipple is the _____.

7. The adult female breast contains _____ to _____ lobes.

8. The glandular elements found in the lobules of the female are the _____.

9. As a woman ages, the size of her breast lobules becomes _____.

10. The normal process of change in breast tissues that occurs as the patient ages is termed _____.

11. Normal involution replaces glandular and parenchymal tissues with increased amounts of _____.

12. The ducts that drain milk from the lobes are the _____ ducts.

13. Another term for the suspensory ligaments of the breast is _____ ligaments.

14. Approximately 75% of the lymph drainage is toward the _____.

15. The internal mammary lymph nodes are situated behind the _____.

Section 1: Exercise 3

Match the pathology terms in Column A with the appropriate definition in Column B. Not all choices from Column B should be selected.

Column A	Column B
_____ 1. Cyst	a. Narrowing or contraction of a passage
_____ 2. Paget's disease	b. A lucent area within the breast resulting from trauma, surgery, or radiation therapy
_____ 3. Fat necrosis	c. Collection of blood within the tissue, typically resulting from trauma
_____ 4. Papilloma	d. Complex sclerosing lesion; benign mass with spiculated borders not related to surgery; caused by abnormal cell growth
_____ 5. Galactocele	e. A growth inside the ducts that may cause discharge
_____ 6. Fibroadenoma	f. Solid benign tumors of glandular and connective tissue with clearly defined margins
_____ 7. Radial scar	g. Carcinoma in the skin of the nipple causing a sore, reddened appearance of the nipple and areola
_____ 8. Hematoma	h. Fluid-filled sac with distinct edges and round or oval in shape
	i. Milk-filled cyst typically found in lactating women

RADIOGRAPHY OF THE BREAST

Section 2: Exercise 1

Mammography is used to demonstrate diseases of the breast. This exercise pertains to mammographic procedures. Provide a short answer or select from a list for each question.

1. Why should the breast be bared for the examination?

2. The patient must remove deodorant and powder from the axilla before mammography because these substances can resemble _____ on the images.

3. Name the two standard projections routinely performed to demonstrate the breast.

4. What condition requires that a nipple marker be placed on the patient?

5. What procedure should a radiographer perform to help produce uniform breast thickness?

6. What procedure should a radiographer perform to identify the location of a palpable mass?

7. Why should the posterior nipple line be measured and compared between two projections?

8. The posterior nipple line is measured in craniocaudal projections between the _____ and the _____, or the _____, whichever comes first.

9. What is the maximum difference for the length of the posterior nipple line when comparing images of craniocaudal and mediolateral oblique projections?

10. Between examinations, the _____ and _____ should be cleaned with an approved disinfectant.

11. The routine projection of the breast that should demonstrate the pectoral muscle is the _____.

12. The imaging modality most commonly used for diagnostic imaging of an augmented breast is _____.

Identify each of the following four mammography projections in Figs. 18.3 through 18.15 by selecting the best choice from the list provided for each figure.

1. Fig. 18.3
    a. Craniocaudal
    b. Mediolateral
    c. Mediolateral oblique
    d. Exaggerated craniocaudal
    e. Lateromedial
    f. Craniocaudal for cleavage
    g. Craniocaudal with roll lateral
    h. Craniocaudal with roll medial
    i. Tangential
    j. Caudocranial
    k. Mediolateral oblique for axillary tail
    l. Lateromedial oblique
    m. Superolateral to inferomedial oblique

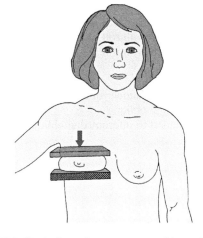

Fig. 18.3 Illustration of a mammographic projection.

2. Fig. 18.4
    a. Craniocaudal
    b. Mediolateral
    c. Mediolateral oblique
    d. Exaggerated craniocaudal
    e. Lateromedial
    f. Craniocaudal for cleavage
    g. Craniocaudal with roll lateral
    h. Craniocaudal with roll medial
    i. Tangential
    j. Caudocranial
    k. Mediolateral oblique for axillary tail
    l. Lateromedial oblique
    m. Superolateral to inferomedial oblique

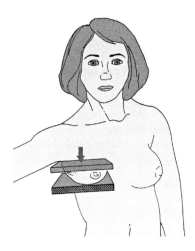

Fig. 18.4 Illustration of a mammographic projection.

3. Fig. 18.5
    a. Craniocaudal
    b. Mediolateral
    c. Mediolateral oblique
    d. Exaggerated craniocaudal
    e. Lateromedial
    f. Craniocaudal for cleavage
    g. Craniocaudal with roll lateral
    h. Craniocaudal with roll medial
    i. Tangential
    j. Caudocranial
    k. Mediolateral oblique for axillary tail
    l. Lateromedial oblique
    m. Superolateral to inferomedial oblique

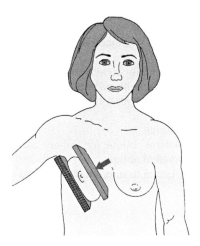

Fig. 18.5 Illustration of a mammographic projection.

507

4. Fig. 18.6
   a. Craniocaudal
   b. Mediolateral
   c. Mediolateral oblique
   d. Exaggerated craniocaudal
   e. Lateromedial
   f. Craniocaudal for cleavage
   g. Craniocaudal with roll lateral
   h. Craniocaudal with roll medial
   i. Tangential
   j. Caudocranial
   k. Mediolateral oblique for axillary tail
   l. Lateromedial oblique
   m. Superolateral to inferomedial oblique

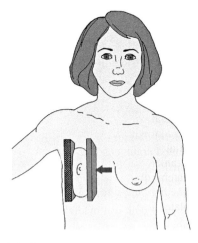

Fig. 18.6 Illustration of a mammographic projection.

5. Fig. 18.7
   a. Craniocaudal
   b. Mediolateral
   c. Mediolateral oblique
   d. Exaggerated craniocaudal
   e. Lateromedial
   f. Craniocaudal for cleavage
   g. Craniocaudal with roll lateral
   h. Craniocaudal with roll medial
   i. Tangential
   j. Caudocranial
   k. Mediolateral oblique for axillary tail
   l. Lateromedial oblique
   m. Superolateral to inferomedial oblique

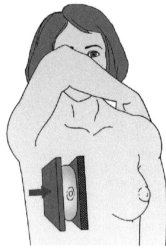

Fig. 18.7 Illustration of a mammographic projection.

6. Fig. 18.8
   a. Craniocaudal
   b. Mediolateral
   c. Mediolateral oblique
   d. Exaggerated craniocaudal
   e. Lateromedial
   f. Craniocaudal for cleavage
   g. Craniocaudal with roll lateral
   h. Craniocaudal with roll medial
   i. Tangential
   j. Caudocranial
   k. Mediolateral oblique for axillary tail
   l. Lateromedial oblique
   m. Superolateral to inferomedial oblique

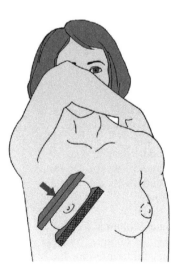

Fig. 18.8 Illustration of a mammographic projection.

7. Fig. 18.9
   a. Craniocaudal
   b. Mediolateral
   c. Mediolateral oblique
   d. Exaggerated craniocaudal
   e. Lateromedial
   f. Craniocaudal for cleavage
   g. Craniocaudal with roll lateral
   h. Craniocaudal with roll medial
   i. Tangential
   j. Caudocranial
   k. Mediolateral oblique for axillary tail
   l. Lateromedial oblique
   m. Superolateral to inferomedial oblique

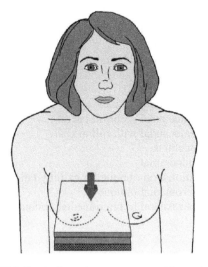

Fig. 18.9 Illustration of a mammographic projection.

8. Fig. 18.10
   a. Craniocaudal
   b. Mediolateral
   c. Mediolateral oblique
   d. Exaggerated craniocaudal
   e. Lateromedial
   f. Craniocaudal for cleavage
   g. Craniocaudal with roll lateral
   h. Craniocaudal with roll medial
   i. Tangential
   j. Caudocranial
   k. Mediolateral oblique for axillary tail
   l. Lateromedial oblique
   m. Superolateral to inferomedial oblique

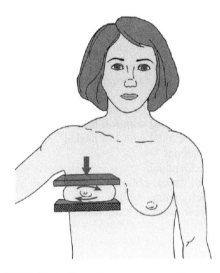

Fig. 18.10 Illustration of a mammographic projection.

9. Fig. 18.11
   a. Craniocaudal
   b. Mediolateral
   c. Mediolateral oblique
   d. Exaggerated craniocaudal
   e. Lateromedial
   f. Craniocaudal for cleavage
   g. Craniocaudal with roll lateral
   h. Craniocaudal with roll medial
   i. Tangential
   j. Caudocranial
   k. Mediolateral oblique for axillary tail
   l. Lateromedial oblique
   m. Superolateral to inferomedial oblique

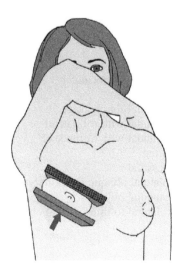

Fig. 18.11 Illustration of a mammographic projection.

10. Fig. 18.12
  a. Craniocaudal
  b. Mediolateral
  c. Mediolateral oblique
  d. Exaggerated craniocaudal
  e. Lateromedial
  f. Craniocaudal for cleavage
  g. Craniocaudal with roll lateral
  h. Craniocaudal with roll medial
  i. Tangential
  j. Caudocranial
  k. Mediolateral oblique for axillary tail
  l. Lateromedial oblique
  m. Superolateral to inferomedial oblique

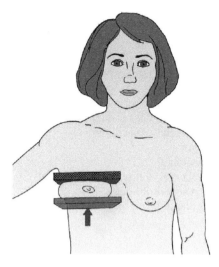

Fig. 18.12 Illustration of a mammographic projection.

11. Fig. 18.13
  a. Craniocaudal
  b. Mediolateral
  c. Mediolateral oblique
  d. Exaggerated craniocaudal
  e. Lateromedial
  f. Craniocaudal for cleavage
  g. Craniocaudal with roll lateral
  h. Craniocaudal with roll medial
  i. Tangential
  j. Caudocranial
  k. Mediolateral oblique for axillary tail
  l. Lateromedial oblique
  m. Superolateral to inferomedial oblique

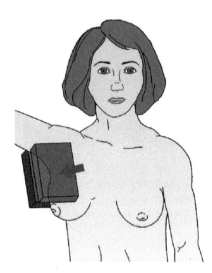

Fig. 18.13 Illustration of a mammographic projection.

12. Fig. 18.14
  a. Craniocaudal
  b. Mediolateral
  c. Mediolateral oblique
  d. Exaggerated craniocaudal
  e. Lateromedial
  f. Craniocaudal for cleavage
  g. Craniocaudal with roll lateral
  h. Craniocaudal with roll medial
  i. Tangential
  j. Caudocranial
  k. Mediolateral oblique for axillary tail
  l. Lateromedial oblique
  m. Superolateral to inferomedial oblique

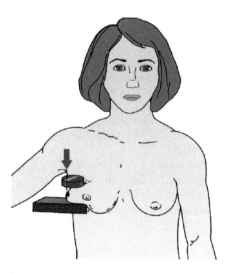

Fig. 18.14 Illustration of a mammographic projection.

13. Fig. 18.15
    a. Craniocaudal
    b. Mediolateral
    c. Mediolateral oblique
    d. Exaggerated craniocaudal
    e. Lateromedial
    f. Craniocaudal for cleavage
    g. Craniocaudal with roll lateral
    h. Craniocaudal with roll medial
    i. Tangential
    j. Caudocranial
    k. Mediolateral oblique for axillary tail
    l. Lateromedial oblique
    m. Superolateral to inferomedial oblique

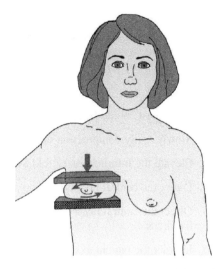

Fig. 18.15 Illustration of a mammographic projection.

Section 2: Exercise 3

Items 1 to 10 are statements that refer to mammography positioning procedures. Examine each statement in Column A and identify the mammography projection from Column B that most closely relates to the statement. Some statements pertain to more than one projection.

Column A

_____ 1. The breast should be perpendicular to the chest wall.

_____ 2. Slowly apply compression until the breast feels taut.

_____ 3. Elevate the inframammary fold to its maximum height.

_____ 4. Direct the central ray perpendicularly to the base of the breast.

_____ 5. Direct the central ray 5 degrees mediolaterally to the craniocaudal base of the breast.

_____ 6. Instruct the patient to stand or be seated facing the IR holder.

_____ 7. Rotate the C-arm to direct the central ray to the medial side of the breast.

_____ 8. Adjust the height of the IR to the level of the inferior surface of the breast.

_____ 9. Adjust the height of the IR so that the superior border is level with the axilla.

_____ 10. Pull the breast tissue superiorly and anteriorly, ensuring that the lateral rib margin is firmly pressed against the IR.

Column B

a. Mediolateral

b. Craniocaudal

c. Mediolateral oblique

d. Exaggerated

Section 2: Exercise 4

Items 1 to 8 are statements that refer to structures that are demonstrated with various mammography projections. Examine each statement in Column A and identify the mammography projection from Column B that most closely relates to the statement.

Column A

_____ 1. Demonstrates air-fluid and fat-fluid levels in breast structures

_____ 2. Resolves superimposed structures seen on the mediolateral oblique projection

_____ 3. Demonstrates the pectoral muscle approximately 30% of the time

_____ 4. Demonstrates all breast tissue with emphasis on the lateral aspect and axillary tail

_____ 5. The central, subareolar, and medial fibroglandular breast tissue should be demonstrated

_____ 6. Demonstrates lesions on the lateral aspect of the breast in the superior or inferior aspects

_____ 7. Demonstrates a sagittal orientation of a lateral lesion located in the axillary tail of the breast

_____ 8. Demonstrates a superoinferior projection of the lateral fibroglandular breast tissue and posterior aspect of the pectoral muscle

Column B

a. Mediolateral

b. Craniocaudal

c. Mediolateral oblique

d. Exaggerated craniocaudal

Answer the following questions by selecting the best choice.

1. The lymphatic vessels of the breast drain laterally into which of the following lymph nodes?
   a. Axillary
   b. Thoracic
   c. Abdominal
   d. Internal mammary chain

2. Where is the tail of the breast located?
   a. Adjacent to the nipple
   b. Along the lateral side to the axilla
   c. Along the medial aspect of the breast
   d. In the glandular tissue against the chest wall

3. Which ducts drain milk from the lobes of the breast?
   a. Axillary
   b. Thoracic
   c. Lymphatic
   d. Lactiferous

4. How do breast tissues change after involution?
   a. Glandular tissues become dense and opaque.
   b. Parenchymal tissues become dense and opaque.
   c. Fatty tissues are replaced with glandular tissues.
   d. Glandular tissues are replaced with fatty tissues.

5. The standard examination for demonstrating the breasts comprises which two projections?
   a. Craniocaudal and lateromedial
   b. Craniocaudal and mediolateral oblique
   c. Caudocranial and lateromedial
   d. Caudocranial and mediolateral oblique

6. Which projection requires that the central ray pass through the breast at an angle of 30 to 60 degrees?
   a. Axillary
   b. Caudocranial
   c. Craniocaudal
   d. Mediolateral oblique

7. Which muscle is often demonstrated with the craniocaudal projection?
   a. Pectoralis major
   b. Serratus anterior
   c. Rectus abdominis
   d. Lateral abdominal oblique

8. What is the primary objective of compressing the breast for mammography?
   a. To reduce exposure time
   b. To decrease geometric distortion
   c. To produce uniform breast thickness
   d. To produce uniform radiographic density

9. Where should the radiopaque marker, used to indicate which side is being examined, be seen on the image of craniocaudal projections?
   a. On the nipple
   b. On the chest wall
   c. Along the lateral side of the breast
   d. Along the medial side of the breast

10. How should a radiographer identify the location of a palpable mass?
    a. Draw a circle around the mass on the resultant mammogram.
    b. Use an ink marker to draw a circle on the skin overlying the mass.
    c. Place a radiopaque marker such as a BB on the breast overlying the mass.
    d. Place a radiopaque arrow marker alongside the breast to point to the mass.

11. What is the maximum difference for the length of the posterior nipple line when comparing images of craniocaudal and mediolateral oblique projections?
    a. 0.2 inch (0.5 cm)
    b. 0.3 inch (1.0 cm)
    c. 0.6 inch (1.5 cm)
    d. 0.8 inch (2.0 cm)

12. Between which two projections should the posterior nipple lines be measured and compared?
    a. Craniocaudal and mediolateral oblique
    b. Craniocaudal and 90-degree mediolateral
    c. Exaggerated craniocaudal and mediolateral oblique
    d. Exaggerated craniocaudal and 90-degree mediolateral

13. In which body position should the patient be placed for craniocaudal or mediolateral oblique projections?
    a. Prone
    b. Supine
    c. Upright
    d. Lateral recumbent

14. Which projection demonstrates all breast tissue with an emphasis on the lateral aspect and axillary tail?
    a. Mediolateral
    b. Craniocaudal
    c. Mediolateral oblique
    d. Exaggerated craniocaudal

15. Which projection requires that the central ray be moved to a horizontal position?
    a. Mediolateral
    b. Craniocaudal
    c. Mediolateral oblique
    d. Exaggerated craniocaudal

19 Mobile Radiography

EQUIPMENT, TECHNICAL CONSIDERATIONS, AND PATIENT CARE

There are many instances in which the technologist has to bring the imaging procedure to the patient, rather than the patient reporting to the radiology department. Mobile radiography is widely used to image patients who are unable to come to the department for routine imaging examinations. Answer the following questions regarding mobile equipment, technical considerations, and patient care concerns.

1. List the common areas in which mobile radiography is performed.

2. What technical controls are typically available on mobile equipment?

3. What is the typical range of milliampere-seconds (mAs) available on mobile x-ray machines?

4. What is the typical range of kilovolt peak (kVp) available on mobile x-ray machines?

5. What is the range of total power for most mobile units? How does this compare with stationary radiographic equipment?

6. What three technical matters must be understood to be competent in mobile radiography?

7. For optimal mobile images, a grid must be:

   A. _____

   B. _____

   C. _____

8. Anode heel effect is more pronounced when using short _____, larger _____, and small _____.

9. Where should the cathode be positioned when performing a femur examination with a mobile x-ray machine?
   a. At the proximal femur
   b. At the distal femur

514

10. What is the preferred source-to-image receptor distance (SID) for mobile examinations? Why?

11. True or false. Mobile radiography produces some of the highest occupational radiation exposures for radiographers.

12. Radiographers performing mobile examinations should wear a _____ for proper radiation protection.

13. The most effective means of radiation protection is:
    a. the shortest exposure time.
    b. the maximum distance from the x-ray source.
    c. a smaller field size.
    d. a lower grid ratio.

14. What is the recommended minimum distance between the radiographer and the x-ray tube?

15. Circle the five clinical situations in which gonadal shielding should be provided.
    a. Mobile examination on a child
    b. Mobile chest examination on a 28-year-old woman in an intensive care unit
    c. Mobile pelvis and hip examination on a 75-year-old woman in a surgical (postoperative) recovery unit
    d. Patient in the emergency department requesting shielding during a mobile knee examination
    e. Cross-table lateral lumbar spine image performed with a mobile unit on a 22-year-old man in the emergency department
    f. Routine hand examination on a 30-year-old patient
    g. Mobile kidney, ureter, and bladder (KUB) image in the emergency department on a 32-year-old woman with blunt abdominal trauma

16. What two types of patients are often cared for in isolation units?

17. Because of the confidentiality of patient records, a radiographer may not know the specific disease of a patient in an isolation unit. All patients should be handled using _____.

18. Which of the following protective apparel should be worn when performing a mobile examination on a patient in strict isolation? Circle all that apply.
    a. Gown
    b. Gloves
    c. Mask
    d. Cap
    e. Shoe covers

19. What should be done to protect the IR when performing a mobile examination on a patient isolated with drainage secretion precautions?

20. What should be done to mobile equipment after performing an examination on a patient in an isolation unit?

MOBILE RADIOGRAPHIC EXAMINATIONS

The following exercises pertain to the performance of specific mobile radiographic procedures. Answer each question regarding the specific mobile examination.

1. Which of the following are preliminary steps for the radiographer before performing mobile radiography? Check all that apply.

    _____ a. Gather all necessary equipment.

    _____ b. Announce your presence to the nursing staff.

    _____ c. Confirm that you have the correct patient.

    _____ d. Introduce yourself to patient and family.

    _____ e. Explain the examination to the patient.

    _____ f. Process the images.

    _____ g. Observe medical equipment in room and move, if necessary.

    _____ h. Disconnect unnecessary medical equipment to remove artifacts.

Questions 2 to 6 pertain to the AP projection of the chest, with the patient in an upright or supine position.

2. Which position would be best to obtain a mobile AP chest image on a conscious and alert patient?
   a. Sitting as upright as is tolerable by the patient
   b. Supine position
   c. Lateral decubitus position
   d. Trendelenburg position

3. The IR should be placed about _____ above the shoulders for the AP projection of the chest performed with a mobile unit.

4. The central ray should be directed _____ to the

   _____ on the mobile AP projection of the chest.

5. The central ray should enter the patient about

   _____ below the _____ on the mobile AP projection of the chest.

6. What device should be used if the kVp is above 90 for a mobile computed radiography AP projection of the chest?

Questions 7 to 10 pertain to the AP projection of the chest with the patient in a right or left lateral decubitus position.

7. When using the lateral decubitus position for a mobile chest examination, which position would be used if fluid was suspected in the left lung?

8. Describe the proper patient position to prevent rotation of the anatomy in an image of a lateral decubitus position.

9. What pathologic conditions would be demonstrated by the right lateral decubitus position?

10. True or false. Proper image ID should be demonstrated to indicate the decubitus position was used.

Questions 11 to 15 pertain to the *AP projection of the abdomen with the patient in a supine position.*

11. The grid IR should be centered at the level of

    _____.

12. If the emphasis is on the upper abdomen, how does the grid IR center change?

13. What anatomy must be visualized on the image if the lower abdomen is of primary interest?

14. The _____ must be seen at the top of the image if the upper abdomen is of primary interest.

15. What error might occur if the patient is not in a true supine position, but the central ray is centered as if he or she is properly positioned?

Questions 16 to 18 pertain to the *AP projection of the abdomen with the patient in the left lateral decubitus position.*

16. How does one check for rotation on an image of the abdomen taken in a left lateral decubitus position?

17. How long should the patient be in the left lateral decubitus position before exposure? Why?

18. The center of the grid IR should be centered

    _____ to include the _____ on the image.

Questions 19 to 21 pertain to the *AP projection of the pelvis.*

19. Where should the center of the grid IR be placed relative to the patient?

20. What possible contraindications prohibit proper positioning of the lower limbs for this examination?

21. What is the rationale for the position of the lower limbs for this examination?

Questions 22 to 25 pertain to the *AP and lateral projections of the femur.*

22. The grid IR should be placed _____ to the plane of the femoral condyles for the AP projection.

23. List the anatomy that must be included on a mobile femur examination.

24. When performing the mediolateral projection of the femur, the unaffected limb should be:
    a. flexed at the knee for support.
    b. parallel to the grid IR.
    c. elevated and supported at a nearly vertical position.
    d. used to support the grid IR in a vertical position.

25. When performing the lateromedial projection of the femur, the grid IR is placed:
    1. perpendicularly to the epicondylar plane.
    2. between the patient's legs.
    3. against the lateral aspect of the affected femur.

    a. 1 and 2 only
    b. 2 and 3 only
    c. 1 and 3 only
    d. 1, 2, and 3

Questions 26 to 28 pertain to the *lateral projection of the cervical spine with the patient in the dorsal decubitus position.*

26. The top of the grid IR should be placed

    _____.

27. Proper alignment of the central ray with the grid IR

    prevents _____.

28. What anatomic structures must be demonstrated on the image?

Questions 29 to 32 pertain to procedures performed with neonates, with the *AP projection of the chest and abdomen.*

29. Chest and abdomen combined projections are typically ordered on:
    a. full-term infants.
    b. toddlers.
    c. adolescents.
    d. premature infants.

30. Who should hold the infant during the radiographic examination?

31. True or false. A covering should be placed over the IR if it is placed directly under the infant.

32. Explain the risks of straightening the head of a neonate with an endotracheal tube.

Questions 33 to 35 pertain to procedures performed with neonates, *with the lateral projection of a patient in the dorsal decubitus position.*

33. True or false. The infant does not need to be elevated for the dorsal decubitus position.

34. What anatomy is of special interest in this position?

35. What pathologic condition, if present, can be demonstrated in this position?

CHAPTER 19: SELF-TEST: MOBILE RADIOGRAPHY

Answer the following questions by selecting the best choice.

1. Mobile radiography is defined as:
   a. using digital equipment to transmit images to remote sites.
   b. using transportable radiographic equipment to bring imaging services to the patient.
   c. using radiographic imaging to increase patient mobility.
   d. using picture archiving and communication systems (PACSs) to transmit images to patients in their homes.

2. Which of the following are common sites in which mobile radiography is performed?
   1. Intensive care units
   2. Patient hospital rooms
   3. Surgery

   a. 1 and 2 only
   b. 2 and 3 only
   c. 1 and 3 only
   d. 1, 2, and 3

3. The typical mAs range on a mobile unit is:
   a. 0.04 to 320 mAs
   b. 1 to 10 mAs
   c. 1 to 100 mAs
   d. 0.5 to 500 mAs

4. The typical kVp range on a mobile unit is:
   a. 1 to 100 kVp
   b. 10 to 500 kVp
   c. 40 to 130 kVp
   d. 50 to 150 kVp

5. What is the grid ratio of focused grids commonly used with mobile radiography?
   a. 5:1 or 10:1
   b. 6:1 or 8:1
   c. 10:1 or 12:1
   d. 12:1 or 16:1

6. What are the primary advantages of a battery-powered mobile unit?
   a. They are lightweight and easy to maneuver.
   b. They are cordless and provide constant kVp and mAs levels.
   c. They do not require much time to charge before the exposure.
   d. They are inexpensive and low maintenance.

7. Which of the following are acceptable projections/positions when performing the lateral femur?
   1. Mediolateral
   2. Lateromedial
   3. Ventral decubitus
   4. Dorsal decubitus

   a. 1, 2, 3, 4
   b. 1, 2, 4
   c. 2, 3, 4
   d. 1, 3, 4

8. When performing a mobile examination of the abdomen, where should the cathode be placed for the AP projection?
   a. The down side of the abdomen
   b. Over the symphysis pubis
   c. Over the diaphragm
   d. No designation for cathode placement

9. The anode heel effect is more pronounced with:
   1. larger field sizes.
   2. larger anode angles.
   3. shorter SID.

   a. 1 and 2 only
   b. 1 and 3 only
   c. 2 and 3 only
   d. 1, 2, and 3

10. If the SID is increased, what risk is also increased?
    a. Imaging of patient motion
    b. Tube overload
    c. Imaging of patient artifacts
    d. Grid cutoff

11. For optimum radiation safety, the radiographer should stand:
    a. at a right angle to the patient.
    b. at a right angle to the x-ray tube.
    c. anywhere, as long as a lead apron is worn.
    d. at least 6 feet away from the patient and x-ray tube.

12. At what kVp level should a grid be employed for mobile chest examinations?
    a. Above 60 kVp
    b. Above 75 kVp
    c. Above 90 kVp
    d. Above 100 kVp

13. Which of the following evaluation criteria for the mobile AP chest is used to evaluate adequate penetration?
    a. Medial portion of clavicles equidistant from the vertebral column
    b. Ribs and thoracic intervertebral disk spaces faintly visible through the heart shadow
    c. Psoas muscles, lower margin of liver, and kidney margins demonstrated
    d. Symmetric appearance of the vertebral column and iliac wings

14. Which of the following evaluation criteria for the mobile AP chest is used to evaluate patient rotation?
    a. Medial portion of clavicles equidistant from the vertebral column
    b. Ribs and thoracic intervertebral disk spaces faintly visible through the heart shadow
    c. Psoas muscles, lower margin of liver, and kidney margins demonstrated
    d. Symmetric appearance of the vertebral column and iliac wings

15. What is the proper position of the median coronal plane for the right lateral decubitus position of the chest?
    a. Horizontal
    b. Perpendicular to the IR
    c. Vertical
    d. Aligned to the center of the IR

16. When performing a mobile lateral decubitus chest examination, how long should the patient be in position before exposure?
    a. 1 minute
    b. 5 minutes
    c. 8 minutes
    d. 20 minutes

17. What is the danger of straightening the head and neck of a neonate during a mobile AP projection of the chest and abdomen?
    a. Risk of physical injury to the underdeveloped vertebrae
    b. Risk of transmission of infectious organisms
    c. Risk of increased occupational exposure
    d. Risk of advancing the endotracheal tube too far into the trachea

18. Which position would be used to demonstrate fluid in the right lung of a patient in an intensive care unit?
    a. Right lateral decubitus
    b. Left lateral decubitus
    c. Supine
    d. Prone

19. Which position would be used to demonstrate free air or fluid levels in a neonate?
    a. Right lateral decubitus
    b. Left lateral decubitus
    c. Dorsal decubitus
    d. Supine

20. Which of the following are contraindications to positioning the feet of a trauma patient during a mobile AP projection of the pelvis?
    a. Decreased level of consciousness
    b. Suspicion of hip fracture
    c. No one available to hold the patient
    d. Increased risk of occupational exposure

21. Patients should be shielded with appropriate radiation protection devices for which of the following situations? (List all that apply.)
    1. X-ray examinations performed on children
    2. X-ray examinations performed on patients of reproductive age
    3. Examinations in which the gonads lie far away from the useful beam
    4. Examinations in which shielding would not interfere with imaging of the anatomy that must be shown

    a. 1 and 2 only
    b. 1, 2, and 3 only
    c. 1, 2, 3, and 4
    d. 1, 2, and 4

22. The source-to-skin distance (SSD) cannot be less than how many inches in accordance with federal safety regulations?
    a. 5 inches (12 cm)
    b. 10 inches (25 cm)
    c. 12 inches (30 cm)
    d. 15 inches (38 cm)

23. At what level should the central ray enter the patient when performing a right lateral decubitus chest?
    a. Midsagittal plane and at the level of the iliac crests
    b. Midcoronal plane and at the level of the iliac crests
    c. 3 inches (7.6 cm) below the jugular notch
    d. 3 inches (7.6 cm) above the jugular notch

24. At what level should the central ray enter the patient when performing an AP abdomen?
    a. Midsagittal plane and at the level of the iliac crests
    b. Midcoronal plane and at the level of the iliac crests
    c. 3 inches (7.6 cm) below the jugular notch
    d. 3 inches (7.6 cm) above the jugular notch

25. At what level should the central ray enter the patient when performing a left lateral decubitus abdomen?
    a. Midsagittal plane and at the level of the iliac crests
    b. Midcoronal plane and at the level of the iliac crests
    c. Midsagittal plane, 2 inches (5 cm) below the iliac crests
    d. Midsagittal plane, 2 inches (5 cm) above the iliac crests

20 Surgical Radiography

EXERCISE 1

Personnel are listed who may be found working within an operating room (OR) during surgical procedures. In the space provided, write S if that person is a sterile team member or N if that person is a nonsterile team member.

_____ 1. Surgeon

_____ 2. Circulator

_____ 3. Radiographer

_____ 4. Anesthesiologist

_____ 5. Surgical assistant

_____ 6. Physician's assistant

_____ 7. Monitoring technologist

_____ 8. Scrub nurse

_____ 9. Certified surgical technologist

_____10. Certified registered nurse anesthetist

Exercise 2

Answer the following questions. For true or false statements, explain any statement you believe is false.

1. Who is the nonsterile surgical team member responsible for monitoring and coordinating all activities within the OR, providing supplies to the certified surgical technologist during the surgical procedure, and managing the care of the patient?
   a. Surgeon
   b. Scrub nurse
   c. Circulator
   d. Monitoring technologist

2. During the surgical procedure, the _____ is responsible for monitoring physiologic functions, maintaining fluid and electrolyte balance, and performing blood replacements.

3. True or false. Street clothes should never be worn within semirestricted areas of the surgical suite.

4. True or false. It takes two people—a radiographer and a sterile team member—to place an IR into a sterile IR cover.

5. True or false. The floor of the OR is always considered contaminated before a surgical procedure begins.

6. True or false. A radiographer may touch only nonsterile items within the OR.

7. True or false. Items of doubtful sterility must be considered nonsterile.

8. True or false. Sterile gowns are considered sterile in front from the shoulder to the level of the knees.

9. True or false. The sleeves of gowns are considered to be sterile from the cuff to the shoulder.

10. True or false. Lifting sterile drapes on a table above table level compromises the sterile field.

11. True or false. The radiographer should place sterile drapes over both ends of the C-arm before entering the OR.

12. True or false. When a mobile x-ray unit becomes contaminated, it should never be cleaned while still inside the OR.

13. During surgical procedures, the most effective means of radiation protection is _____.

14. All of the following provide optimum radiation protection during surgical procedures for the radiographer except:
    a. Standing a minimum of 6 feet from the x-ray source
    b. Standing at a right angle to the patient
    c. Standing at a right angle to the primary beam
    d. Placing the tube side of the C-arm above the patient

15. True or false. The radiographer should be the person who places sterile drapes over both ends of the C-arm.

16. List the reasons operative cholangiography is performed.

    a. _____

    b. _____

    c. _____

17. For the PA projection of the cervical spine ACDF surgical procedure, the C-arm should be:
    a. Directed perpendicular
    b. Angled 15 degrees caudal
    c. Angled 15 degrees cephalic
    d. Angled according to surgeon preference

18. Images of the hip during surgical fixation procedures must demonstrate from the lateral side of the

    _____ to the _____
    to ensure the hardware did not enter the joint.

19. True or false. When lining up the screw holes in the nail during a retrograde femoral nailing procedure, the hole should be imaged perfectly round and centered on the monitor.

20. During a femoral nailing procedure, which surgical team member may manipulate the patient's leg to align the screw holes in the C-arm image?

21. True or false. When positioning the C-arm for imaging a tibial nail insertion, the C-arm should be tilted to match the angle of the affected leg.

22. True or false. When positioning the C-arm for use during a chest line placement, the C-arm enters the sterile field perpendicular to the patient demonstrating a PA projection.

23. True or false. The femur and the tibia should be seen in the image after the subtraction technique is performed during femoral and tibial arteriography.

24. True or false. When performing a radiograph of an extremity during surgical procedures to install reduction hardware, the radiographer should remove sterile draping from the affected extremity to ensure proper centering.

25. *Strike-through* refers to:
    a. moisture from a nonsterile surface soaking through to a sterile surface, causing bacteria to reach a sterile area.
    b. fixation hardware that has been driven too far through the bone.
    c. movement of the C-arm into the "rainbow" position.
    d. a surgical case that requires imaging.

26. When the patient is supine during an antegrade femoral nailing, how should the patient's legs be positioned?

27. When the patient is in the lateral position during an antegrade femoral nailing, how should the patient's legs be positioned?

28. Describe the position of the C-arm relative to the patient when imaging a lateral projection cervical spine (ACDF).

29. Describe the position of the C-arm relative to the patient when imaging a PA projection of the humerus.

30. Describe the position of the C-arm relative to the patient when imaging a hip pinning.

523

Answer the following questions by selecting the best choice.

1. Which of the following personnel is a member of the sterile team during a surgical procedure?
   a. Circulator
   b. Radiographer
   c. Anesthesia provider
   d. Physician's assistant

2. Which of the following personnel is not a member of the sterile team during a surgical procedure?
   a. Surgeon
   b. Radiographer
   c. Surgical assistant
   d. Certified surgical technologist

3. What is the accepted protocol for the wearing of street clothes within the semirestricted and restricted areas of a surgical suite?
   a. They should never be worn in either area.
   b. They can be worn only in the semirestricted areas.
   c. They can be worn in either area only before the surgical procedure begins.
   d. They can be worn in either area only after the surgical procedure is completed.

4. What is the accepted protocol for the wearing of surgical caps within the semirestricted and restricted areas of a surgical suite?
   a. They should always be worn in either area.
   b. They should be worn only in the restricted areas.
   c. They should be worn in either area only after the surgical procedure begins.
   d. They should be worn in either area only before the surgical procedure begins.

5. What should a radiographer do with shoe covers after radiography services are no longer needed in the surgical suite?
   a. Remove them and hand them to the circulator.
   b. Remove and dispose of them before leaving the surgical area.
   c. They should be saved for use during the next visit to the surgical suite.
   d. Wear them until after returning to the radiology department and then properly dispose of them.

6. What procedure should be followed if the radiographer who routinely performs surgical radiography has an acute infection or a sore throat, and radiography services are requested within the operating room (OR)?
   a. Send a different radiographer to the surgical suite.
   b. Ensure that the sick radiographer changes into proper OR attire.
   c. Send another radiographer to assist the sick radiographer inside the OR.
   d. Ensure that the sick radiographer wears gloves and a facemask when inside restricted areas of the surgical suite.

7. What procedure should a radiographer do if the sterile field is accidentally compromised?
   a. Immediately notify a member of the OR staff.
   b. Wipe down the mobile unit and repeat the procedure.
   c. Quickly finish the procedure and leave the OR.
   d. Change into clean OR attire and finish the procedure

8. What is the proper procedure for placing an IR into a sterile IR cover?
   a. A radiographer should hand the IR to the surgeon so that he or she can put it into a sterile IR cover.
   b. A radiographer should open the sterile IR cover and place the IR into it.
   c. A surgical technologist should open the sterile IR cover and hold it open for the radiographer to insert the IR into it.
   d. A radiographer should open the sterile IR cover and hold it open for the surgical technologist to insert the IR into it.

9. Which article of his or her OR attire should a radiographer remove before handling the IR after performing a surgical radiography procedure?
   a. Cap
   b. Mask
   c. Gloves
   d. Shoe covers

10. What procedure should a radiographer perform if an exposed IR becomes contaminated in the OR?
    a. Leave the contaminated IR in the OR.
    b. Repeat the examination with a clean IR.
    c. Wrap the contaminated IR in a sterile drape.
    d. Clean the IR with a hospital-approved disinfectant before leaving the OR.

11. When cleaning contaminated x-ray equipment within the OR suite, why is it preferred that cleaning solutions be poured instead of sprayed onto a rag?
    a. To conserve cleaning solutions
    b. To prevent possible contamination from the spray
    c. To reduce the amount of time it takes to clean the equipment
    d. To enable the cleaning of x-ray equipment while using only one hand

12. What is the position of the C-arm relative to the patient when imaging the humerus?
    a. Perpendicular
    b. Parallel or at a 45-degree angle
    c. Perpendicular or at a 45-degree angle
    d. Parallel or at a 30-degree angle

13. Where should the C-arm be centered for an operative cholangiogram?
    a. Over the left side of the abdomen and superior to the rib line
    b. Over the left side of the abdomen and inferior to the rib line
    c. Over the right side of the abdomen and superior to the rib line
    d. Over the right side of the abdomen and inferior to the rib line

14. Why is it necessary to demonstrate a catheter from its insertion point to its terminal end with a C-arm unit when performing a line placement examination?
    a. To ensure there are no kinks in the catheter and to ensure that it is in the proper position
    b. To ensure there are no kinks in the catheter and to measure the length of the catheter accurately
    c. To measure the depth of penetration accurately and to ensure that it is in the proper position
    d. To measure the depth of penetration accurately and to measure the length of the catheter accurately

15. How many degrees and in which direction should the C-arm be tilted for the AP projection of the cervical spine during an ACDF procedure?
    a. 15 degrees caudad
    b. 15 degrees cephalad
    c. 25 degrees caudad
    d. 25 degrees cephalad

16. When using a C-arm unit to perform the lateral projection of the cervical spine, what procedure should be accomplished to place the spine into the center of the monitor?
    a. Raise or lower the C-arm.
    b. Remove padding from under the patient.
    c. Raise or lower the surgery table and patient.
    d. Place radiolucent cushions under the patient.

17. After obtaining a PA projection when using the C-arm during a hip pinning procedure, what procedure should be done to obtain a lateral image?
    a. Rotate the image intensifier 90 degrees.
    b. Rotate the C-arm under the leg and table.
    c. Rotate the patient's leg to the lateral position.
    d. Rotate the patient into a lateral recumbent position.

18. Where should a radiographer position the C-arm for use during a hip pinning procedure?
    a. Alongside the upper torso
    b. Between the patient's legs
    c. At right angles to the patient on the affected side
    d. At right angles to the patient on the unaffected side

19. When using the C-arm during a hip pinning procedure, what structures should be visualized to determine a starting point and to ensure no hardware enters the joint?
    a. Distal end of the femur and acetabular rim
    b. Distal end of the femur and intercondylar fossa
    c. Lateral side of the femur and acetabular rim
    d. Lateral side of the femur and intercondylar fossa

20. When using the C-arm during a tibial nailing procedure, how is it determined that the C-arm is correctly positioned over the patient's affected leg?
    a. Tilt the tube and image intensifier to match the angle of the leg.
    b. Tilt the tube and image intensifier to match the angle of the femur.
    c. Turn the wheels of the machine parallel with the patient to move the machine longitudinally.
    d. Turn the wheels of the machine perpendicular to the patient to move the machine toward the patient.

21. When using the C-arm during a tibial nailing procedure, what is the purpose for turning the wheels of the C-arm parallel with the long axis of the affected tibia?
    a. To prevent the C-arm from tilting during the procedure
    b. To prevent the C-arm from moving during the procedure
    c. To enable the C-arm to move toward the midline of the patient
    d. To enable the C-arm to move longitudinally alongside the patient

22. Why should a sterile drape not be allowed to remain on the tube of the C-arm for a long time?
    a. The tube may overheat.
    b. The drape may become contaminated.
    c. The drape may cause artifacts on the image.
    d. The drape may contaminate the sterile field.

23. How should the C-arm be positioned relative to the patient when imaging the patient during a bronchoscopy?
    a. Lateral
    b. Perpendicular
    c. AP axial with 30 degrees caudal angulation
    d. AP axial with 30 degrees cephalad angulation

24. Which surgical procedure will most likely require subtraction technique with C-arm imaging?
    a. Hip pinning
    b. Femoral nailing
    c. Chest line placement
    d. Femoral arteriography

25. What are two reasons for performing a lateral projection of thoracic or lumbar spine inside the OR?
    a. To identify specific vertebrae and to show the position of hardware
    b. To identify specific vertebrae and to perform an operational check of the portable unit
    c. To demonstrate intervertebral foramina and to show the position of hardware
    d. To demonstrate intervertebral foramina and to perform an operational check of the portable unit

21 Pediatric Imaging

Students must be prepared to meet the challenges of specific patient populations. Children are not just smaller versions of adults, so unique and specific skills are required to image pediatric patients successfully. The following questions provide a review of necessary skills to work with pediatric patients successfully.

1. List artifacts unique to digital imaging of pediatric patients.

2. Children are more sensitive to radiation exposure than adults.
   a. True
   b. False

3. Within the imaging room, which of the following can reduce patient anxiety and the need for immobilization?
   1. Provide age-appropriate videos.
   2. Perform the procedure in a room with a good view.
   3. Align the imaging equipment before bringing the patient in the room.

   a. 1 and 2 only
   b. 1 and 3 only
   c. 2 and 3 only
   d. 1, 2, and 3

4. When communicating with a child, it is important to (circle all that apply):
   a. Use language that the child can understand.
   b. Bend down and talk to the child at the child's eye level.
   c. Provide plenty of options to allow the child freedom of choice.
   d. Threaten the child to intimidate him or her to cooperate.
   e. Employ distraction techniques, such as talking to the child about school, TV shows, or siblings.
   f. Use sincere praise.

5. Which age group is eager to please but is also modest and embarrasses easily?

6. In dealing with a child with special needs, the imaging professional should speak and provide instructions only to the adult caregiver.
   a. True
   b. False

7. Which condition is the invagination or telescoping of the bowel into itself?

8. Which condition manifests with the presence of air or gas in the peritoneal cavity as a result of disease or for the treatment of certain conditions?

9. Which of the following is one of the most dangerous causes of acute upper airway obstruction in children and is treated as an emergency?
   a. Osteogenesis imperfecta
   b. Epiglottitis
   c. Omphalocele
   d. Hypothermia

10. Which pediatric disease makes children more prone to spontaneous fractures?

11. What is the first course of action for a radiographer who suspects child abuse of a pediatric patient?

12. According to the American College of Radiology, what are the three indications for performing a skeletal survey on pediatric patients?

13. Which of the following are measures to protect pediatric patients from unnecessary radiation exposure? Check all that apply.

_____ a. Place lead shielding on the upper torso and gonads during upper limb radiography.

_____ b. Include multiple parts within the collimated field to reduce individual exposures.

_____ c. Have older children wear child-sized full lead aprons or adult aprons.

_____ d. Use strategic placement of gonadal and breast shielding, and employ effective immobilization techniques to reduce the need for repeat examinations.

_____ e. Employ diagonal placement of small gonadal aprons along the thorax and abdomen to protect the sternum and gonads of infants and toddlers during supine radiography.

_____ f. Use low kVp and high mAs techniques for optimum diagnostic images.

14. The _____ is a commonly used immobilization device for pediatric chest radiography on patients from birth to age 3 years.

15. For skull radiography, the _____ immobilization technique is often employed.

16. True or false. The Pigg-O-Stat can be used for effective immobilization when performing abdominal images on newborns and children up to 3 years of age.

17. Which of the following is the most reliable method of detecting inspiration on chest radiography for patients from birth to age 3 years?
a. Wait until the child stops crying
b. Watching the rise and fall of the chest and abdomen
c. Rely on the parent to tell you
d. All of these methods

18. List immobilization techniques that could be employed if there is not another adult available to assist throughout the procedure?

19. Which of the following are true regarding gonadal shielding during pelvis/hip radiography of pediatric patients? Check all that apply.

_____ a. Always use on boys.

_____ b. Girls may be shielded after the initial examination has ruled out sacral problems.

_____ c. Always use on girls.

_____ d. Place shielding on boys in midline at the level of the anterior superior iliac spine (ASIS).

_____ e. Place shielding on girls in midline at the level of the ASIS.

_____ f. Place shielding on boys at the level of greater trochanters.

20. In imaging the limbs of a pediatric patient, it is often necessary to examine the side for _____.

21. What type of fracture occurs through the epiphysis?

22. What are some indications for ordering hip examinations on children?

23. When examining a pediatric patient for a possible aspirated foreign body, the routine protocol should include the following:

    a. _____

    b. _____

    c. _____

    d. _____

24. Which of the following are important radiation protection practices for scoliosis images?
    1. Accurate collimation
    2. Breast shields
    3. Gonadal shield

    a. 1 and 2 only
    b. 1 and 3 only
    c. 2 and 3 only
    d. 1, 2, and 3

25. _____ is often required to perform an MRI examination on a pediatric patient, greatly

    increasing the _____ of the procedure.

26. List some difficulties to consider when imaging children with autism spectrum disorders.

27. True or false. Children with autism spectrum disorder process information in their brain similar to the average person.

28. Does autism spectrum disorder affect boys or girls more commonly?

29. List some tips to consider when imaging children with autism spectrum disorder.

30. True or false. Children with autism spectrum disorders often have trouble interpreting facial expressions, body language, and tone of voice.

Answer the following questions by selecting the best choice.

1. One of the ways to obtain the cooperation of a pediatric patient is to:
   a. make sure you explain everything to the parents.
   b. talk to the child at his or her eye level.
   c. talk to the child in "baby talk."
   d. give the child plenty of options to choose from.

2. In communicating with an adolescent patient, it is important to assess the individual's:
   a. maturity level.
   b. intelligence level.
   c. sensitivity level.
   d. level of independence.

3. One of the greatest dangers facing a premature infant is:
   a. radiation exposure.
   b. exposure to contagions.
   c. hyperthermia.
   d. hypothermia.

4. Whenever possible, a premature infant should be examined:
   a. within the isolette or infant warmer.
   b. in an upright position.
   c. with the diaper in place.
   d. within the imaging department.

5. Pediatric patients with a sinusitis must be examined in the _____ position.
   a. upright
   b. supine
   c. prone
   d. Trendelenburg

6. Which congenital anomaly manifests with imperfectly formed bone, short stature, and a triangular-shaped face?
   a. Myelomeningocele
   b. Omphalocele
   c. Osteogenesis imperfecta
   d. Spina bifida

7. When performing a soft tissue neck examination on a pediatric patient who has a suspected swollen epiglottis, what is the recommended body position?
   a. Supine
   b. Upright
   c. Dorsal
   d. Prone

8. Which pediatric fracture usually occurs in the forearm when bending resistance is exceeded but the bone does not break?
   a. Supracondylar
   b. Salter-Harris
   c. Greenstick
   d. Bowing

9. Which of the following is characteristic of osteogenesis imperfecta?
   a. Acute respiratory distress
   b. Increased risk of hypothermia
   c. Increased susceptibility to fractures
   d. Increased dependency on parents

10. In a case of suspected child abuse, the radiographer's first course of action is to:
    a. talk with the parents.
    b. call the police.
    c. consult with a radiologist or other attending physician.
    d. submit a written report to the social work department.

11. Which of the following radiologic findings indicate high specificity of physical child abuse?
    1. Posterior rib fractures
    2. Scapular fractures
    3. Sternal fracture

    a. 1 and 2 only
    b. 1 and 3 only
    c. 2 and 3 only
    d. 1, 2, and 3

12. One of the most commonly used immobilizers for pediatric chest and abdominal radiography is the:
    a. Pigg-O-Stat
    b. octagonal infant immobilizer
    c. "bunny" wrap
    d. conscious sedation

13. A voiding cystourethrogram is used to help rule out which of the following?
    a. Foreign object
    b. Reflux
    c. Perforation
    d. Constipation

14. The most reliable method to detect inspiration for chest radiography on patients from birth to age 3 years is to:
    a. watch the rise and fall of the chest and abdomen.
    b. rely on the parent to tell you.
    c. expose in between gasps when crying.
    d. wait until the child stops crying.

15. What type of immobilization is recommended for skull radiography of patients age 3 years or younger?
    a. Pigg-O-Stat
    b. Conscious sedation
    c. "Bunny" wrap
    d. Velcro straps and adult physical restraint

16. Which of the following is the recommended method of limb radiography of preschool-age patients?
    a. Sitting on a parent's lap
    b. Modified "bunny" wrap immobilization
    c. Octagonal infant immobilizer
    d. Velcro straps and adult restraint

17. Which of the following is often required for limb radiography of a pediatric patient?
    a. Conscious sedation
    b. Examination of the contralateral limb
    c. Neurologic assessment
    d. Stress positions

18. Which type of fracture occurs through the epiphysis?
    a. Salter-Harris fractures
    b. Bucket-handle fractures
    c. Greenstick fractures
    d. Torus or buckle fractures

19. Hip examinations on children are most often ordered to assess for:
    a. fractures
    b. Legg-Calvé-Perthes disease
    c. osteogenesis imperfecta
    d. Osgood-Schlatter disease

20. Which of the following statements is true regarding shielding of female patients during hip and pelvic radiography?
    a. Female patients are always shielded.
    b. The top of the shield is placed at the level of the greater trochanters.
    c. Female patients can be shielded after the initial examination has ruled out sacral problems.
    d. Female patients can never be shielded for pelvis/hip radiographs.

21. Which of the following body parts may be imaged for bone age studies?
    1. Left hand and wrist
    2. Right knee
    3. Bilateral hips

    a. 1 only
    b. 1 and 3 only
    c. 2 and 3 only
    d. 1, 2, and 3

22. Which type of immobilization is most versatile for imaging chest, abdomen, pelvis, and hips among the different pediatric age groups?
    a. "Bunny" wrap technique
    b. Velcro straps
    c. Pigg-O-Stat
    d. Baby box

23. Which of the following should be part of the routine protocol when imaging a pediatric patient for a suspected aspirated foreign body?
    1. PA chest on inspiration
    2. PA chest on expiration
    3. Lateral chest

    a. 1 and 2 only
    b. 1 and 3 only
    c. 2 and 3 only
    d. 1, 2, and 3

24. Where is an aspirated foreign body more likely to lodge?
    a. The upper esophagus
    b. Just superior to the cricoid cartilage of the trachea
    c. The right primary bronchus
    d. The left primary bronchus

25. What is the primary hindrance for the use of MRI on pediatric patients?
    a. Length and nature of the examination requires general anesthesia to avoid patient motion, increasing the risk.
    b. Magnet strength has not been proven safe for persons with premature skeletons and organs.
    c. Pediatric patients do not have sufficient hydrogen atom content to provide quality, diagnostic images.
    d. Computer algorithms cannot compensate for smaller patients with less body mass, so image quality is compromised.

26. Which of the following are recommendations for imaging children with autism spectrum disorder?
    a. Schedule the examination at a time when the department is not busy.
    b. Reduce loud noises and visual distractions.
    c. Adjust lighting.
    d. All of the above.

27. Which of the following are examples of social stories that could be used when imaging children with autism spectrum disorder? (Circle all that apply.)
    a. Written or visual guide describing various social interactions or situations
    b. Flash cards
    c. Illustrations of shopping in a grocery store
    d. Pictures of the parking garage, waiting room, imaging room

531

28. Identify some difficulties to consider when imaging children with autism spectrum disorders. (Circle all that apply.)
    a. Sensitivity to touch
    b. Communication
    c. Overstimulation
    d. Identifying the correct patient

29. When performing needle-sticks on children with autism spectrum disorder, which of the following are true?
    a. Child could be oversensitive to pain
    b. Child could be undersensitive to pain
    c. Child may feel pain acutely
    d. Child may not feel any pain
    e. All of the above

30. Technologists should consider the following patient responses among children with autism spectrum disorder EXCEPT:
    a. assume that a nonverbal patient is not understanding what you are saying.
    b. patients are still listening even if there is no eye contact.
    c. extra time is needed to assure the patient processes instructions.
    d. laughter and singing is a possible response to pain.

22 Geriatric Radiography

GERIATRIC PATIENTS

Section 1: Exercise 1

Students must be prepared to meet the challenges of specific patient populations. The increasing number of elderly persons demands that radiographers be prepared to meet their unique needs. The following questions provide a review of necessary skills to work with geriatric patients successfully.

1. Define *geriatrics*.

2. To work successfully with elderly patients, the radiographer must be able to differentiate between:
   a. age-related changes and disease processes.
   b. senility and dementia.
   c. senior citizens and elderly persons.
   d. cognitive impairments and dementia.

3. List the top 10 chronic conditions of people age 65 years and older.

4. What are the most common health complaints of elderly patients?

5. Progressive cognitive impairment that eventually interferes with daily functioning is termed

   _____.

6. True or false. All elderly persons develop dementia.

7. What is the most common form of dementia?

8. The Joint Commission has a standard that requires radiographers to demonstrate competency in working with geriatric patients when it is applicable.
   a. True
   b. False

9. Which of the following are reasons to educate the geriatric patient and his or her family members about imaging procedures?
   1. Obtain their confidence
   2. Decrease patient stress
   3. Improve patient compliance

   a. 1 and 2 only
   b. 2 and 3 only
   c. 1 and 3 only
   d. 1, 2, and 3

10. How should the radiographer adjust his or her communication skills to accommodate an elderly patient who has a hearing loss?

533

11. Elimination of _____ will improve the listening environment for an elderly patient.

12. List three ways to increase the security for a geriatric patient when transporting him or her from the wheelchair to the examination table.

13. To reduce the risk of tearing the fragile skin of a geriatric patient, the use of _____ for immobilization should be avoided.

14. The amount of contrast media administered to an elderly patient varies because of

_____.

15. Knowledge of age-related changes and disease processes _____ the radiographer's ability to meet the special care needs of the elderly patient.
    a. Improves
    b. Decreases
    c. Does not affect

Section 1: Exercise 2

This exercise will increase your medical vocabulary of terms and disease processes that are common to geriatric patients. Match the age-associated condition with the organ system in which it manifests or affects. Some systems may be used more than once, and some conditions may be linked to more than one system.

Column A

_____ 1. Anemia

_____ 2. Incontinence

_____ 3. Hearing loss

_____ 4. Postural hypotension

_____ 5. Difficulty swallowing

_____ 6. Graying and thinning hair

_____ 7. Increases vulnerability to nosocomial infections

_____ 8. Increased risk of falls

_____ 9. Osteoporosis

_____ 10. Osteoarthritis

_____ 11. Dementia

_____ 12. Diverticulosis

_____ 13. Increased vulnerability to abrasions

_____ 14. Presbyopia

_____ 15. Atherosclerosis

_____ 16. Autoimmune diseases

_____ 17. Decreased elasticity of alveoli

_____ 18. Diabetes mellitus

_____ 19. Kyphosis

_____ 20. Contractures

Column B

a. Integumentary system

b. Endocrine system

c. Gastrointestinal system

d. Immune system

e. Sensory system

f. Urinary system

g. Cardiovascular system

h. Nervous system

i. Musculoskeletal system

j. Respiratory system

k. Hematologic system

GERIATRIC RADIOGRAPHY

Section 2: Exercise 1: Chest and Spine Adaptations

1. For the PA projection of the chest, how should the position of the upper limbs be altered to increase comfort and adapt to the abilities of a geriatric patient?

2. The lateral projections of the chest never require positioning adaptation for geriatric patients.
   a. True
   b. False

3. When kyphosis is present, the image receptor should be centered _____ and the central ray should be centered _____ to accommodate changes in positioning of the anatomy of interest.

4. During spine imaging on geriatric patients, _____ is a common consideration in terms of increased discomfort and pain during positioning.

5. If the geriatric patient's safety is not compromised, obtaining spine images in the _____ position may be a more comfortable accommodation.

Section 2: Exercise 2: Pelvis, Upper Limb, and Lower Limb Adaptations

1. Hip pathologies in geriatric patients are often caused by:
   a. _____.
   b. _____.
   c. _____.

2. What positioning adaptation is made for the AP projection of the pelvis and hips if trauma is an indication?

3. Contractures of the upper limb are often seen in geriatric patients who have experienced a _____.

4. Contracted limbs must be forced into the correct position to obtain accurate images.
   a. True
   b. False

5. In the upper limb, the _____ is a common site for reduced mobility and flexibility, fractures, and dislocations.

6. AP projections of the forearm, humerus, and elbow can be difficult to obtain in geriatric patients because _____ is often impaired by contractures, paralysis, and fractures.

7. If a geriatric patient cannot turn on his or her side for a lateral projection of the lower limb, what accommodation may be used?

8. Radiography of the foot and ankle on geriatric patients may be performed more safely with the patient in a wheelchair, rather than risking transfer to the radiographic table.
   a. True
   b. False

9. To maintain sufficient contrast in skeletal radiography on geriatric patients, a _____ kilovolt peak is often required.

10. Maintaining the proper position is a consideration with geriatric patients, so the _____ _____ _____ should always be used to reduce the risk of imaging voluntary or involuntary motion.

CHAPTER 22: SELF-TEST: GERIATRIC RADIOGRAPHY

Answer the following questions by selecting the best choice.

1. The branch of medicine dealing with elderly people and the problems of aging is termed:
   a. pediatrics.
   b. geriatrics.
   c. psychiatry.
   d. endocrinology.

2. To provide quality images and work well with the geriatric patient, the radiographer must be able to:
   a. adapt procedures to accommodate disabilities and diseases unique to the geriatric population.
   b. speak loudly and eliminate background noises.
   c. adapt technical factors to ensure proper radiation protection.
   d. calculate necessary contrast media adjustments.

3. It is important for the health care professional not only to know diseases and disorders common to specific age groups but also to know:
   a. the associated economic status.
   b. most popular social activities.
   c. a particular ethnic group.
   d. the effects on different genders.

4. Which of the following are among the top 10 chronic conditions for people older than age 65 years?
   1. Visual impairment
   2. Cancer
   3. Diabetes

   a. 1 and 2 only
   b. 1 and 3 only
   c. 2 and 3 only
   d. 1, 2, and 3

5. A term used to describe the stereotyping of and discrimination against elderly persons is:
   a. ageism.
   b. elderism.
   c. geriatricism.
   d. racism.

6. What is one of the common psychological effects of aging?
   a. Gray hair
   b. Wrinkles
   c. Depression
   d. Alzheimer disease

7. One of the most common health complaints of elderly patients is:
   a. hair loss.
   b. depression.
   c. diabetes.
   d. fatigue.

8. Which of the following can slow the progress of age-related joint stiffness, fatigue, weight gain, and bone mass loss?
   a. Vitamin supplements
   b. Nonsteroidal antiinflammatory drugs (NSAIDs)
   c. Mental games
   d. Low-impact exercise

9. Which of the following can cause cognitive impairment in elderly persons?
   1. Disuse
   2. Aging
   3. Disease

   a. 1 and 2 only
   b. 1 and 3 only
   c. 2 and 3 only
   d. 1, 2, and 3

10. Which of the following terms is defined as progressive cognitive impairment that eventually interferes with normal daily functioning?
    a. Dementia
    b. Senility
    c. Alzheimer disease
    d. Depression

11. Alzheimer disease is the most common form of:
    a. depression.
    b. senility.
    c. dementia.
    d. ageism.

12. Which body system is usually the first to show apparent signs of aging?
    a. Gastrointestinal system
    b. Integumentary system
    c. Cardiovascular system
    d. Musculoskeletal system

13. Which body system is responsible for most of the disabilities in people older than 65 years?
    a. Integumentary system
    b. Nervous system
    c. Immune system
    d. Cardiovascular system

538

14. Hearing and visual impairments associated with aging are classified as disorders of the:
    a. sensory system.
    b. integumentary system.
    c. nervous system.
    d. musculoskeletal system.

15. What is the predominate age-related change in the blood vessels?
    a. Loss of elasticity
    b. Ulcerations
    c. Atherosclerosis
    d. Degeneration

16. The major hematologic concern in geriatric patients is:
    a. ischemia.
    b. atherosclerosis.
    c. diabetes.
    d. anemia.

17. Which of the following is crucial to obtain an elderly patient's compliance and confidence?
    a. Education about imaging procedures
    b. Demonstration of empathy
    c. Knowledge of imaging procedures
    d. Demonstration of self-confidence and personal hygiene

18. Elimination of _____ will aid in listening and communications with geriatric patients.
    a. extraneous words
    b. body language
    c. background noise
    d. facial expressions

19. An elderly patient often experiences _____ when going from a recumbent position to a sitting position.
    a. nausea
    b. vertigo
    c. fear
    d. depression

20. The amount of contrast media used for imaging procedures varies for elderly patients because of:
    a. incontinence.
    b. anemia.
    c. age-related changes in cardiovascular system.
    d. age-related changes in liver and kidney functions.

21. To obtain an accurate PA projection of the chest, a geriatric patient is likely to be more comfortable with the upper limbs positioned:
    a. low, with the backs of the hands resting on the hips, shoulders rolled forward.
    b. wrapped around the chest stand.
    c. resting on top of the head.
    d. straight by the sides of the body.

22. Supination of the upper limb is often impaired in geriatric patients because of all of the following except:
    a. cognitive impairment.
    b. contractures.
    c. paralysis.
    d. fractures.

23. When performing lower limb images, what projection(s) can be substituted for the routine lateral when the patient is unable to lie on his or her side?
    a. Both internal and external obliques
    b. AP
    c. Cross-table lateral
    d. Axial

24. Because radiographic landmarks can change with age, centering for the chest in a geriatric patient with extreme kyphosis may need to be:
    a. more medial than normal.
    b. more lateral than normal.
    c. higher than normal.
    d. lower than normal.

25. To obtain sufficient contrast in geriatric radiography, kVp may need to be:
    a. decreased.
    b. increased.
    c. the same as for pediatric patients.
    d. the same, but mAs must be increased.

539

23 Sectional Anatomy for Radiographers

REVIEW

It is essential that the radiographer have an understanding of the relationships between organ and skeletal structures to perform computed tomography (CT), magnetic resonance imaging (MRI), and diagnostic medical sonography examinations because all three modalities create images of sectional anatomy. This exercise is a review of sectional anatomy. Identify structures for each item.

Fig. 23.1A and B show CT and MR localizers, or scout, images of the skull. Figs. 23.2 through 23.5 pertain to the imaging planes shown in Fig. 23.1.

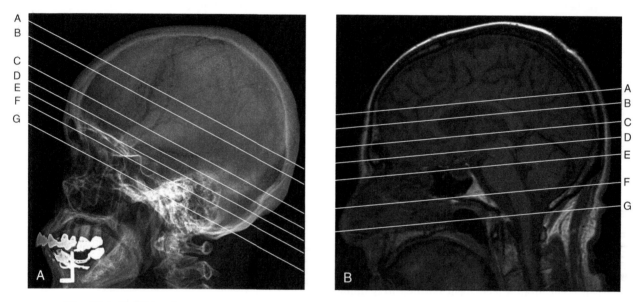

Fig. 23.1 (A) CT localizer, or scout, image of the skull. (B) Sagittal localizer for MR images of the brain.

1. Identify each lettered structure shown in Fig. 23.2.

   A. _____

   B. _____

   C. _____

   D. _____

   E. _____

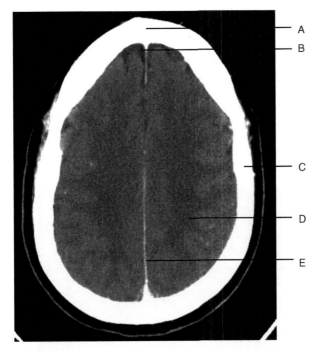

Fig. 23.2 CT image corresponding to level A in Fig. 23.1A.

Refer to Fig. 23.2 and answer the following questions.

2. The central tract of white matter in the cerebrum that is demonstrated in the CT image as darker than the surrounding cortex is called the

   _____.

3. Which letter in Fig. 23.2 labels the structure defined in question 2?

4. The fold of dura mater that lines the longitudinal fissure is the _____.

5. Identify each lettered structure shown in Fig. 23.3.

   A. _____

   B. _____

   C. _____

   D. _____

   E. _____

   F. _____

   G. _____

   H. _____

   I. _____

   J. _____

   K. _____

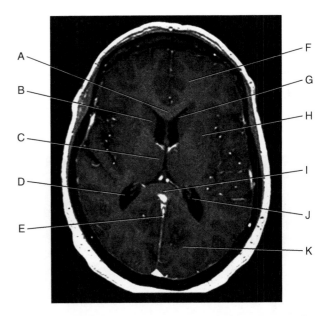

Fig. 23.3 MR image corresponding to level C in Fig. 23.1B.

Refer to Fig. 23.3 and answer the following questions.

6. Which structure labeled in Fig. 23.3 forms the lateral walls of the third ventricle?

Chapter **23 Sectional Anatomy for Radiographers**

7. Which structures labeled in Fig. 23.3 are parts of the basal nuclei?

8. The function of the choroid plexus is to _____ _____.

9. Identify each lettered structure shown in Fig. 23.4.

A. _____

B. _____

C. _____

D. _____

E. _____

F. _____

G. _____

H. _____

I. _____

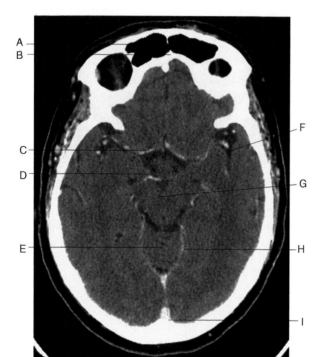

Fig. 23.4 CT image corresponding to level D in Fig. 23.1A.

10. The structures labeled as C, D, and F in Fig. 23.4 are part of the _____.

11. Identify each lettered structure shown in Fig. 23.5.

A. _____

B. _____

C. _____

D. _____

E. _____

F. _____

G. _____

H. _____

I. _____

J. _____

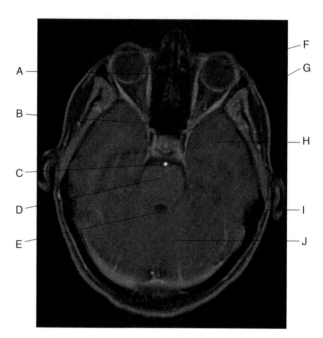

Fig. 23.5 MR image corresponding to level E in Fig. 23.1B.

Examine Fig. 23.5 and answer the following questions.

12. True or false. The optic nerves can also be seen in this image.

13. Which portions of the cerebrum are seen on the lateral sides of the sella turcica in Fig. 23.5?

14. Corresponding to level A in Fig. 23.6, identify each lettered structure shown in Fig. 23.7.

A. _____

B. _____

C. _____

D. _____

E. _____

F. _____

G. _____

H. _____

I. _____

J. _____

K. _____

L. _____

M. _____

N. _____

O. _____

P. _____

Q. _____

R. _____

S. _____

T. _____

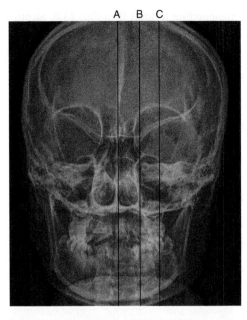

Fig. 23.6 PA projection of skull for localization of sagittal images.

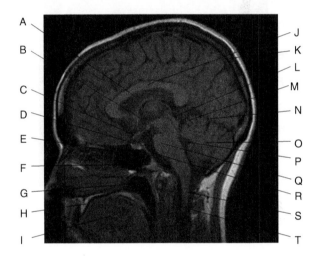

Fig. 23.7 Sagittal MR image of brain through the midsagittal plane.

Chapter **23 Sectional Anatomy for Radiographers**

15. Corresponding to level B in Fig. 23.6, identify each lettered structure shown in Fig. 23.8.

A. _____

B. _____

C. _____

D. _____

E. _____

F. _____

G. _____

H. _____

I. _____

J. _____

Fig. 23.9 shows a CT localizer, or scout, image of the skull. Figs. 23.10 to 23.12 pertain to the imaging planes shown in Fig. 23.9.

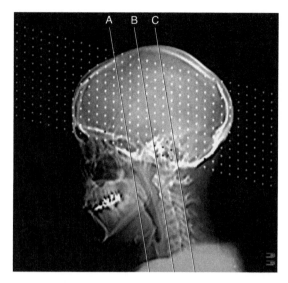

Fig. 23.9 CT localizer, or scout, image of the skull.

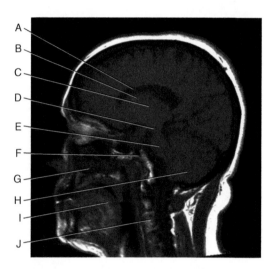

Fig. 23.8 Sagittal MR image through medial wall of orbit corresponding to level B in Fig. 23.6.

16. Identify each lettered structure shown in Fig. 23.10.

A. _____

B. _____

C. _____

D. _____

E. _____

F. _____

G. _____

H. _____

I. _____

J. _____

K. _____

L. _____

M. _____

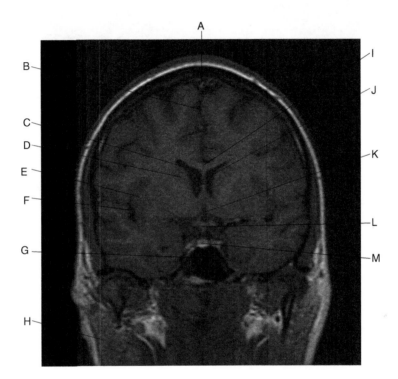

Fig. 23.10 MR image corresponding to level A in Fig. 23.9.

17. What connecting membrane can be seen in this image between the lateral ventricles in Fig. 23.10?

18. True or false. The external carotid arteries are visible in the parotid salivary glands in Fig. 23.10.

Chapter **23 Sectional Anatomy for Radiographers**

19. Identify each lettered structure shown in Fig. 23.11.

A. _____

B. _____

C. _____

D. _____

E. _____

F. _____

G. _____

H. _____

I. _____

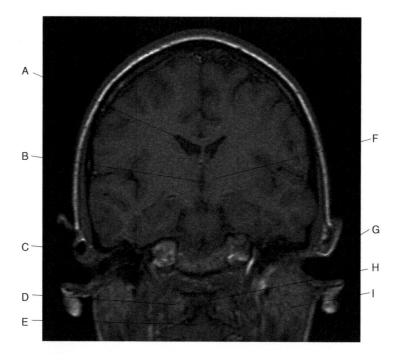

Fig. 23.11 MR image corresponding to level B in Fig. 23.9.

20. Identify each lettered structure shown in Fig. 23.12.

A. _____

B. _____

C. _____

D. _____

E. _____

F. _____

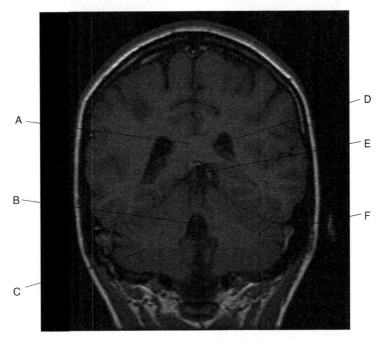

Fig. 23.12 MR image corresponding to level C in Fig. 23.9.

21. What portion of the corpus callosum is labeled as A in Fig. 23.12?

22. Identify each lettered structure shown in Fig. 23.13.

A. _____   C. _____

B. _____   D. _____

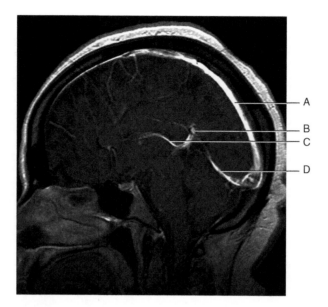

Fig. 23.13 Mid-sagittal contrast enhanced MR of the brain.

23. Identify each lettered structure shown in Fig. 23.14.

A. _____   C. _____

B. _____

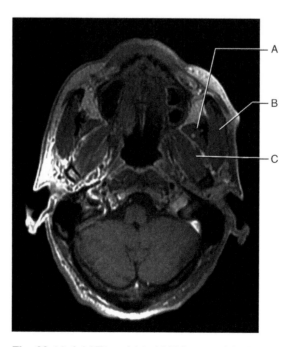

Fig. 23.14 Axial T1-weighted MR image of the brain.

Fig. 23.15 shows a CT localizer, or scout, image of the thorax. Figs. 23.16 to 23.18 pertain to the imaging planes shown in Fig. 23.15.

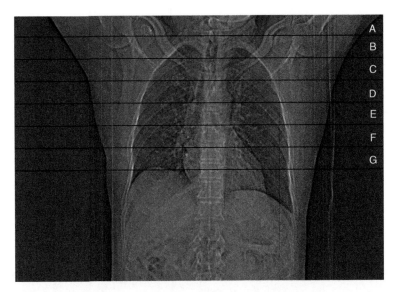

Fig. 23.15 CT localizer, or scout, image of the thorax.

24. Identify each lettered structure shown in Fig. 23.16.

A. _____

B. _____

C. _____

D. _____

E. _____

F. _____

G. _____

H. _____

I. _____

J. _____

K. _____

L. _____

M. _____

N. _____

O. _____

P. _____

Q. _____

R. _____

S. _____

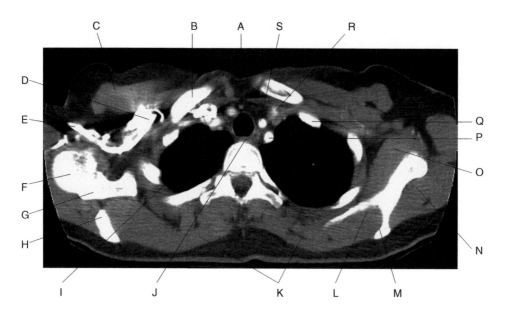

Fig. 23.16 CT image corresponding to level B in Fig. 23.15 through the jugular notch.

25. Identify each lettered structure shown in Fig. 23.17.

A. _____

B. _____

C. _____

D. _____

E. _____

F. _____

G. _____

H. _____

I. _____

J. _____

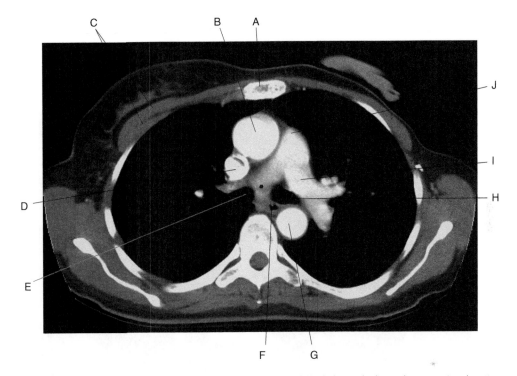

Fig. 23.17 CT image corresponding to level E of Fig. 23.15 through the pulmonary trunk.

26. Identify each lettered structure shown in Fig. 23.18.

A. _____

B. _____

C. _____

D. _____

E. _____

F. _____

G. _____

H. _____

I. _____

J. _____

K. _____

L. _____

M. _____

N. _____

O. _____

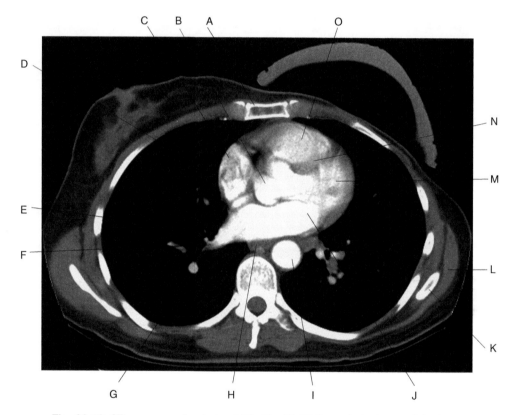

Fig. 23.18 CT corresponding to level F in Fig. 23.15 through the base of the heart.

Fig. 23.19 shows a CT localizer image representing levels of sagittal sections through the thorax. Figs. 23.20 and 23.21 pertain to the imaging planes shown in Fig. 23.19.

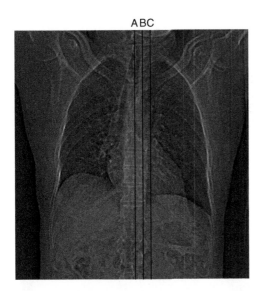

ABC

Fig. 23.19 CT localizer image representing levels of sagittal sections through the thorax.

27. Identify each lettered structure in Fig. 23.20.

A. _____

B. _____

C. _____

D. _____

E. _____

F. _____

G. _____

H. _____

I. _____

J. _____

K. _____

L. _____

M. _____

N. _____

O. _____

P. _____

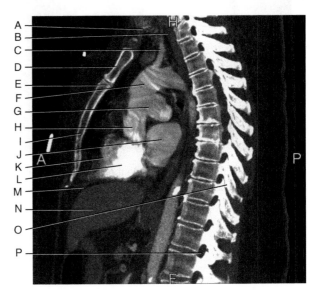

Fig. 23.20 Sagittal CT image of the thorax corresponding to level A in Fig. 23.19.

Chapter **23 Sectional Anatomy for Radiographers**

28. Identify each lettered structure shown in Fig. 23.21.

A. _____

B. _____

C. _____

D. _____

E. _____

F. _____

G. _____

H. _____

I. _____

J. _____

29. What large vessel is seen just anteriorly to the thoracic vertebrae in Fig. 23.21?

Fig. 23.22 shows a lateral chest image representing the levels of coronal sections through the thorax. Figs. 23.23 and 23.24 pertain to the imaging planes shown in Fig. 23.22.

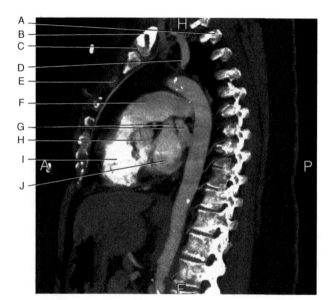

Fig. 23.21 Sagittal CT image of the thorax corresponding to level C in Fig. 23.19.

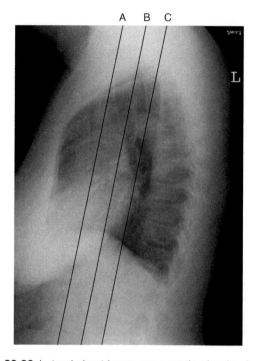

Fig. 23.22 Lateral chest image representing levels of coronal sections through the thorax.

30. Identify each lettered structure shown in Fig. 23.23.

A. _____

B. _____

C. _____

D. _____

E. _____

F. _____

G. _____

H. _____

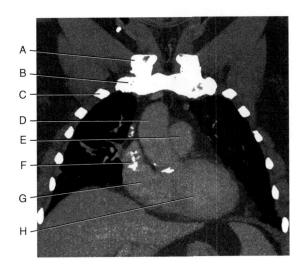

Fig. 23.23 Coronal CT image of the thorax corresponding to level A in Fig. 23.22.

31. Identify each lettered structure shown in Fig. 23.24.

A. _____

B. _____

C. _____

D. _____

E. _____

F. _____

G. _____

H. _____

I. _____

J. _____

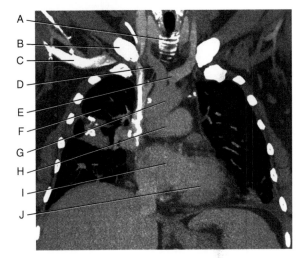

Fig. 23.24 Coronal CT image of the thorax corresponding to level B in Fig. 23.22.

Chapter **23 Sectional Anatomy for Radiographers**

Fig. 23.25 shows a CT localizer, or scout, image of the abdominopelvic region. Figs. 23.26 through 23.31 pertain to the imaging planes shown in Fig. 23.25.

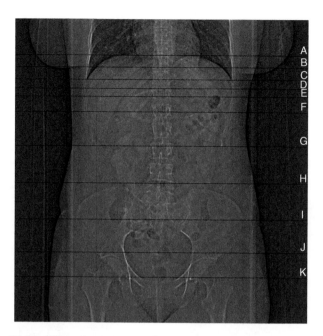

Fig. 23.25 CT localizer, or scout, image of the abdominopelvic region.

32. Identify each lettered structure shown in Fig. 23.26.

A. _____

B. _____

C. _____

D. _____

E. _____

F. _____

G. _____

H. _____

I. _____

J. _____

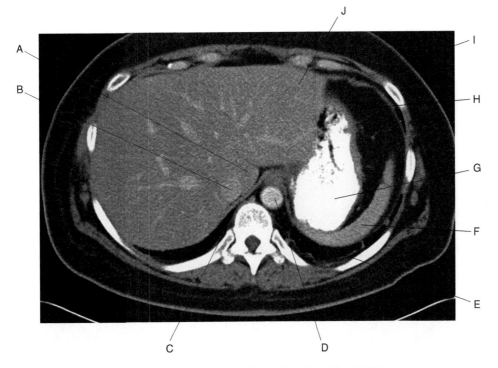

Fig. 23.26 CT corresponding to level B in Fig. 23.25.

33. Identify each lettered structure shown in Fig. 23.27.

A. _____

B. _____

C. _____

D. _____

E. _____

F. _____

G. _____

H. _____

I. _____

J. _____

K. _____

L. _____

M. _____

N. _____

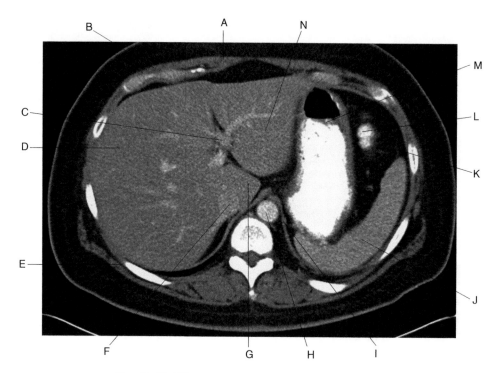

Fig. 23.27 CT corresponding to level C in Fig. 23.25.

34. Identify each lettered structure shown in Fig. 23.28.

A. _____

B. _____

C. _____

D. _____

E. _____

F. _____

G. _____

H. _____

I. _____

J. _____

K. _____

L. _____

M. _____

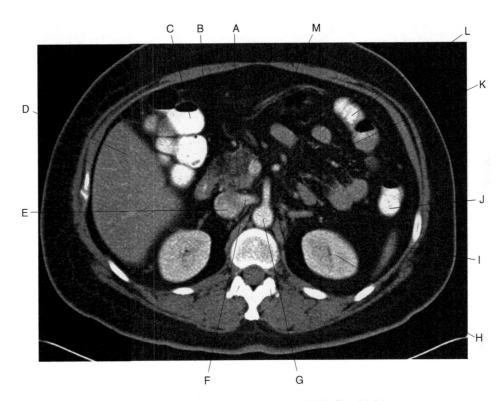

Fig. 23.28 CT corresponding to level F in Fig. 23.25.

35. Identify each lettered structure shown in Fig. 23.29.

A. _____   F. _____

B. _____   G. _____

C. _____   H. _____

D. _____   I. _____

E. _____   J. _____

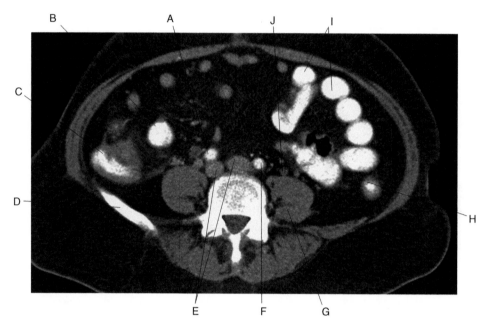

Fig. 23.29 CT image corresponding to level H in Fig. 23.25.

36. Identify each lettered structure shown in Fig. 23.30.

A. _____   G. _____

B. _____   H. _____

C. _____   I. _____

D. _____   J. _____

E. _____   K. _____

F. _____   L. _____

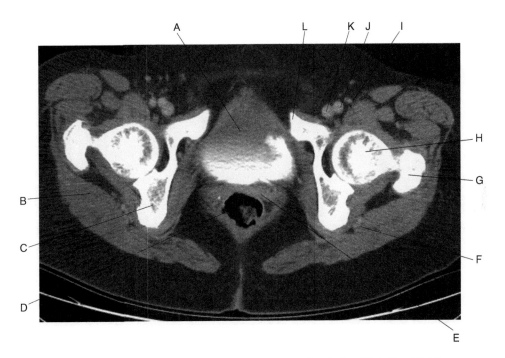

Fig. 23.30 CT image of female pelvis corresponding to level K in Fig. 23.25.

37. Identify each lettered structure shown in Fig. 23.31.

A. _____

B. _____

C. _____

D. _____

E. _____

F. _____

G. _____

H. _____

I. _____

J. _____

K. _____

L. _____

M. _____

N. _____

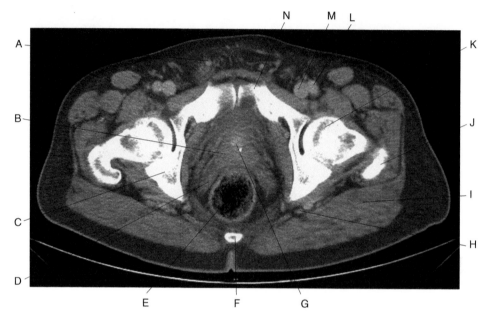

Fig. 23.31 CT image of male pelvis corresponding to level K in Fig. 23.25.

38. Identify each lettered structure shown in Fig. 23.32.

A. _____

B. _____

C. _____

D. _____

E. _____

F. _____

G. _____

H. _____

I. _____

J. _____

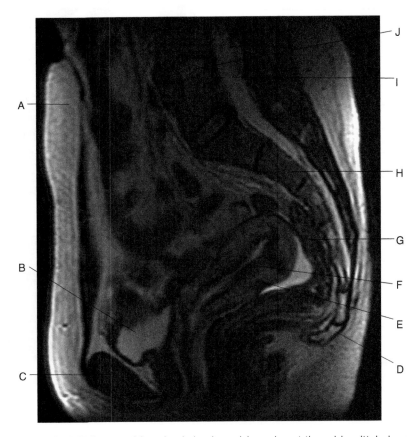

Fig. 23.32 MR image of female abdominopelvic region at the midsagittal plane.

Chapter **23 Sectional Anatomy for Radiographers**

39. Identify each lettered structure shown in Fig. 23.33.

A. _____

B. _____

C. _____

D. _____

E. _____

F. _____

G. _____

H. _____

I. _____

J. _____

K. _____

L. _____

M. _____

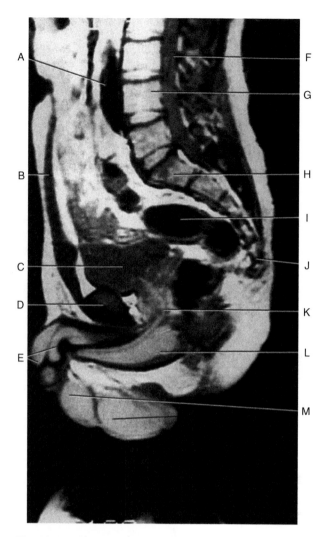

Fig. 23.33 MR image of the male abdominopelvic region at the median sagittal plane.

40. Identify each lettered structure shown in Fig. 23.34.

A. _____

B. _____

C. _____

D. _____

E. _____

F. _____

G. _____

H. _____

I. _____

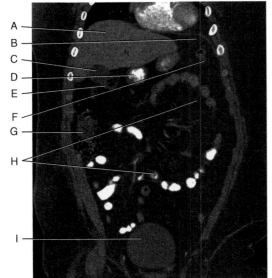

Fig. 23.34 Coronal CT image through the anterior abdomen.

41. Identify each lettered structure shown in Fig. 23.35.

A. _____

B. _____

C. _____

D. _____

E. _____

F. _____

G. _____

H. _____

I. _____

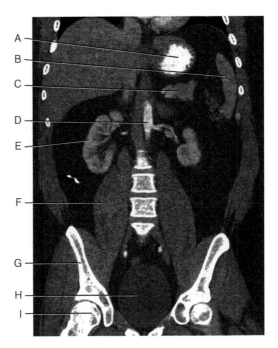

Fig. 23.35 Coronal CT image of the abdomen posterior to midcoronal plane.

Chapter **23 Sectional Anatomy for Radiographers**

24 Computed Tomography

Computed tomography (CT) is used so extensively that an understanding of this modality is becoming essential information for all radiographers. The following questions provide a brief review of CT. Answer the following fill-in-the-blank, short answer, true or false (explaining any statement you believe to be false), and multiple choice questions.

1. Define *computed tomography*.

2. Fill in the blanks to describe the basic scanning steps in CT. The x-ray tube _____ around the patient or part. A _____ measures the radiation exiting the patient and feeds the data to a computer. The computer compiles and calculates the data according to a preselected _____ and assembles it into an _____. The image is displayed on a _____.

3. List the three major components of a CT scanner.

a. _____

b. _____

c. _____

4. Match the terms in Column A to the definition in Column B.

Column A

_____ 1. Detector assembly

_____ 2. Matrix

_____ 3. Hounsfield unit

_____ 4. Data acquisition system (DAS)

_____ 5. Field of view (FOV)

_____ 6. Voxel

_____ 7. Window level

_____ 8. Gantry

_____ 9. Window width

_____ 10. Pixel

Column B

a. Number used to describe average density of tissue

b. Area of anatomy displayed by the monitor

c. Volume element; determined by slice thickness

d. Part of detector assembly that converts analog signals to digital signals

e. Determines the midpoint of the range of gray levels displayed

f. The range of CT numbers used to map signals into shades of gray

g. Part of scanner that houses the x-ray tube, cooling system, detector assembly, and DAS

h. One individual cell surface within an image matrix used for CRT image display; picture element

i. Electronic component of scanner that measures remnant radiation exiting the patient and converts it to a proportional analog signal

j. Array of numbers arranged in a grid; comprises the digital image

5. What is multiplanar reconstruction?

6. What are the three most commonly requested CT procedures?

7. By what three routes is contrast introduced for CT procedures?

8. Why are power injectors needed for CT contrast procedures?

9. The four main factors that affect CT image quality are:

a. _____

b. _____

c. _____

d. _____

10. The amount of blurring in a CT image is described

as _____.

11. The ability to differentiate between small differences in density within the image is termed

_____.

12. The most common cause of noise in a CT image arises from the random variation in photon detection,

or _____.

13. Why would it be best to schedule a CT scan of the abdomen on a patient several days after the patient's gastrointestinal (GI) fluoroscopy procedure?

For items 14 to 22, indicate the image quality factor(s) affected by the scan parameter or item listed by writing *S* for spatial resolution, *C* for contrast resolution, *N* for noise, and *A* for artifacts.

_____14. FOV

_____15. Matrix size

_____16. Slice thickness

_____17. Dental fillings

_____18. X-ray beam energy

_____19. Focal spot size

_____20. Residual barium

_____21. Reconstruction algorithm

_____22. Patient size

23. List four image quality factors that are under the technologist's control.

24. Which new CT data acquisition method involves the continuous rotation of the gantry as the table moves through the gantry?

25. Which new CT data acquisition technology has detector arrays containing multiple rows of elements along the *z*-axis, instead of a single row of detectors?

26. List three advantages of CT angiography (CTA) over conventional angiography.

27. The three common techniques used for creating three-dimensional (3-D) images from CT data are

_____, _____, and

_____.

28. Which 3-D imaging technique is commonly used for CTA?

29. To ensure proper operation, most CT systems require

preventive maintenance _____ or

_____.

30. What method was first used to describe a CT dose as a result of multiple scan locations?

31. List the factors that directly influence the CT radiation dose to the patient.

    a. _____

    b. _____

    c. _____

    d. _____

    e. _____

    f. _____

    g. _____

    h. _____

32. Indicate the preferred or more useful imaging modality by writing *CT* or *MRI* in the blank beside each item listed.

    _____ a. Bony structures

    _____ b. Less scan time

    _____ c. Soft tissue

    _____ d. Claustrophobic patients

    _____ e. Better low-contrast resolution

    _____ f. Less costly

For items 33 to 38, fill in the CT scan parameters.

33. Anatomic scan range for a basic head CT scan:

    _____

34. Typical scan slice thickness for a basic head CT scan:

    _____

35. Anatomic scan range for a cervical spine CT scan:

    _____

36. Typical scan slice thickness for a cervical spine CT scan:

    _____

37. Anatomic scan range for a CT scan of the abdomen:

    _____

38. Typical scan slice thickness for a CT scan of the abdomen: _____

39. Which of the following should be considered for CT imaging of pediatric patients? (Circle all that apply.)
    a. Use multiple scanning phases to ensure most diagnostic information is obtained.
    b. Radiation dose should be "child size."
    c. Scan only when necessary.
    d. Scan beyond indicated areas to avoid repeat scans.
    e. Use shielding whenever possible.
    f. Multiple scanning phases are seldom indicated.

40. CT protocols for pediatric patients are based on:
    a. age.
    b. weight.
    c. suspected pathologic condition.
    d. all of the above.

Radiographers are expected to recognize CT images from other modalities, identify basic anatomic structures, and identify the imaging plane. Answer each question related to the images provided to aid in your ability to analyze CT images.

1. Which image in Fig. 24.1 (A or B) is the CT image?

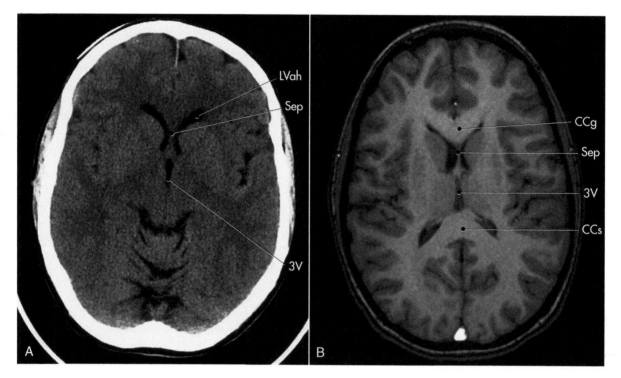

Fig. 24.1 A, B

2. Identify each lettered structure shown in Fig. 24.2.

A. _____

B. _____

C. _____

D. _____

E. _____

F. _____

G. _____

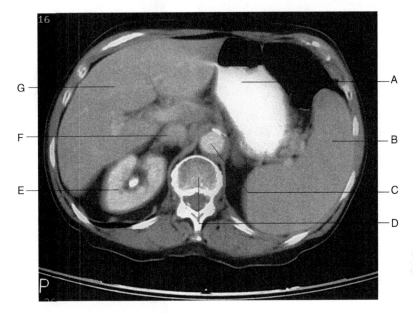

Fig. 24.2 Axial CT image of abdomen.

3. Label each image in Fig. 24.3 as a soft tissue window or a bone window.

A. _____

B. _____

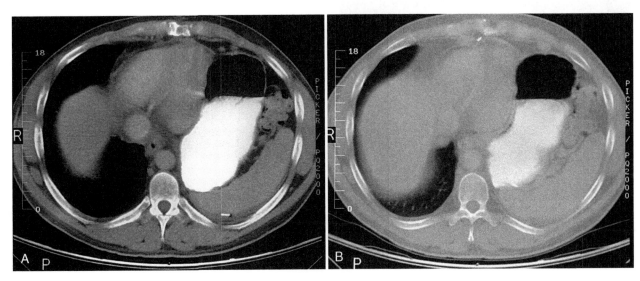

Fig. 24.3 A, B

Indicate the imaging plane, coronal or axial, for Figs. 24.4 to 24.7.

4. Fig. 24.4: _____ plane

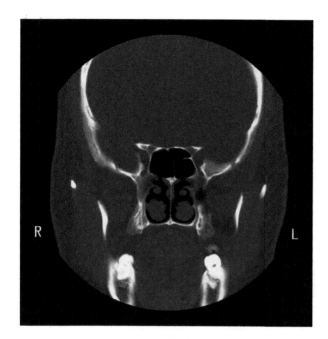

Fig. 24.4

5. Fig. 24.5: _____ plane

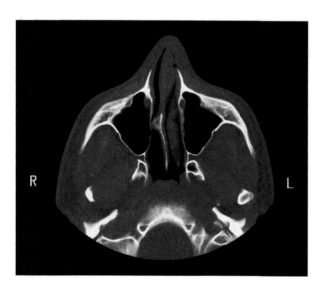

Fig. 24.5

6. Fig. 24.6: _____ plane

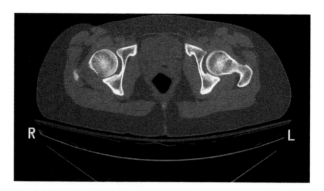

Fig. 24.6

7. Fig. 24.7: _____ plane

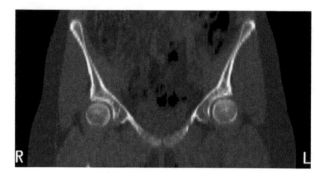

Fig. 24.7

Which of the following images demonstrate contrast media administration? Indicate by circling your answer above each image.

8. Fig. 24.8:

Contrast   Noncontrast

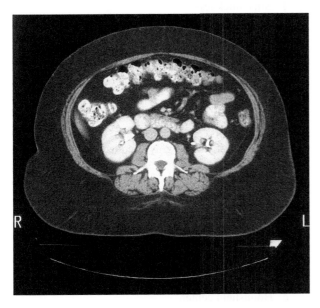

Fig. 24.8

9. Fig. 24.9:

Contrast   Noncontrast

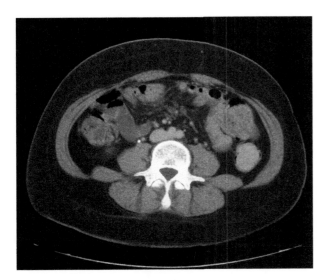

Fig. 24.9

10. Fig. 24.10:

Contrast   Noncontrast

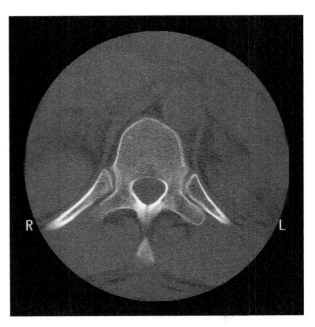

Fig. 24.10

Answer the following questions by selecting the best choice.

1. What term is applied to a single square, or picture element, in the image display matrix?
   a. CT number
   b. Hounsfield unit
   c. Pixel
   d. Raw data

2. What determines the amount of data displayed on the monitor?
   a. Number of volume elements
   b. Pixel size
   c. Tissue density
   d. FOV

3. A volume element is called a:
   a. pixel.
   b. voxel.
   c. matrix.
   d. CT number.

4. A relative comparison of x-ray attenuation of a voxel of tissue to an equal volume of water is a(n):
   a. CT number.
   b. matrix.
   c. FOV.
   d. scan profile.

5. What is the CT number of water?
   a. −1000
   b. −1500
   c. 0
   d. 1000

6. Which of the following are the major system components of a CT scanner?
   a. Gantry, computer and operator's console, and patient table
   b. Monitor, gantry, and aperture
   c. Computer and operator's console, patient table, and DAS
   d. Patient table, computer, and 3-D reconstruction algorithms

7. A circular device that houses the x-ray tube, DAS, and detector array is called the:
   a. gantry.
   b. computer.
   c. aperture.
   d. algorithm.

8. X-ray tubes used in advanced CT scanners can tolerate:
   a. 0.5 to 1.5 million heat units (MHU)
   b. 2 to 3 MHU
   c. 4 to 5 MHU
   d. 6 to 10 MHU

9. Which of the following can be selected at the operator's console?
   1. Slice thickness
   2. Table index
   3. Imaging technique factors

   a. 1 and 2 only
   b. 1 and 3 only
   c. 2 and 3 only
   d. 1, 2, and 3

10. The range of CT numbers that are used to map signals into shades of gray is called the:
    a. window level.
    b. window width.
    c. image registration.
    d. matrix display.

11. The midpoint of the range of gray levels to be displayed on the monitor is the:
    a. window level.
    b. window width.
    c. Hounsfield center.
    d. algorithm point.

12. A narrow window width would display:
    a. a long gray scale.
    b. many shades of gray.
    c. low contrast.
    d. high contrast.

13. The window level should be set to:
    a. one half of the algorithm point.
    b. the Hounsfield center.
    c. one fourth of the window width.
    d. the CT number of the tissue of interest.

14. CT is the examination of choice for:
    a. limb fractures.
    b. head trauma.
    c. the GI tract.
    d. the genitourinary system.

15. The amount of blurring in a CT image is termed:
    a. noise.
    b. artifact.
    c. spatial resolution.
    d. contrast resolution.

16. The ability to differentiate between small differences in density within the CT image is called:
    a. spatial resolution.
    b. contrast resolution.
    c. windowing.
    d. gray level mapping.

17. Which of the following is the most significant geometric factor that contributes to spatial resolution?
    a. Detector aperture width
    b. Focal spot size
    c. Slice thickness
    d. Detector array

18. Random variation in photon detection results in:
    a. quantum noise.
    b. streak artifacts.
    c. beam hardening.
    d. image misregistration.

19. Which of the following contribute to image noise in CT?
    1. Detector aperture width
    2. Matrix size
    3. Patient size

    a. 1 and 2 only
    b. 1 and 3 only
    c. 2 and 3 only
    d. 1, 2, and 3

20. Metallic objects, such as dental fillings, can cause:
    a. image misregistration.
    b. quantum noise.
    c. windowing gauss.
    d. artifacts.

21. High-resolution CT scans are made using:
    a. shorter scan times.
    b. thinner sections or slices.
    c. wider window widths.
    d. volume rendering algorithms.

22. Which of the following quality factors is affected by x-ray beam energy?
    1. Contrast resolution
    2. Spatial resolution
    3. Noise

    a. 1 and 2 only
    b. 1 and 3 only
    c. 2 and 3 only
    d. 1, 2, and 3

23. Which image quality factor is affected by focal spot size?
    a. Noise
    b. Artifacts
    c. Spatial resolution
    d. Contrast resolution

24. Tissue density differences of less than _____ can be distinguished by CT.
    a. 0.01%
    b. 0.1%
    c. 0.5%
    d. 1.0%

25. Reconstruction algorithm affects all of the image quality factors EXCEPT for:
    a. artifacts.
    b. contrast resolution.
    c. spatial resolution.
    d. noise.

26. The image that appears on the monitor depends on the:
    a. focal spot size.
    b. detector array.
    c. detector aperture width.
    d. display field of view.

27. What is based on the principle that different structures enhance at different rates after contrast administration?
    a. Dynamic scanning
    b. 3-D imaging
    c. Spiral CT
    d. Image misregistration

28. What new CT data acquisition method involves continuous gantry rotations combined with constant table movement through the aperture?
    a. Dynamic scanning
    b. Maximum intensity projection
    c. Volume rendering
    d. Spiral or helical CT

29. Which 3-D imaging technique is commonly used for CTA?
    a. Dynamic scanning
    b. Maximum intensity projection
    c. Shaded surface display
    d. Volume rendering

30. All of the following are methods of 3-D reconstruction EXCEPT:
    a. maximum intensity projection.
    b. volume rendering.
    c. segmentation.
    d. shaded surface display.

31. How often do most CT systems require preventive maintenance to ensure proper operation?
    a. Twice a day to daily
    b. Weekly to biweekly
    c. Monthly to quarterly
    d. Quarterly to annually

32. All of the following affect radiation dose in CT EXCEPT:
    a. FOV.
    b. beam energy.
    c. tube current.
    d. section/slice thickness.

33. The anatomic scan range for a basic head CT is from the _____ to the _____.
    a. sella turcica; occipital condyles
    b. glabella; inion
    c. bottom of C2; skull vertex
    d. base of skull; vertex of head

34. What is the anatomic scan range for a CT of the cervical spine?
    a. Foramen magnum to T1
    b. Occipital condyles to below T2
    c. Sella turcica to below T1
    d. Mastoid process to below T2

35. What is the typical scan slice thickness for a CT scan of the abdomen?
    a. 1.5 mm
    b. 2.5 mm
    c. 3 mm
    d. 5 mm

25 Vascular, Cardiac, and Interventional Radiography

ANATOMY OF THE CIRCULATORY SYSTEM

Section 1: Exercise 1

This exercise pertains to the anatomy of the circulatory system. Identify structures for each item.

1. Identify each lettered structure shown in Fig. 25.1.

A. _____

B. _____

C. _____

D. _____

E. _____

F. _____

G. _____

H. _____

I. _____

J. _____

K. _____

L. _____

M. _____

N. _____

O. _____

P. _____

Q. _____

R. _____

S. _____

T. _____

U. _____

V. _____

W. _____

X. _____

Y. _____

Z. _____

AA. _____

BB. _____

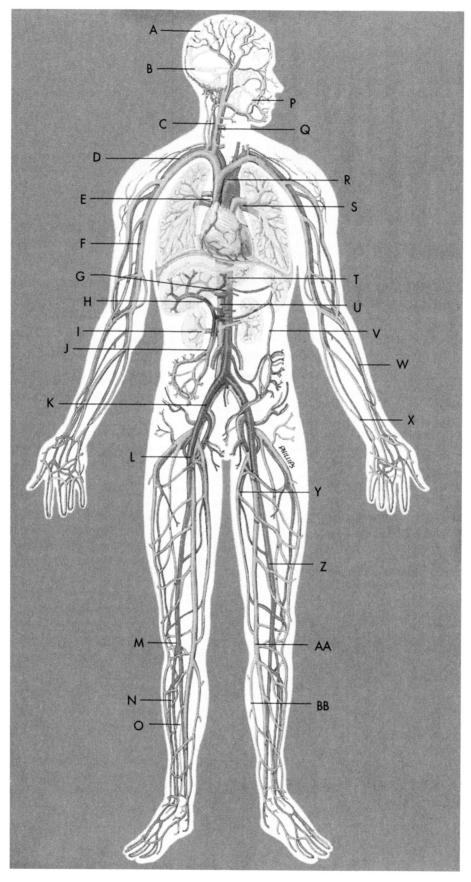

Fig. 25.1 Major arteries and veins.

2. Identify each lettered structure shown in Fig. 25.2.

A. _____

B. _____

C. _____

D. _____

E. _____

F. _____

G. _____

H. _____

I. _____

J. _____

K. _____

L. _____

M. _____

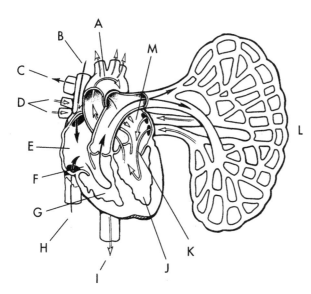

Fig. 25.2 The heart and greater vessels. *Black arrows* indicate deoxygenated blood flow. *White arrows* indicate oxygenated blood flow.

3. Identify each lettered structure shown in Fig. 25.3.

A. _____

B. _____

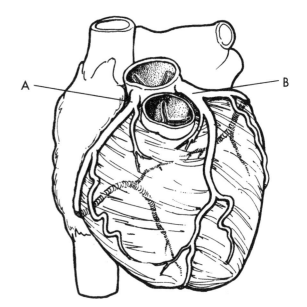

Fig. 25.3 Anterior view of the coronary arteries.

4. Identify each lettered structure shown in Fig. 25.4.

A. _____

B. _____

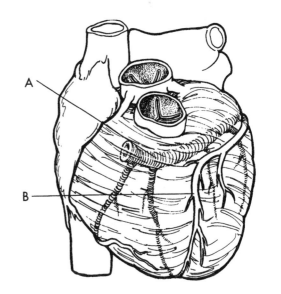

Fig. 25.4 Anterior view of the coronary veins.

579

5. Identify each lettered structure shown in Fig. 25.5.

A. _____   G. _____

B. _____   H. _____

C. _____   I. _____

D. _____   J. _____

E. _____   K. _____

F. _____   L. _____

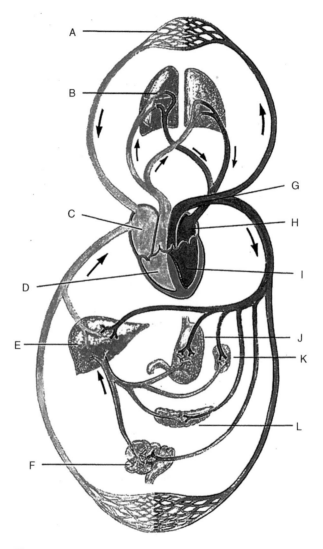

Fig. 25.5 The pulmonary, systemic, and portal circulation.

6. Identify each lettered structure shown in Fig. 25.6.

A. _____

B. _____

C. _____

D. _____

E. _____

F. _____

G. _____

H. _____

I. _____

J. _____

K. _____

L. _____

M. _____

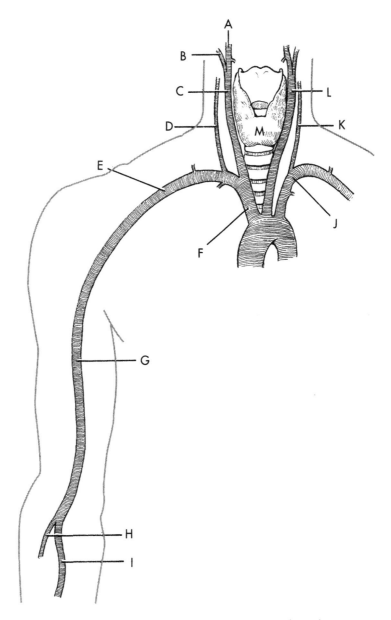

Fig. 25.6 Major arteries of the upper chest, neck, and arm.

7. Identify each lettered structure shown in Fig. 25.7.

A. _____

B. _____

C. _____

D. _____

E. _____

F. _____

G. _____

H. _____

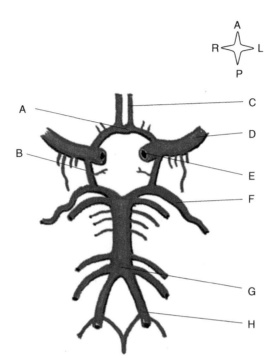

Fig. 25.7 Circle of Willis. (From Thibodeau GA, Patton KP: *Anatomy and physiology*, ed 6, St Louis, 2007, Mosby.)

8. Identify each lettered structure show in Fig. 25.8.

A. _____   E. _____

B. _____   F. _____

C. _____   G. _____

D. _____

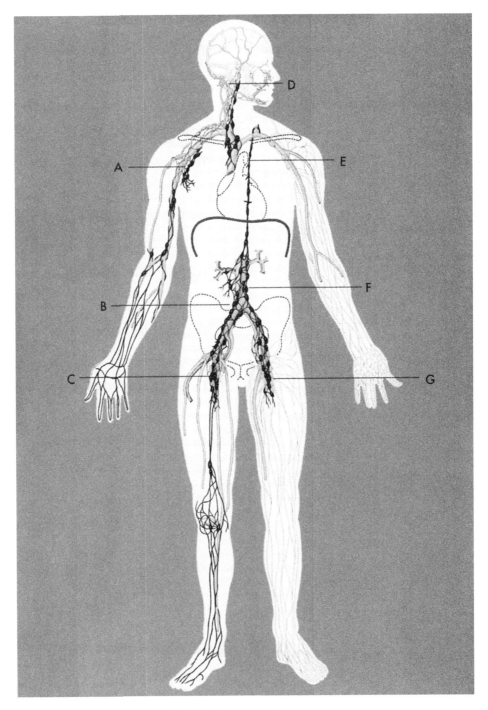

Fig. 25.8 The lymphatic system.

Section 1: Exercise 2

This exercise is a comprehensive review of the circulatory system. Fill in missing words for each item.

1. The circulatory system comprises two systems of related vessels, the _____ system and the _____ system.

2. The two systems that make up the blood-vascular system are _____ circulation and _____ circulation.

3. The system that traverses the lungs to discharge carbon dioxide and take up oxygen is _____ circulation.

4. The vessels that carry blood away from the heart are collectively called _____.

5. The vessels that carry blood back toward the heart are collectively called _____.

6. Arteries subdivide to form _____.

7. Arterioles subdivide to form _____.

8. Capillaries unite to form _____.

9. The beginning branches for veins are _____.

10. Blood is transported to the left atrium by _____ veins.

11. The major vein that returns blood from the upper parts of the body to the heart is the _____.

12. The major vein that returns blood from the lower parts of the body to the heart is the _____.

13. The muscular wall of the heart is the _____.

14. The membrane that lines the chambers of the heart is the _____.

15. The membrane that covers the heart is the _____.

16. The chamber of the heart where the myocardium is the thickest is the _____.

17. The space between the two walls of the pericardial sac is the _____.

18. The two upper chambers of the heart are the _____.

19. The two lower chambers of the heart are the _____.

20. The receiving chambers of the heart are the _____.

21. The distributing chambers of the heart are the _____.

22. Another name for the right atrioventricular valve is the _____ valve.

23. Two other terms that refer to the left atrioventricular valve are the _____ valve and the _____ valve.

24. The side of the heart that pumps venous (deoxygenated) blood is the _____ (right or left) side.

25. The side of the heart that pumps arterial (oxygenated) blood is the _____ (right or left) side.

26. The chamber of the heart that pumps blood through the aortic valve is the _____.

27. The vessels that supply blood to the myocardium are the right and left _____ arteries.

28. The coronary sinus receives blood from the _____ veins.

29. The coronary sinus empties blood into the _____ (right or left) atrium.

30. The great vessel that arises from the left ventricle to transport blood to the body is the _____.

31. The abdominal aorta divides into the right and left common _____ arteries.

32. The external iliac artery enters the lower limb and becomes the _____ artery.

33. The femoral artery passes blood into the _____ artery.

34. The popliteal artery bifurcates into the anterior and posterior _____ arteries.

35. The vessel that drains blood into the liver is the _____ vein.

36. The vessels that drain blood from the liver are the _____ veins.

37. Hepatic veins transport blood to the _____.

38. The large vessel that arises from the right atrium is the _____ artery.

39. The only arteries of the body that transport deoxygenated blood are the _____ arteries.

40. The only veins of the body that transport oxygenated blood are the _____ veins.

41. The contraction phase of the heart is called the _____.

42. The relaxation phase of the heart is called the _____.

43. The four arteries that supply the brain are the right and left _____ arteries and the right and left _____ arteries.

44. Of the four trunk arteries that supply the brain, the one that arises directly from the arch of the aorta is the _____ artery.

45. The right and left vertebral arteries arise from the _____ arteries.

46. The right and left vertebral arteries unite to form the _____ artery.

47. Each common carotid artery bifurcates into the _____ and _____ carotid arteries.

48. Each internal carotid artery bifurcates into anterior and middle _____ arteries.

49. The basilar artery bifurcates into the right and left _____ arteries.

50. Blood is drained from the head by the _____ veins.

51. To reach the right subclavian artery, blood passes from the aorta through the _____ artery.

52. Blood passes from the brachiocephalic artery to the right _____ artery.

53. A subclavian artery supplies blood to the axillary artery and then to the _____ artery.

54. The brachial arteries bifurcate into the _____ arteries.

55. The part of the body in which the cephalic vein originates is the _____.

56. The renal arteries arise from the _____.

57. The circle of Willis is located within the _____.

58. The central organ of the blood-vascular system is the _____.

59. The main terminal trunk of the lymphatic system is the _____ duct.

60. The thoracic duct drains its contents at the junction of the left vein and the internal _____ vein.

RADIOGRAPHY OF THE CIRCULATORY SYSTEM

Section 2: Exercise 1

This exercise pertains to various radiographic examinations for the circulatory system. Because many of these procedures depend on the preferences of the radiologist, most of the following exercise items are general in content rather than emphasizing a specific procedure. Identify structures, fill in missing words, select from a list, or provide a short answer for each item.

1. List four reasons that catheterization is preferred over direct injection of the contrast media through a needle.

2. The *preferred* method of catheterization is the _____ technique.

3. The most common site for insertion of the catheter for selective angiography is the _____ artery.

4. What is the purpose of side holes near the tip of the pigtail catheter?
   a. To draw fluid into the catheter
   b. To reduce whiplash, stabilizing the catheter
   c. To maintain positive pressure inside the catheter

5. From the following list, circle the three symptoms of a vasovagal reaction that are caused by the injection of the contrast media.
   a. Hives
   b. Nausea
   c. Sweating
   d. Difficult breathing
   e. Increase in pulse rate
   f. Increase in blood pressure
   g. Decrease in blood pressure

6. From the following list, circle the three symptoms of shock.
   a. Low pulse rate
   b. High pulse rate
   c. Rapid breathing
   d. Shallow breathing
   e. Loss of consciousness
   f. Rise in body temperature

7. What treatment should be given to patients experiencing low blood pressure because of a vasovagal reaction?

8. In preparation for angiography, why should the patient be instructed not to consume solid food?

9. In preparation for angiography, why should the patient be allowed to drink clear liquids?

10. For thoracic aortography, to which vertebra should the perpendicular central ray be directed?

11. Identify each lettered structure shown in Fig. 25.9.

A. _____   E. _____

B. _____   F. _____

C. _____   G. _____

D. _____   H. _____

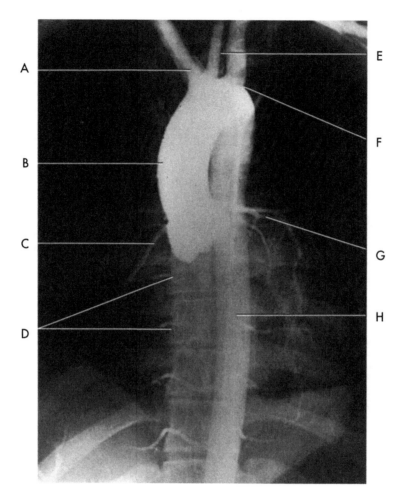

Fig. 25.9 AP thoracic aortogram.

12. How much of the aorta should be imaged for abdominal aortography?

13. For abdominal aortography, which projection of the abdominal aorta (anteroposterior [AP] or lateral) best demonstrates the celiac and superior mesenteric artery origins?

14. Identify each lettered structure shown in Fig. 25.10.

A. _____

B. _____

C. _____

D. _____

E. _____

F. _____

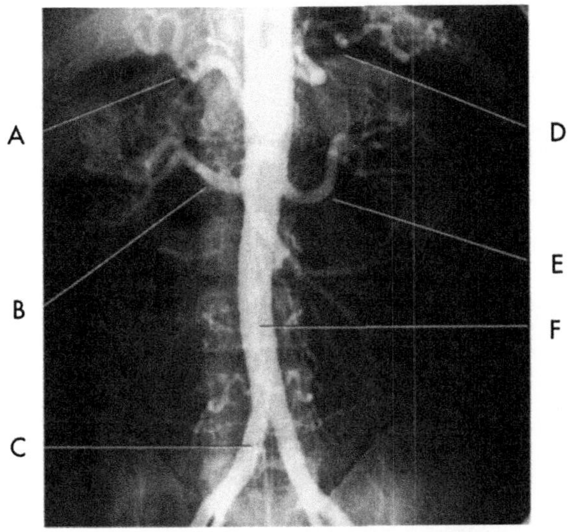

Fig. 25.10 AP abdominal aortogram.

15. Identify each lettered structure shown in Fig. 25.11.

A. _____

B. _____

C. _____

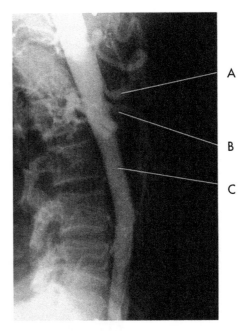

Fig. 25.11 Lateral abdominal aortogram.

16. All images for selective abdominal visceral arteriography should be exposed when the patient has suspended

_____

(inspiration or expiration).

17. Identify each lettered structure shown in Fig. 25.12.

A. _____

B. _____

C. _____

D. _____

E. _____

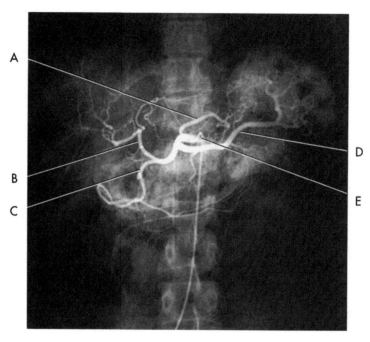

Fig. 25.12 Selective AP celiac arteriogram.

18. The renal arteries arise from the right and left side of the abdominal aorta between _____ and _____.

19. For renal venography, the renal vein is most easily catheterized using the _____ approach.

20. Into which vein should a catheter be positioned for the best demonstration of the superior vena cava?
    a. Subclavian
    b. Common iliac
    c. Inferior vena cava

21. Into which vein should a catheter be positioned for the best demonstration of the inferior vena cava?
    a. Portal
    b. Common iliac
    c. Superior vena cava

22. Into which artery should the catheter be positioned for the best demonstration of the arteries of an entire upper limb with a single injection of contrast medium?
    a. Femoral
    b. Subclavian
    c. Common iliac

23. Identify each lettered structure shown in Fig. 25.13.

    A. _____

    B. _____

    C. _____

    D. _____

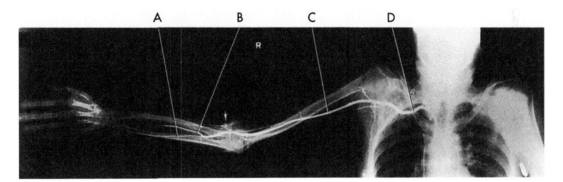

Fig. 25.13 Right upper limb arteriogram. (The radial artery is not demonstrated because of occlusion.)

24. Where is the injection site for the introduction of contrast media for upper limb venography?

25. Identify each lettered structure shown in Fig. 25.14.

A. _____

B. _____

C. _____

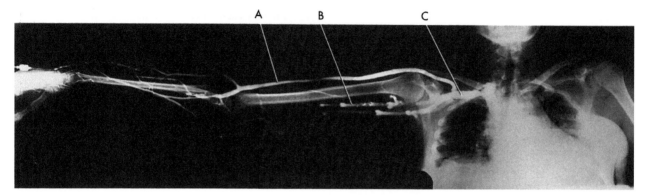

Fig. 25.14 Right upper limb venogram.

26. For simultaneous bilateral femoral arteriograms, how should the patient's legs be positioned?

27. Identify each lettered structure shown in Fig. 25.15.

A. _____

B. _____

C. _____

D. _____

E. _____

F. _____

G. _____

H. _____

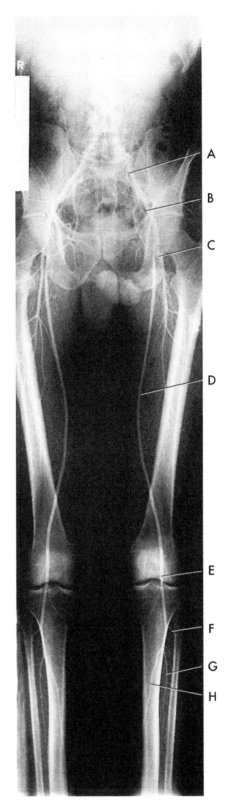

Fig. 25.15 Normal aortofemoral arteriogram in the late arterial phase.

28. Identify each lettered structure shown in Fig. 25.16.

A. _____

B. _____

C. _____

D. _____

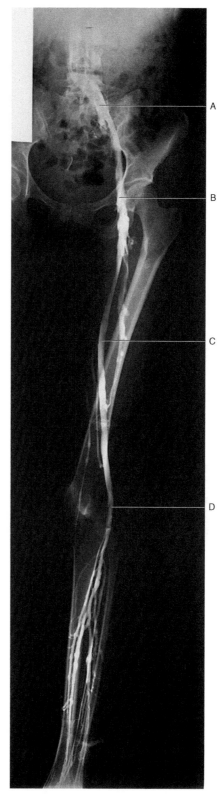

Fig. 25.16 Normal left lower venogram.

29. List the indications for performing abdominal visceral arteriography studies.

30. List the indications for performing thoracic aortography studies.

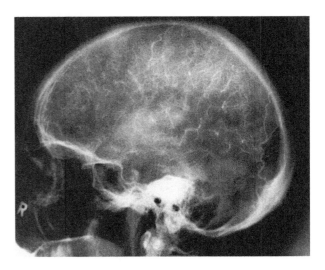

Fig. 25.17 Cerebral angiogram.

31. Approximately how many seconds does it take for blood to flow from the internal carotid artery to the jugular vein in cerebral angiography?
    a. 3 seconds
    b. 6 seconds
    c. 9 seconds

32. Why should the first image of a cerebral arteriography series be made before the arrival of the contrast media?
    a. To check exposure factors
    b. To confirm patient positioning
    c. To serve as a subtraction mask
    d. To demonstrate soft tissue abnormalities

33. What is the visualization sequence for the three phases of blood flow that should be seen in cerebral angiography?
    a. Arterial, capillary, and venous
    b. Arterial, venous, and capillary
    c. Capillary, arterial, and venous
    d. Capillary, venous, and arterial
    e. Venous, arterial, and capillary
    f. Venous, capillary, and arterial

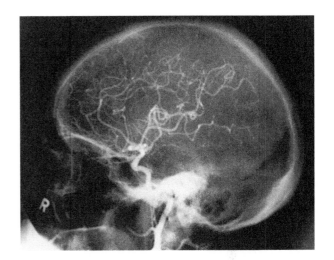

Fig. 25.18 Cerebral angiogram.

34. Figs. 25.17 to 25.19 are cerebral angiograms, and each shows a phase of blood flow. Examine each image and identify which phase of blood flow— arterial, capillary, or venous—the image represents.

    a. Fig. 25.17: 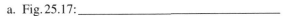_____

    b. Fig. 25.18: _____

    c. Fig. 25.19: _____

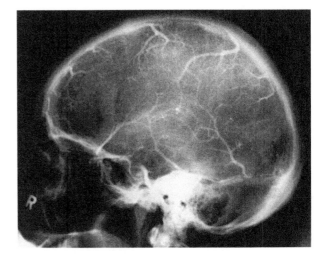

Fig. 25.19 Cerebral angiogram.

35. For the basic AP projection during cerebral angiography, what positioning line of the skull should be perpendicular to the horizontal plane?

36. For the AP axial oblique projection (transorbital) demonstrating anterior circulation during cerebral angiography, in which direction (toward the injected side or away from the injected side) should the head be rotated?

INTERVENTIONAL RADIOGRAPHY

Section 3: Exercise 1

This exercise pertains to interventional radiography. Fill in missing words, select from a list, or provide a short answer for each item.

1. Percutaneous transluminal angioplasty, abbreviated as

   _____, is a therapeutic radiologic proce-

   dure designed to _____ stenotic or oc-
   cluded areas within a vessel.

2. A metal device that is placed and left in a vessel to

   hold open a stenotic area is a _____.

3. _____ involves the therapeutic introduction of various substances to occlude or reduce drastically blood flow within a vessel.

4. List the three main purposes of embolization.

5. Check all of the following lesions or conditions that
   may be treated with embolization.

   _____ Aneurysm   _____ Neoplasm

   _____ Hemorrhage   _____ Angina

   _____ Aortic   _____ Arteriovenous
           dissection   malformation

6. The interventional procedure for the treatment of

   portal hypertension is the _____.

7. A transjugular intrahepatic portosystemic shunt (TIPS)
   creates an artificial pathway between the:
   a. portal and hepatic veins.
   b. portal and hepatic arteries.
   c. venous and biliary circulation.
   d. hepatic artery and inferior vena cava.

8. A blood clot, or _____, that has broken
   free of a vessel wall and migrates into the circulating

   blood is termed a(n) _____.

9. The primary source of a pulmonary embolus is

   _____.

10. An interventional procedure used to reduce the risk
    of pulmonary embolism when anticoagulant therapy

    is contraindicated is _____ placement.

CARDIAC CATHETERIZATION

Section 4: Exercise 1

1. The most definitive procedure for visualizing the arteries of the heart is _____.

2. According to the American College of Cardiology and the American Heart Association, relative contraindications for cardiac catheterization include the following. (Check all contraindications.)

    _____ Known cardiac disease

    _____ Acute or chronic renal failure

    _____ Recent stroke

    _____ Asthma and/or chronic bronchitis

    _____ Fever

    _____ Short life expectancy because of other illness

    _____ Severe uncontrolled hypertension

    _____ Bleeding disorders

    _____ Previous cardiac interventional procedure

    _____ Uncontrolled ventricular arrhythmias

    _____ Previous anaphylactic contrast agent reaction

3. The most frequent percutaneous access site for cardiac catheterization is the _____ area.

On questions 4 to 8, match the cardiac procedures to the reason for the procedure.

4. ____ Left ventriculography

5. ____ Aortic root angiography

6. ____ Selective coronary angiography

7. ____ Endomyocardial biopsy

8. ____ Electrophysiology

A. Evaluates the extent of coronary artery stenosis
B. Checks the competence of the aortic valve
C. Provides a tissue sample for pathologic evaluation of cardiac muscle
D. Facilitates detailed mapping of the electrical conduction system within the heart
E. Provides information about valvular competence, interventricular septal integrity, and ejection fraction

9. What are the two most common cardiac interventional procedures?

10. The cardiac interventional procedure that uses mechanical devices that cut away or remove the fatty deposit or thrombus material from the artery lumen is _____.

CHAPTER 25: SELF-TEST: VASCULAR, CARDIAC, AND INTERVENTIONAL RADIOGRAPHY

Answer the following questions by selecting the best choice.

1. Which vessels have exceedingly thin walls through which the essential functions of the blood-vascular system take place?
   a. Veins
   b. Venules
   c. Arterioles
   d. Capillaries

2. In which part of the body is the basilic vein located?
   a. Head
   b. Abdomen
   c. Lower limb
   d. Upper limb

3. Which chamber of the heart receives deoxygenated blood?
   a. Left atrium
   b. Left ventricle
   c. Right atrium
   d. Right ventricle

4. Which chamber of the heart receives blood from the pulmonary veins?
   a. Left atrium
   b. Left ventricle
   c. Right atrium
   d. Right ventricle

5. The circuit for blood flow from the left ventricle to the right atrium is _____ circulation.
   a. deep
   b. systemic
   c. superficial
   d. pulmonary

6. Which arteries are the first to branch from the ascending aorta?
   a. Coronary
   b. Vertebral
   c. Subclavian
   d. Common carotid

7. Through which valve does blood pass when it exits the heart for systemic circulation?
   a. Aortic
   b. Mitral
   c. Bicuspid
   d. Tricuspid

8. If the atrial septum does not contain a preexisting opening, an artificial defect can be created using by which of the following approach?
   a. Percutaneous
   b. Transseptal system
   c. Antecubital
   d. Transcatheter

9. Which of the following is used when multiple catheters will be used during an angiographic procedure?
   a. General anesthesia
   b. Introducer sheath
   c. Larger needle
   d. Cut-down technique

10. Which procedure should be performed to reduce the magnification of structures for lateral projections during thoracic aortography?
    a. Use an IR changer.
    b. Use the smallest available focal spot.
    c. Increase the source-to-image receptor distance (SID).
    d. Increase the object-to-image receptor distance (OID).

11. To which level of the patient should the IR and central ray be centered for AP abdominal aortograms?
    a. T6
    b. T10
    c. L2
    d. Iliac crests

12. To which level of the patient should the IR and central ray be centered for celiac arteriograms?
    a. T2
    b. T6
    c. L1
    d. S1

13. To which level of the patient should the IR be centered for hepatic arteriograms?
    a. Left and upper margins of the spleen
    b. Right and lower margins of the spleen
    c. Upper and right margins of the liver
    d. Lower and left margins of the liver

14. To which level of the patient should the IR be centered for splenic arteriograms?
    a. Upper and right margins of the liver
    b. Lower and left margins of the liver
    c. Right and lower margins of the spleen
    d. Left and upper margins of the spleen

15. The most common form of arterial stenosis treated by transluminal angioplasty is caused by which of the following conditions?
    a. Metastatic hepatic lesions
    b. Atherosclerosis
    c. Vein thrombosis
    d. Gastric varices

16. Why should an image be taken before the arrival of contrast media for cerebral angiography?
    a. To serve as a subtraction mask
    b. To ensure that collimation is adequate
    c. To check for proper positioning of the patient
    d. To verify that the correct exposure factors are used

17. Which phase of blood flow should have the most images exposed during cerebral angiography?
    a. Venous
    b. Arterial
    c. Capillary
    d. Parenchymal

18. Which positioning line of the skull should be perpendicular to the horizontal plane for basic AP projections during cerebral arteriography?
    a. Orbitomeatal
    b. Glabellomeatal
    c. Acanthiomeatal
    d. Infraorbitomeatal

19. Which interventional procedure involves the use of various substances to occlude or reduce drastically blood flow within a vessel?
    a. Transcatheter embolization
    b. Stents
    c. PTCA
    d. Atherectomy

20. The percutaneous intervention that creates an artificial low-pressure pathway between the portal and hepatic veins to relieve portal hypertension is:
    a. PTCA.
    b. electrophysiology.
    c. angioplasty.
    d. transjugular intrahepatic portosystemic shunt (TIPS).

21. The therapeutic intervention used to reduce the risk of pulmonary embolism is:
    a. TIPS.
    b. atherectomy.
    c. stents.
    d. inferior vena cava filter placement.

22. The most common disease that necessitates cardiac catheterization is:
    a. myocardial infarction.
    b. coronary artery disease.
    c. hypertension.
    d. uncontrolled ventricular arrhythmias.

23. All of the following are relative contraindications for cardiac catheterization EXCEPT:
    a. previous cardiac interventional procedures.
    b. coagulopathy and bleeding disorders.
    c. active gastrointestinal bleeding.
    d. severe anemia.

24. All of the following equipment is readily available during cardiac procedures because of inherent risks EXCEPT:
    a. a defibrillator
    b. a pulse oximeter
    c. electroencephalogram equipment
    d. a temporary pacemaker

25. The vessel commonly accessed to perform a right heart catheterization is the:
    a. femoral artery.
    b. brachial artery.
    c. external jugular vein.
    d. femoral vein.

9780323597043